RUNNER'S WORLD

RUN YOUR BELLY OFF!

CONTENTS

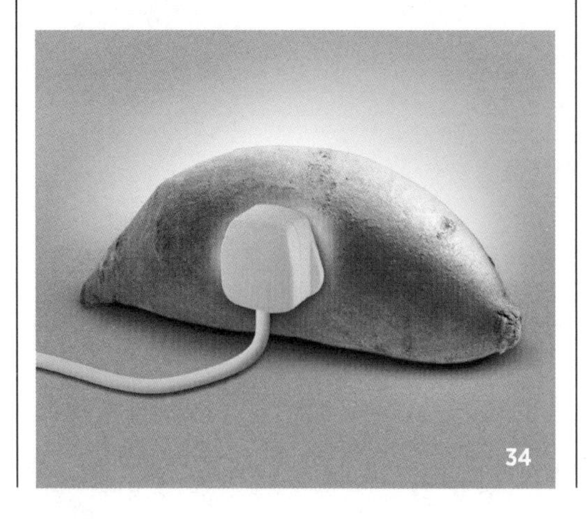

34

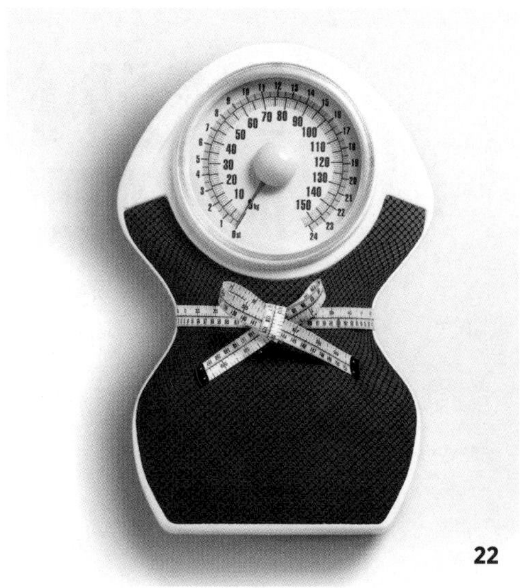

22

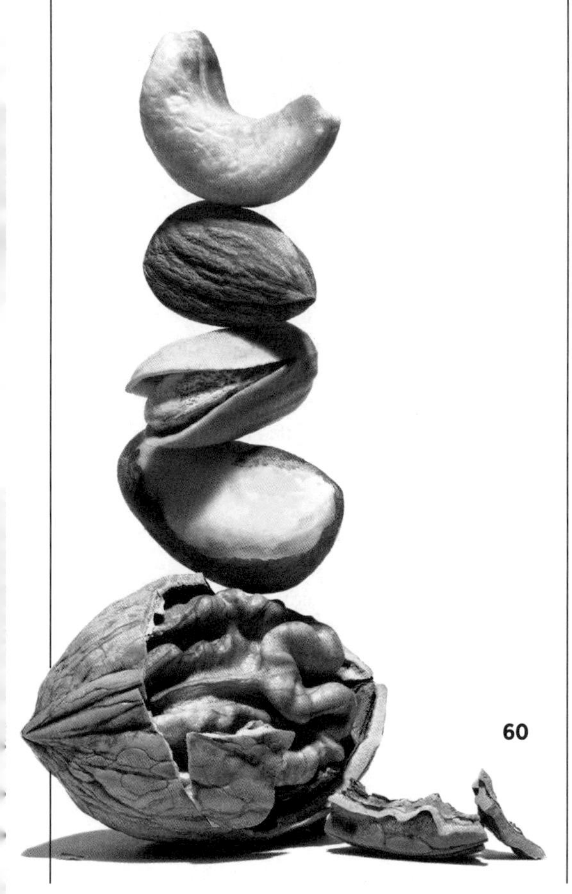

60

110

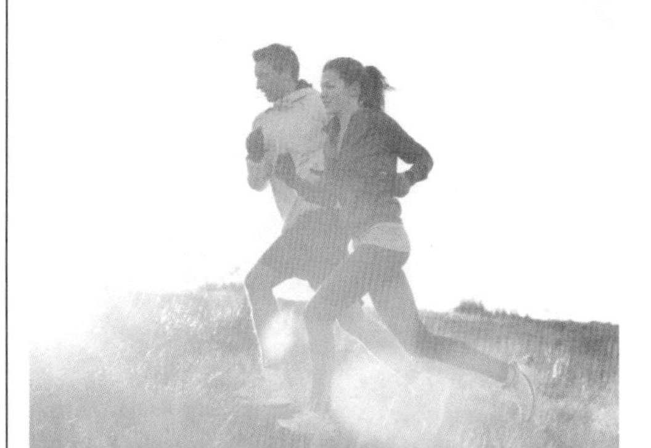

Exactly how much food should you be packing away every day to keep your running and weight-loss targets on track? We show how to work it out according to your needs.

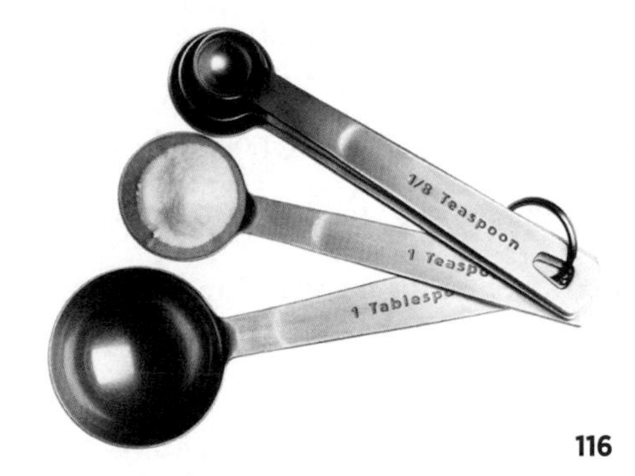

116

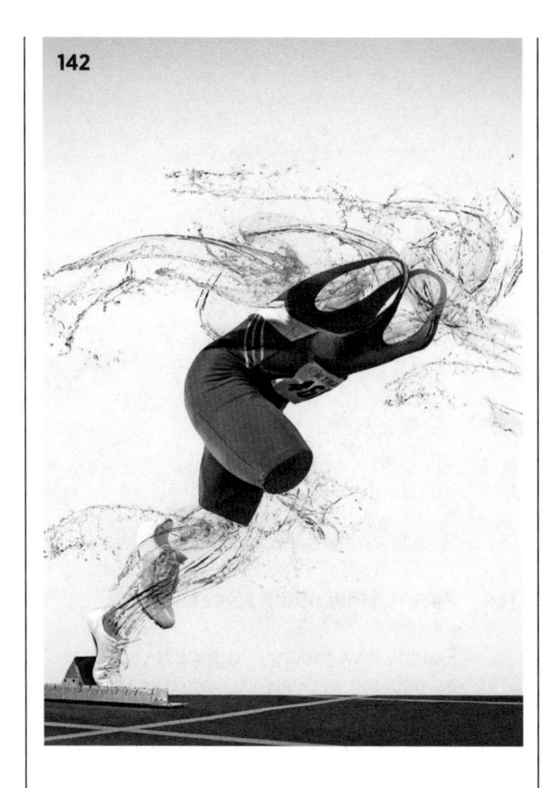
142

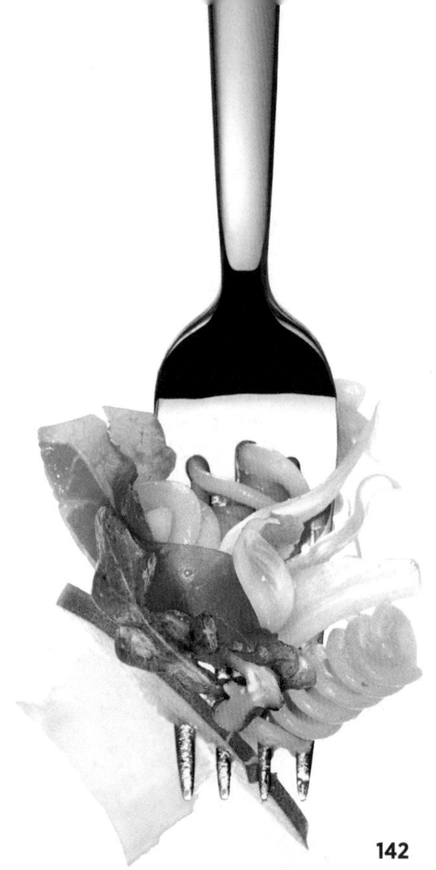
142

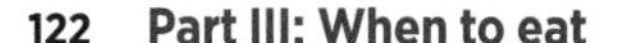

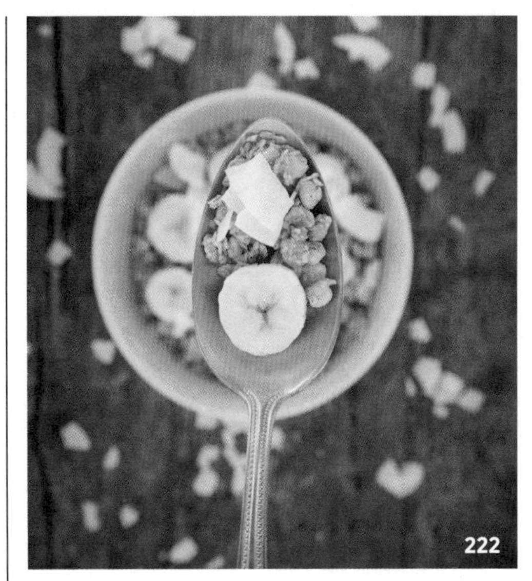
222

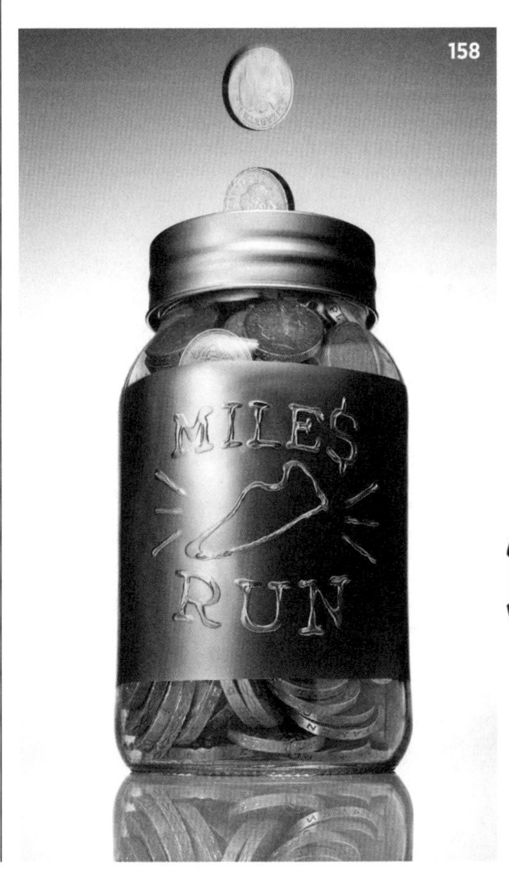

158

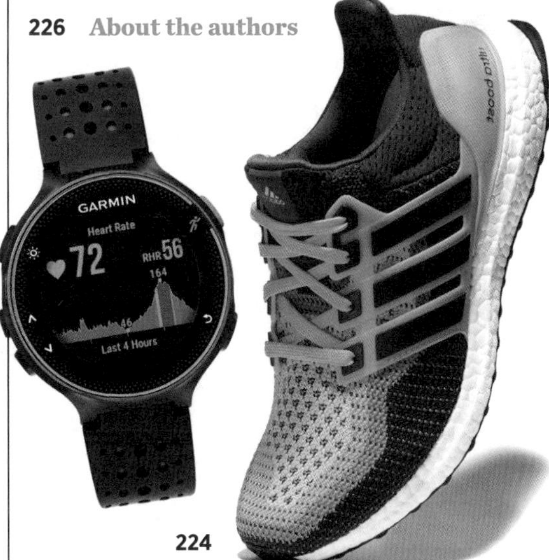

224

Authors
Jennifer Van Allen, Pamela Nisevich Bede

Art Director
Jack Tennant

Chief Sub Editor
David Rothon

Editor
Joe Mackie

Cover illustration
Telegramme

Back cover photograph
Tule Lillegraven

Workflow Director
Terry Barbrook

Group Publishing Director
Alun Williams

HEARST RODALE JOINT BOARD OF DIRECTORS
President and CEO, Hearst Magazines International
Duncan Edwards

Senior Vice President, International Business Development and Partnerships, Rodale International
Robert Novick

RODALE INTERNATIONAL
Rodale Inc, 33 East Minor Street, Emmaus, Pennsylvania 18098, USA

EDITORIAL
Editorial Director, Rodale International
John Ville

Editorial Director, Runner's World International
Veronika Ruff Taylor

Senior Content Manager
Karl Rozemeyer

Editorial Assistant
Natanya Spies

BUSINESS
Executive Director, Business Development and Global Licensing
Kevin LaBonge

Director, Global Marketing
Tara Swansen

Director, Business Development and Global Licensing
Angela Kim

International Finance Manager
Erica Adam

Introduction

It's often said that weight loss is a simple matter of consuming fewer calories than your body burns.

If that sentence made you want to throw this book out of the window, you're probably not alone. Anyone who's tried to lose weight on that basis knows it isn't always so simple. Yes, for a lucky few the unwanted pounds just melt off as soon as they start exercising more and cutting back on calories. But for many more of us, the process of reaching a feel-great weight is much more confusing. And frustrating.

One could get whiplash trying to stay abreast of the barrage of diet trends. It seems every day brings new claims about some sort of superfood – green tea, chia seeds, coconut oil, lemon juice, chillies – and the weight-loss magic it brings. Just as dizzying is the list of ingredients we're told to avoid: gluten, meat, wheat, carbs, fats sugar, fruit... It's hard to keep up – much less figure out how to make the scales move.

It's difficult to wade through the tidal waves of advice

And if you're running to lose weight, or trying to slim down while training for a race, it's even more difficult to wade through the tidal waves of advice in order to shrink your waistline *and* your race times. So often, nutrition guidance for runners contradicts even the most conventional dieting advice.

What's all this about fuelling up for a run, for example? Why would you go out and eat more calories to prepare for a workout designed to burn off those you've already consumed?

And if weight loss is a matter of taking in fewer calories and incinerating more, the idea of consuming calories *during* a run where you're trying to burn them sounds plain ludicrous.

And what about carbs?

Dieters everywhere are cutting them to shed weight. But runners are told to make carbs account for over half of their daily calories.

And running or training for a race introduces so many other questions. Does completing a three-mile run mean you get to eat 300 extra calories that day? If you run six miles, do you deserve a brownie?

No wonder there's so much confusion.

There certainly was for Steve Lambert, 33, who lost more than 7st with the help of Weight Watchers and a half-marathon training programme. "My Weight Watchers mind was telling me not to eat anything while training, but my body was telling me I needed fuel after 90 minutes of running," he says. Ultimately he took the advice of running mates and went for an energy bar during long sessions on the road. "It worked perfectly," he says, "but subconsciously I was still worrying about how many points I was consuming that day."

For others, like 40-year-old Rob Walter, the confusion leads to a frustrating process of training harder and harder, and restricting more and more foods, only to see the scales – and race times – refusing to budge.

Rob was looking to get faster, feel more comfortable in his jeans, and shave about 1½st from his 6ft 1in frame. He tried various high-protein and low-carb approaches while training for half-marathons and marathons, but nothing lasted more than a few weeks. "I'd feel like crap before, during and after workouts," he recalls. "I had zero energy, and my cravings were horrendous because the bread and carbs I loved were discouraged."

Others, like Lynn Ramsey, 45, have found that no matter how many miles they run, the scales only move in the wrong direction. The more Lynn ran, the hungrier she became. "I hate dieting, counting calories and depriving myself," she says. "And I get really hungry as my mileage increases."

She's not alone. In one study [1] of 64 marathon trainees, some runners lost almost 2st; others gained up to 1st. And these people weren't slow; the average finish time was 4:25. Some 63% of the subjects said they ate more during training.

We've heard thousands of similar stories at *Runner's World*; runners who've found that the pain and frustration of having extra lbs to shed are more difficult to cope with than any physical discomfort involved in making their legs and lungs stronger.

As for Steve, after several failed attempts at weight loss, "I just told myself, 'Right, I'm an athletic fat guy; that's what I am.' I pretended that being overweight was OK. I pretended I could just go to the gym a few times a week, and barely doing anything would make a difference."

But eventually it became clear that it wouldn't. "My sleep wasn't efficient, I was out of breath tying my shoes and just everyday stuff was hard," he says. "I realised that I needed to be healthy so I could enjoy life."

The lighter you are, the more efficiently you'll run, the more you'll enjoy it and the faster you'll finish. Research shows [2] weight can affect performance in running more than in other sports, such as cycling and swimming.

Wesley Cure, a 31-year-old runner who lost 5st 5lb to get back to his weight as a school leaver, learnt this first-hand. "When I started running, it really hurt my shins," he says. "After I lost 1-1½st, the pain stopped. After that, my speed increase seemed to be in direct correlation to my weight loss. I generally felt healthier; I had more energy and I was faster."

But losing weight and getting faster don't always happen in this tidy upward progression – not even for those like Wesley, who ran a 3:10 in his first marathon. He struggled to find how treats could fit into his regular diet. After months of swearing off sweets, he says, "I ended up bingeing once and realised there was no way I could go without them. To try to give up the occasional treat just wasn't realistic for me. Now I eat a little so that I don't want a lot."

First you must identify your own personal obstacles

And this isn't just an issue for those who are overweight. Runners at all levels struggle to balance their racing and weight-loss goals. Shedding weight while getting the fuel you need to log a PB just isn't easy.

It certainly wasn't for Olympian and 2015 USA Marathon champ Blake Russell. After becoming a mother, resuming her professional running life meant losing the near-3st she gained with each of her two children, having taken months off with each pregnancy.

Eating for recovery – focusing on carbs, protein and fat to help her recover, as well as hydration – helped Blake regain her fitness and speed without getting injured. But so did a few key phrases: a note on the scales at her doctor's surgery that read, '*These scales measure weight, not worth; you are worthy and beautiful.*' Plus sage words from her coach...

"He always said that talent doesn't go away," she says. "These words echoed in my head and, frankly, I clung to them as I was whipping myself into shape. And it helped that I remembered what it was like to feel fit and fast. I wanted that feeling again."

In *Run Your Belly Off*, you'll learn how to juggle your weight-loss and training goals to see the numbers you want both on the scales and at the finish line. But first you must identify your personal obstacles. Everyone has a unique set of habits, lifestyle, temptations, and time and resource constraints getting in the way of their goals,

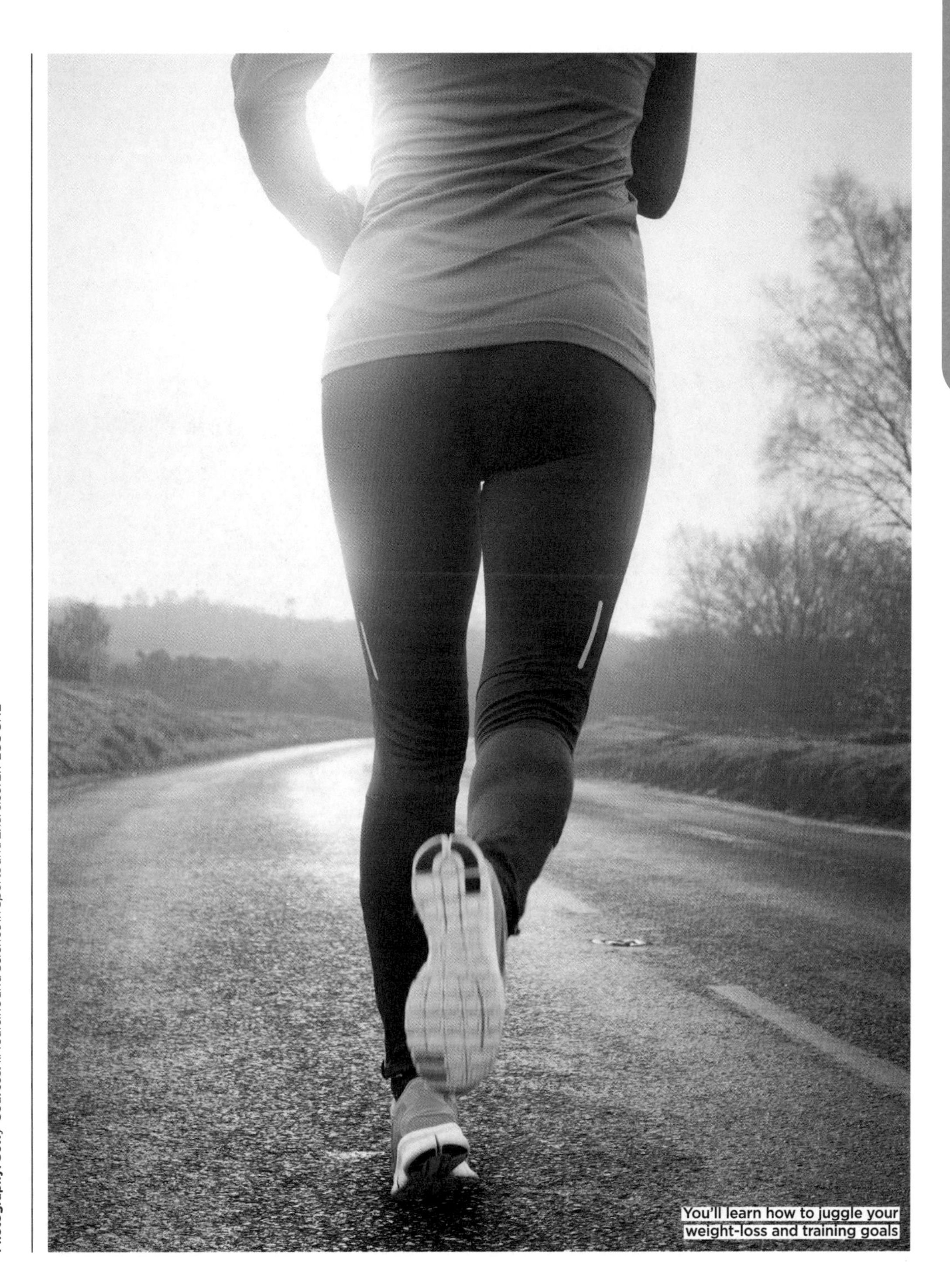

You'll learn how to juggle your weight-loss and training goals

Photography: Getty **Sources:** 1. *Medicine and Science in Sports and Exercise*. 2. *PLOS ONE*

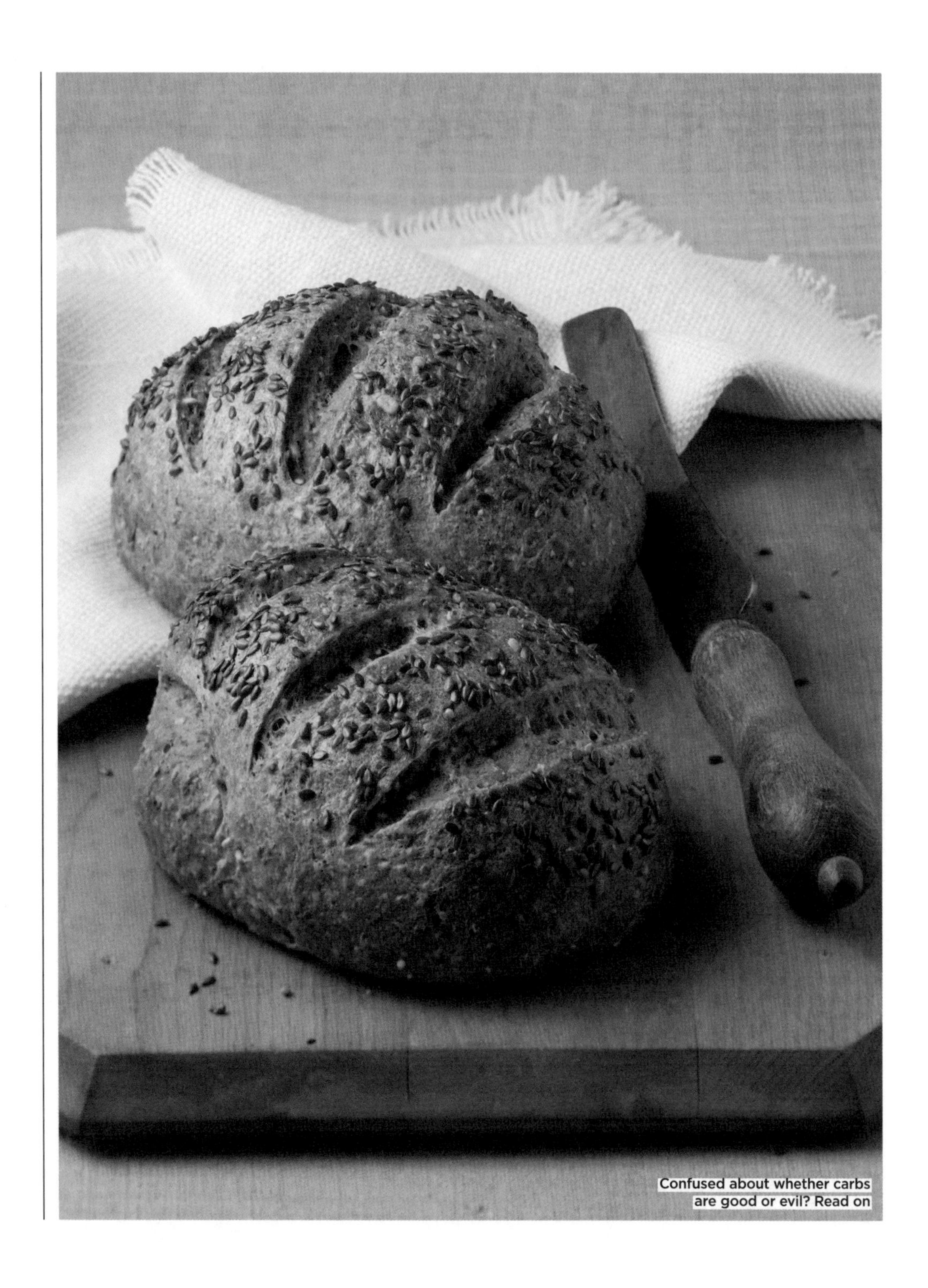

Confused about whether carbs are good or evil? Read on

so your solutions will be unique for you. If you want to lose weight and get faster, only *you* can identify what your challenges are, and what approach will best address them.

For Rob Walter, it wasn't until he started incorporating the carbs back into his diet that he started seeing the results he was after.

Kate McPhail, 31, lost over 7st by making small, incremental changes, such as swapping white bread for whole-grain, and finding healthier items that were still full of flavour. "I never decided to eat x amount of calories; I just started to make smarter food choices," says Kate, 31. "Instead of buying biscuits, I'd make my own, healthier versions."

For Kyle Klaver, 48, it was about eliminating processed foods. "If it comes in a box or a bag, I don't eat it," he says. Because Kyle travels a lot for work, his plan involved finding restaurants with healthy options ahead of time, and 'deconstructing' menu items where necessary. "They'll sometimes let me order a dish the way I want, or I'll order the standard and tear it apart at the table," he says.

You can design your own plan in a way that works for *you*

In this book you'll learn how to identify the obstacles keeping you from reaching your weight-loss and running goals. And you'll find all the tools you need to overcome them.

Start by doing our quiz on page 20 and use the responses to help you navigate the book. Remember, there are no right answers – only honest ones. Redo it periodically for a gut check.

Confused about whether carbs are good or evil? Turn to Chapter 1. Don't know how much to eat? In Part II, you'll find help. Need to rev up your calorie burn while keeping workout times short? Find out how in Chapter 23. Do you feel powerless when a box of doughnuts appears in the office? Turn to Chapter 29. And what about stress eating – when the going gets tough, do the tough turn to chocolate? (Chapter 28 can help you with that, too.) Can green tea boost your calorie burn, even when sat at your desk? (Find out in Chapter 15.) And if you're trying to choose one of the popular conventional diet plans, or you're already on one, we can help you integrate that diet into your life as a runner (turn to Chapter 14). You can apply the information in this book to any conventional diet or training approach – this will ultimately help you design your *own* diet and running programme in a way that works best for you.

That said, there are a few ground rules to follow (see page 14 for those). Your eating and your exercise efforts have to improve the quality of your life, not diminish it. If you can't imagine keeping up a particular training or eating routine forever, it's not right for you. It won't last and the weight will return.

The time you take to work out your own plan will be well worth the investment. The rewards go beyond anything that could be measured on the scales or the finish-line clock. Just ask anyone who's done it themselves.

For Kyle, losing weight has boosted his confidence. He doesn't hide in the background of photos; he doesn't get the constant colds he used to, and at 48, he has more energy than ever.

"My energy level is unbelievable," he says. "I used to take naps on Saturdays and Sundays. Now, even after a long run, I feel I could go and do it again later in the day. And my mind and memory are better, too."

Or take it from Sarah Williarty. She started running to improve her health, but in the process of cutting an hour from her marathon time, breaking two hours in the half-marathon, and finally getting rid of that last 5lbs, she benefited in ways that could never be measured by numbers.

"Getting that much faster made me feel like a rock star, and kind of like an athlete," she says. As a self-described bookworm, "Those were very new feelings." But that wasn't all. "In other parts of life, I stopped being afraid," she says. "I was no longer scared of getting hurt if I tried to run fast. I stopped being afraid of talking to other mums. I even started speaking up a lot more at work. I started organising more social events for my family. The drive to run faster has spilled over into other parts of my life in ways that are very positive. It's given me a lot more confidence."

As you begin your own *Run Your Belly Off* journey, we hope that you gain benefits that are just as enduring. ■

Photography: Getty

Ground rules

We believe strongly that weight loss and running better aren't one-size-fits-all propositions; each person has unique obstacles, and *Run Your Belly Off* is designed to help you learn how to balance your weight-loss and training goals and design strategies that best fit *your* needs, lifestyle, temperament and temptations. At the end of each chapter you'll find steps you can take to overcome your personal obstacles.

That said, certain ground rules have been proven to work for anyone; to help you reach your goals no matter what diet you're on or what your kryptonite food is. Why? Because these behaviours organically foster and nourish the habits that pave the way for weight-loss and running success. Think of them as a healthy version of gateway drugs. They're based on the most enduring lessons we've learnt from experts who spend their lives researching this stuff, and on the strategies we've found to be most powerful in our work with thousands of runners and dieters over the years. So rip these pages from our book or mix, match and make up your own (see rule 14!).

These rules are like a healthy version of gateway drugs

1. You are an experiment of one. Running guru and *Runner's World* contributor George Sheehan said that, and it's true. What works for others may not work for you. No one else has to live your precise life, with your specific challenges, biochemistry, anatomy, injury history, boss, commute, calendar or minefield of family commitments. So yes, reach for guidance from experts (including us), but the organising principle of any diet should be how well it works for your unique life. And it should, in some way, fit into your personal definition of fun and enjoyment. As US author and journalist Anna Quindlen once wrote, 'If your success is not on your own terms, if it looks good to the world but does not feel good in your heart, it is not success at all.'

2. Take good notes. When a run goes well, write it down. When a run goes the opposite of well, write it down. Same goes for weight watching. A day of perfect eating? Write it down. A day of careening completely off the rails? You guessed it. Taking notes can be time consuming, and it can be humiliating to record something you feel ashamed about. But doing so will ultimately help you. Why? You'll draw confidence from seeing all you've accomplished, and when the going gets tough, that'll help you restore faith in yourself and remind you that one day is not destiny. Having a record of the good *and* bad will also help you identify the culprit when you're getting hurt, gaining weight or just feeling low. What's more, research has shown that good notes lead

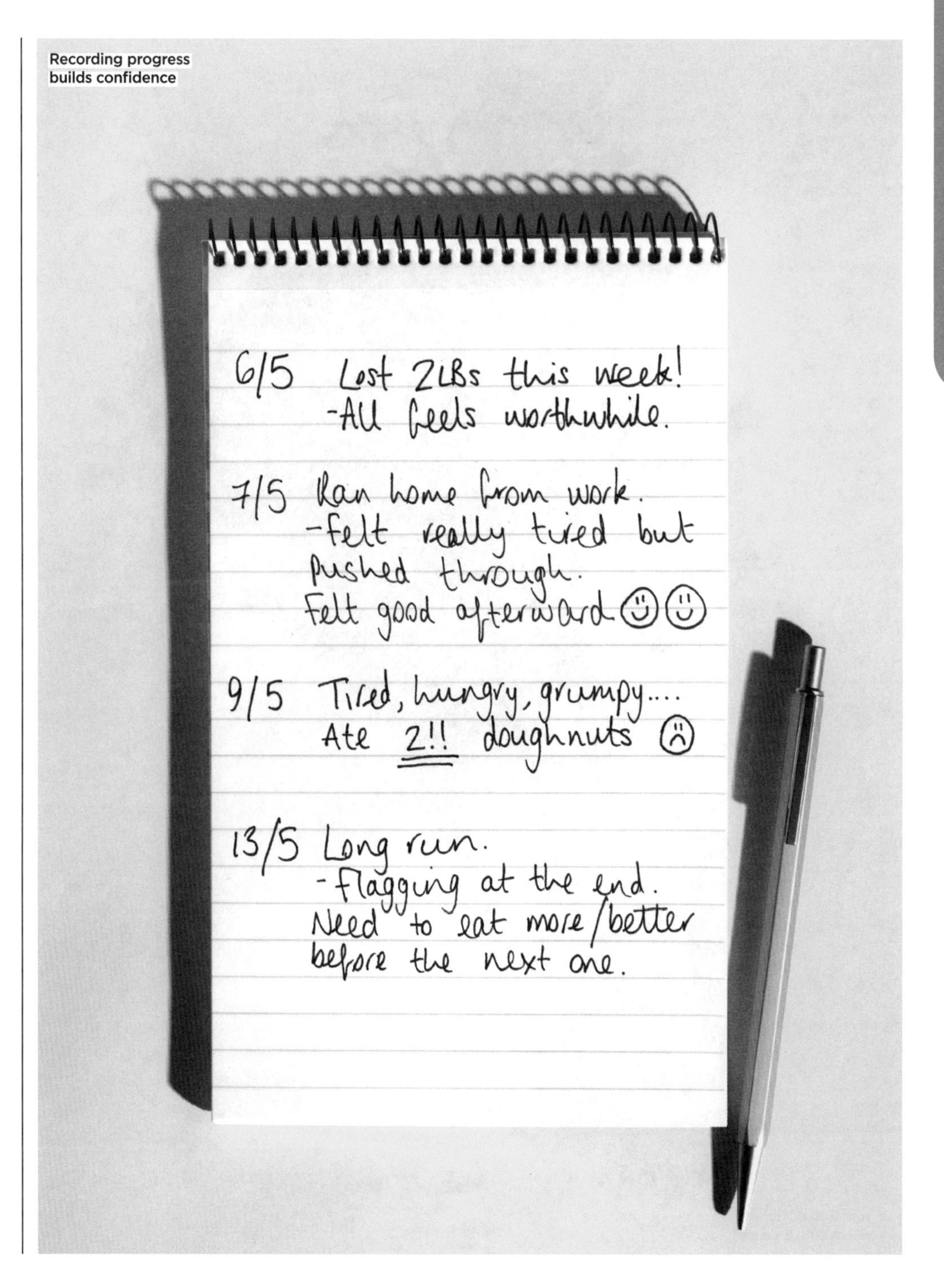

Recording progress builds confidence

Photography: Getty

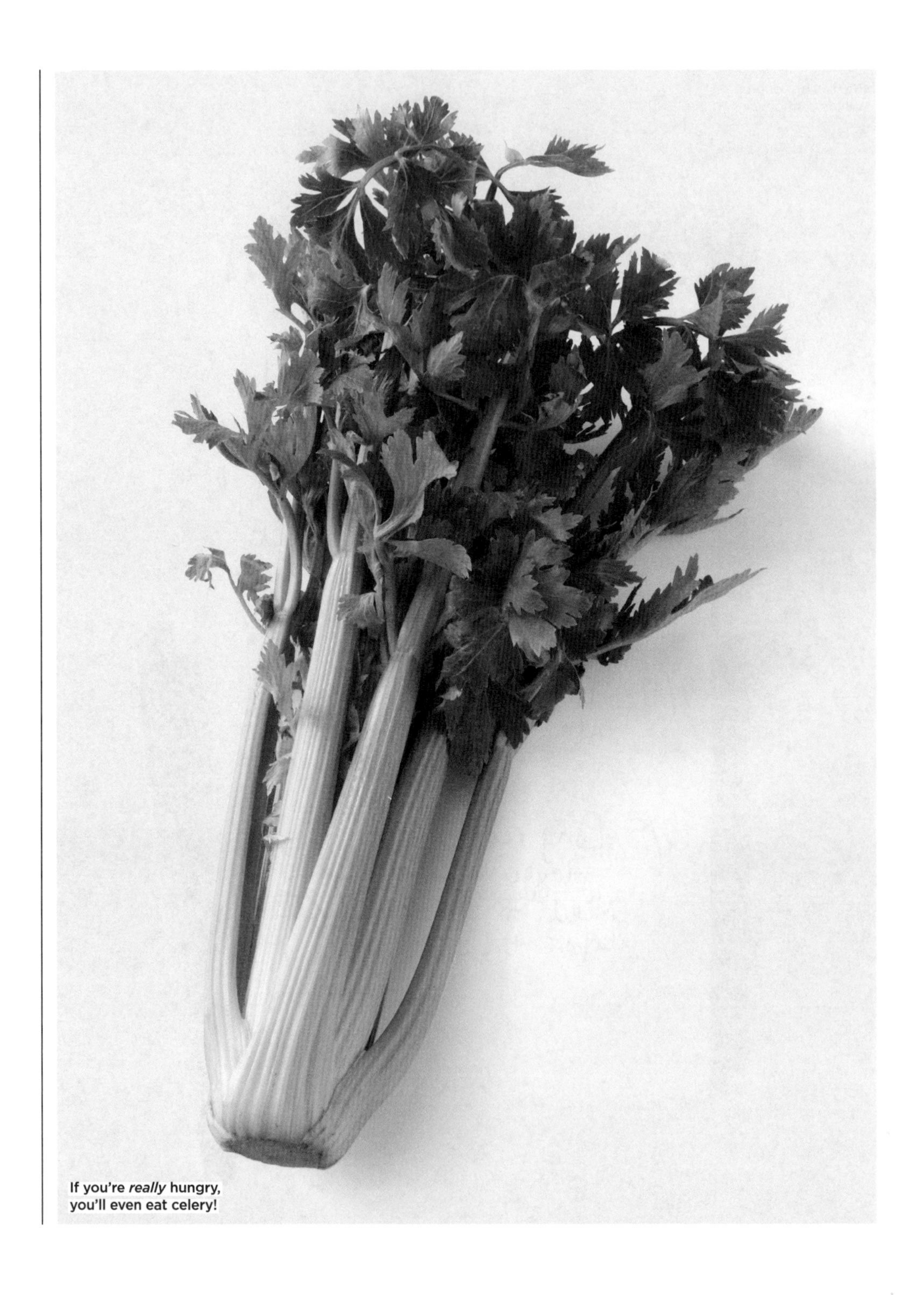

If you're *really* hungry, you'll even eat celery!

to weight loss. A 2008 study in the *American Journal of Preventive Medicine* found that among 1,700 overweight runners, those who kept a food diary more than five days a week lost almost twice weight as much as those who didn't – *and* they kept it off.[1]

3. When something works, excuse-proof it. Running and weight watching are tough enough; make the habits that work for you as easy as possible to practise. Any sort of strategy that requires you to twist your life, your family and other priorities into a pretzel won't last and won't work. So keep tempting foods out of the house, out of sight and out of mind. If you love running at sunrise but worry about waking the kids on your way out, keep your running gear by the front door or in your car. Need a coffee before you go? Invest in a coffee maker that automatically brews in the morning. Splash out on good-quality gear that allows you to get outside in snow, sleet, rain and any other weather. Believe us, you'll get a little extra runner's high from venturing out in conditions that other people won't even drive in.

However much you eat, that feeling will still be there

4. When something stops working, stop working it. Give any new strategy at least a week before you call it quits. But remember, as Albert Einstein (supposedly) said, the definition of insanity is doing the same thing over and over again and expecting different results. Yes, it can be scary to diverge from the known, especially if something *has* worked for you in the past. But if the thought of running the same three-mile loop is boring you and making it more difficult to get out the door, take a different route. If you're not seeing results from the strength-training routine you've been doing for two months, try something else. Likewise, if the same meal that helped you shed the first 5lbs now makes you feel bored, deprived or constipated – or has just stopped tasting good – try something new that fits the right nutrient profile. (The internet is awash with healthy recipes designed by people who share your goals – and your dietary restrictions. And go to runnersworld.co.uk/recipes.)

5. Follow the celery rule. It's often difficult to separate a mental craving from true physical hunger. When you're truly ravenous, even a celery stick will do. When you crave something, it's usually very specific – the rush of a piece of chocolate; the salty crunch of a crisp – and really you're probably hankering for relief from something deeper: boredom, frustration, loneliness, fear, a work deadline, a quandary with a loved one... No matter what you do or how much you eat, that feeling is still going to be there when you finish eating. And it'll be compounded by feelings of remorse about what you just ate.

6. Take time out. Scientists have shown that it can take less than two minutes for an urge, a thought or a craving to disappear from your consciousness. Many mindful-eating experts, such as Dr Susan Albers, psychologist and author of seven books, including *Eat Q: Unlock the Weight-Loss Power of Emotional Intelligence*, have recommended that dieters use this to their advantage. (Read more about mindful eating in Chapter 27.) If you're hammering away at a frustrating work assignment and thinking about that packet of crisps in your drawer, rather than engaging in a wrestling match with your willpower or automatically inserting your hand into the packet, tell yourself you can have the crisps – in two minutes. Set a timer to go off in two minutes, then do something else. (Brushing your teeth, walking around the block or refilling your water bottle are good options.) Chances are, by the time you hear the timer, those crisps won't seem so compelling anymore. Other research has confirmed that distraction works. A study performed by eating-behaviour expert Dr Brian Wansink found that when people were given just a few

Photography: Getty. **Sources:** 1. *American Journal of Preventive Medicine*

bites of a snack they wanted, then distracted for 15 minutes, they were equally as satisfied as others who'd been given bigger portions.[2]

7. Get outside. Research has proved it: time spent among nature relieves stress, boosts mood and combats depression. In a study published in the *Journal of Environmental Psychology*[3] in 2014, participants who spent time in a wooded, natural setting felt more restored and had better moods, more creativity and vitality, and lower levels of cortisol (the stress hormone) than those who spent time in an urban setting. Even if you're not running – and especially on days when you're not scheduled to exercise – it's important to get at least 10 minutes of outside time, enjoying the fresh air, hearing the tweeting birds and looking at trees, grass and flowers. If you set the bar low – 10 minutes is ideal – chances are, by the end of that time you'll want to keep going.

8. Reach out. Cultivate a circle of people who you know will genuinely help you celebrate your successes and commiserate when things don't go so well. It doesn't matter whether they're online or in the 'real world'. Research has shown that social connection helps seal success: a study published in a 2012 issue of *Obesity* found that in a programme where 34% of participants lost at least 5% of their body weight, a powerful factor was 'social influence'. Close friends with similar goals acted as a team, worked out together and exchanged pep-talk emails.[4] With such a support network, however low or lost you feel, you can be assured that someone else out there has felt the same way at some point. (And see rule 10.)

9. Act like the person you want to be. Gandhi said, "Be the change you want to see in the world," and when it comes to weight loss and running, it really does work. Think of the person you'd like to be or someone you admire – who has succeeded in weight loss or reached an amazing personal best. And when you start dithering over whether you should get the heck outside or stick your hand in a packet of crisps for stress relief, consider what that person you aspire to be, or whom you most admire, would do. (For more on this, see Chapter 29.)

10. When you get lost, ask for directions. Connect with others, online or on the ground. There is so much free help out there – not least at runnersworld.co.uk, where you'll find training plans, recipes and much more. Researchers have spent hundreds of years studying what works and what doesn't, and people like us spend our lives helping other people with obstacles like yours to reach a whole variety of specific goals. We're so lucky to live in an age where we can connect with others like you *and* with experts in just a few keystrokes. Take advantage of that.

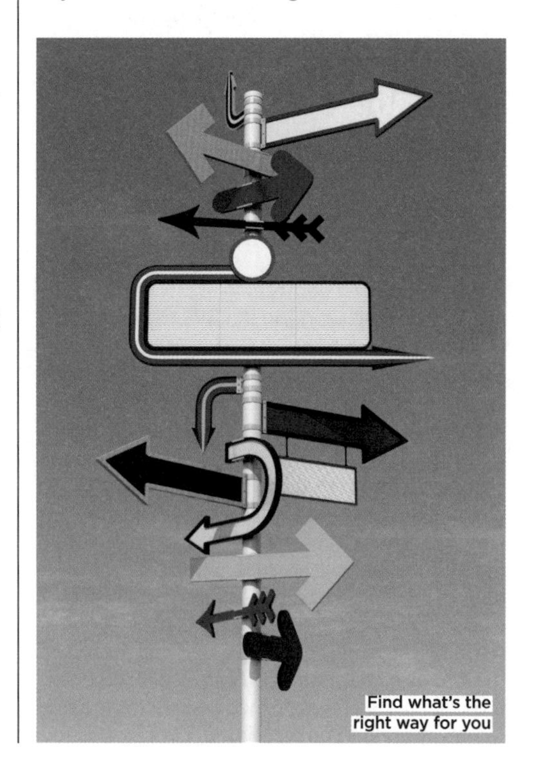
Find what's the right way for you

11. Compromise, don't sacrifice. Any healthy way of eating or exercising will expand your life, not contract it. Yes, long runs will inevitably nibble away at your family – and possibly even your work – time. But on the whole, sustainable eating and exercise habits should help you meet new people, explore places you've never seen, open your perspective and live longer so you can enjoy more quality time with your loved ones. When your eating and exercise habits are contracting your life – making you feel deprived, lonely, isolated and like you're being forced to make uncomfortable sacrifices – those strategies are destined not to work, because they won't last. This is particularly important when it comes to your eating habits. A successful diet should pave the way for you to try new fruits, vegetables, grains, recipes and ways of cooking you've never tried before. If you feel limited and deprived, and your daily meals feel like punishment, something needs to be changed.

12. Be nice. That goes for yourself and others. Trying to flog your body, your will or someone else into submission just doesn't work. Studies have shown that people who are compassionate with others feel better and are more likely to avert binges, compared with those who have a negative attitude towards themselves. A study published in the *Journal of Social and Clinical Psychology* in 2007 found that after indulging in a doughnut, dieters with self-compassion could monitor and hold back on further eating more so than those who focused on the negative implications of their indulgence.[5] If, after an off-the-diet chocolate-chip cookie, you're filled with feelings of hopelessness, self-hatred and regret, chances are you'll resign yourself to failure, throw your hands up and, in an effort to feel better, eat the whole pack. (See Chapter 27 for more on this.) But if you imagine you're counselling a friend who just ate the same cookie, you'd be more likely to assure them that one cookie won't ruin a diet and that everyone goes off the rails sometimes. If you look at your food or training log, you'll see that 99% of the time you're doing great; you can start again and get back on track right away. You can calm down and put the cookies away. The same goes for running. This is why rule 2 is so important. If you hit the wall before finishing one run and have to shuffle home, the demoralisation can be so paralysing it can be days before you find the courage to take to the road again. But if you look at your log and see how many miles you've covered, or days you've run, you'll see that one bad day is no big deal in light of all you've accomplished.

If you're feeling deprived, that strategy isn't going to work

13. Set up non-food rewards. Make a list of five things you can buy or do to celebrate your successes. These all should be completely unrelated to food, as rewarding yourself with a muffin the size of a volleyball is never a good idea. (See Chapter 27 on mindless eating.) Likewise, you don't want to wait until you accomplish some mileage milestone to get new shoes. Buy a book. Buy a new shirt. Get a manicure. Have a massage. Make a date to see friends. Plan a trip. It can be anything.

14. Make your own rules. (See rule 1.) Take the rules on these pages to heart, but set up other ones that suit *your* goals and needs, and help you overcome your unique obstacles. It might be a rule of 'no computers in the kitchen' so you don't get in the habit of eating while you're working. You may decide to make your home a chocolate-free zone to avoid temptation, or impose a 'no eating in the car' rule. A 'fresh air' rule that requires you to go outside every day for emotional and mental benefits is a good idea for everyone (see rule 7). After you do our quiz (pages 20-21), read this book, then do the quiz again, and make up your own ground rules that set you up for success. Think of them as the key pieces of advice you'd give a loved one who was sharing your struggle.

Photography: Getty. **Sources:** 2. Journal of Food Quality and Preference. 3. Journal of Environmental Psychology. 4. Obesity. 5. Journal of Social and Clinical Psychology

Run Your Belly Off self-quiz

Whether or not you know what's stopping you reaching your weight-loss goals, we'll help you identify your weaknesses and figure out how to get stronger. This quiz will help you reflect on where you're getting stalled, so you can more easily find the tools you need to break through. Let your answers guide you to the most relevant chapters in the book.

1. Age:
A. ______________________

2. Current weight:
A. ______________________

3. Goal weight:
A. ______________________

4. Body-fat percentage (if known):
A. ______________________

5. Goal body-fat percentage (if applicable):
A. ______________________

6. Goal race time and distance:
A. ______________________

7. Current race time and distance:
A. ______________________

8. Do you have a chronic medical condition?
A. ______________________

9. Do you take any prescribed medications that may affect your weight?
A. ______________________

10. Any limitations to your physical activity?
A. ______________________

11. Do you have any medical conditions or allergies that affect what you eat?
A. ______________________

12. Do you take any vitamins or supplements? If so, what – and why?
A. ______________________

13. Why do you want to lose weight?
A. ______________________

14. Worst eating habit:
A. ______________________

15. Healthiest eating habit:
A. ______________________

16. How many alcoholic drinks do you consume per week?
A. ______________________

17. How many nights a week do you eat out?
A. ______________________

18. How many nights a week do you cook?
A. ______________________

19. How often do you eat fruit and vegetables?
A. ______________________

20. How often do you skip meals?
A. ______________________

21. How often do you eat breakfast?
A. ______________________

22. Do you track your calories or your intake of carbs, fats and protein?
A. ______________________

23. Do you read the nutrition labels on packaged foods?
A. ______________________

24. Do you keep a food diary?
A. ______________________

25. How often do you weigh yourself?

A. ______________________

26. Do you monitor your weight loss in some other way – say, a favourite pair of trousers?

A. ______________________

27. How many times a week do you work out?

A. ______________________

28. Do you regularly do faster-paced runs, eg, tempo runs and speedwork?

A. ______________________

29. Do you strength train? If so, how often?

A. ______________________

30. Do you cross-train?

A. ______________________

31. Do you measure how fast, how far and how long you run?

A. ______________________

32. What's your favourite type of workout?

A. ______________________

33. What's your least favourite workout?

A. ______________________

34. Do you keep a training diary?

A. ______________________

35. If so, which metrics do you track?

A. ______________________

36. Have you been sidelined for more than two weeks by running-related injuries?

A. ______________________

37. If you answered yes to Q.36, did you eat less, the same or more while sidelined?

A. ______________________

38. How often do you get outside for exercise or otherwise?

A. ______________________

39. How many hours per day do you sit (in a car, at your office, etc)?

A. ______________________

40. Do you do any physical activities other than running on a regular basis?

A. ______________________

41. What diets have you tried?

A. ______________________

42. Which elements of those diets have worked?

A. ______________________

43. Which elements of those diets have not worked?

A. ______________________

44. Have you ever eliminated entire food groups for weight-loss – not medical – reasons?

A. ______________________

45. Do you ever eat when you're not hungry, but due to some negative emotion?

A. ______________________

46. Do you ever eat food just because it's there?

A. ______________________

47. If you could remove one bad eating habit, what would it be?

A. ______________________

48. Do you do any contemplative, self-reflective activities regularly (eg, writing, meditation)?

A. ______________________

49. Do you have anyone in whom you can confide about your weight-loss struggles (whether online or in person)?

A. ______________________

50. Do you have a fitness or running role model? What kinds of eating and exercise habits do they practise?

A. ______________________

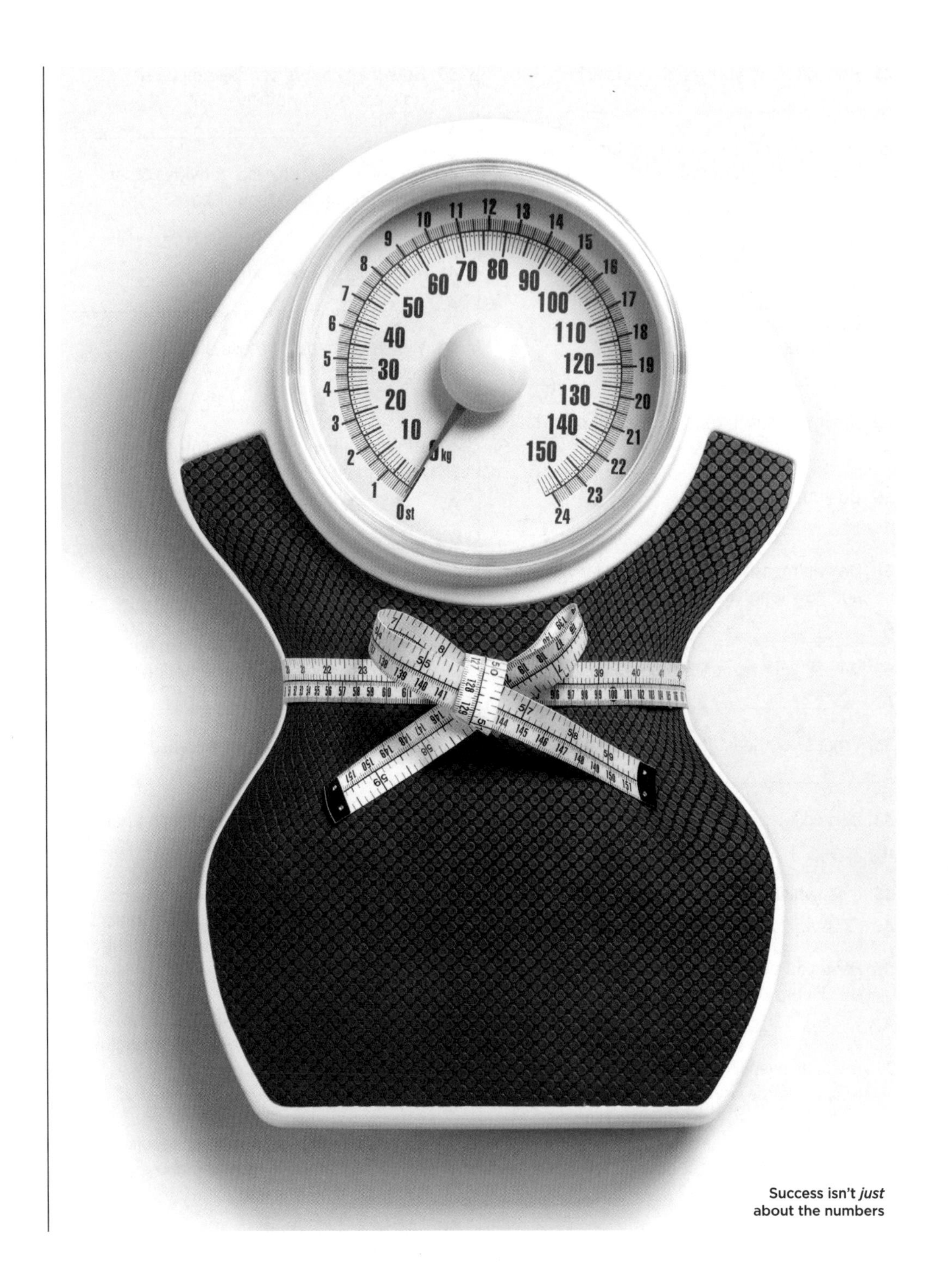

Success isn't *just* about the numbers

Measuring success

When it comes to tracking your progress, the scales shouldn't be the only tool you use. A variety of factors that have nothing to do with your speed or eating habits can drive the scales skyward, throw off your race times, and drive you absolutely nuts. We live and die by these numbers; they can make us swell with confidence we never thought possible, or send us reeling into dark caves of depression. After all, who wants to spend precious hours and days trying to eat right and run better if, according to the numbers, it's not working? The resulting depression can be pretty powerful, driving us to resign ourselves to a 'why bother?' state of mind, skip our next workout and, possibly, drown our sorrows in a bucket of Häagen-Dazs.

When it comes to numbers, here's what we think: tracking progress works, but single tools used in isolation – whether it's the scales, the finish-line clock, your training watch, a body-composition test, blood pressure and cholesterol levels, or even the number next to the word 'size' on your favourite jeans – can't tell the whole story: for example, how much fitter you're becoming and how you feel.

Because each metric has its limitations, and because progress rarely occurs as a straightforward, upward trajectory, it's wise to measure as many metrics as possible without risking obsession and compulsion. That way, your sense of satisfaction and accomplishment from all the hard work you do isn't completely dependent on a single measure, which could be way off for any variety of factors that have nothing to do with what you're consuming or your running progress. Using three to five metrics, which you can take at a variety of different frequencies, is a good place to start.

Here are some key measures of success and how to work with them.

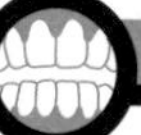

CHEW ON THIS

Looking at your life as a whole, even the highest-tech gadget can't detect some of the most important measures of success – such as your confidence, your effectiveness at work and the happiness of your loved ones. Regardless of what any electronic readout says, the miles you run and the food you eat should improve your quality of life, not diminish it. If your family are feeling neglected, your boss is annoyed or you just feel dissatisfied or deprived, none of those metrics matters. So as you look at the numbers, try not to lose sight of the big picture: your own happiness, the contentment of your loved ones and the causes and work you care about count for a lot.

The scales

Why they matter Trying to change something specific without tracking whether that something is changing is an invitation for frustration and delusion. In one of the key findings of the National Weight Control Registry, a long-term US study of people who'd lost an average of 4st 10lb and kept it off for at least five years, 75% of all participants weighed themselves at least once a week.[1]

Many of the headlines that urge you to throw out the scales are warnings about its limitations – and those should be real considerations. Your body weight can fluctuate throughout the day, and from day to day, due to factors that have nothing to do with what you're eating or how fast you're running. These can include hormones, dehydration, the amount of carbs or sodium in your last meal, or even constipation.

When to measure First thing in the morning, naked, after you've been to the bathroom but before you eat or drink anything.

How often No more than once a day. Given how many factors can make your weight fluctuate, weighing yourself any more often is a waste of time. The exception is if you're using this to take the 'sweat test' (see Chapter 8 on what to drink) to figure out how much fluid you need for your workout.

What they leave out Whether you're getting faster and how much you're improving your body composition by increasing your muscle mass and decreasing your body-fat percentage. The scales also won't measure whether your blood pressure, cholesterol levels and risk of chronic disease are all heading in the right direction.

Your mileage and pace

Why they matter It's important to ramp up mileage and speed very gradually to prevent injury, and allow your body to adapt to new stresses and get stronger. In general you don't want to increase either factor by more than 10% from one week to the next. Taking good notes on how many miles you run, your pace, how you feel, and the shoes you wear can help you detect injuries or signs of burnout before they derail you.

How often Every time you run.

What they leave out What you're eating. If you're consuming all the calories you burned (aka overcompensating) after every workout, you're probably undoing any potential weight-loss benefits you're getting from your workouts. By the same token, if you're restricting your calories or carbs too much, going into every run feeling depleted and hitting the wall before you finish the day's mileage, you're handicapping your workouts before you even hit the road. While a training journal will offer some clues about what's helping – or hurting – your weight-loss efforts, what you're eating is a huge part of it, too.

5K times

Why they matter In a 5K race setting, you're running at the fastest pace you can sustain. This is a great way to measure your aerobic fitness and running performance. It's also an effective means of testing your racing and fuelling tactics. And because the race itself involves a very small time commitment, and the training required can be as little as 20 miles a week, it's a very accessible way to measure your fitness. What's more, because races typically offer aid stations, cheering spectators, a measured course and automated timing, you're set up for success. Try to find races on courses with similar elevation profiles to use throughout the season. Some running clubs have race series on the same course, as do Parkruns, so you can fairly measure your fitness gains. If one 5K race is on a flat course and your next one is hilly, you won't be able to fairly compare your times.

When to measure At the beginning of your fitness programme.

How often Every six to eight weeks.

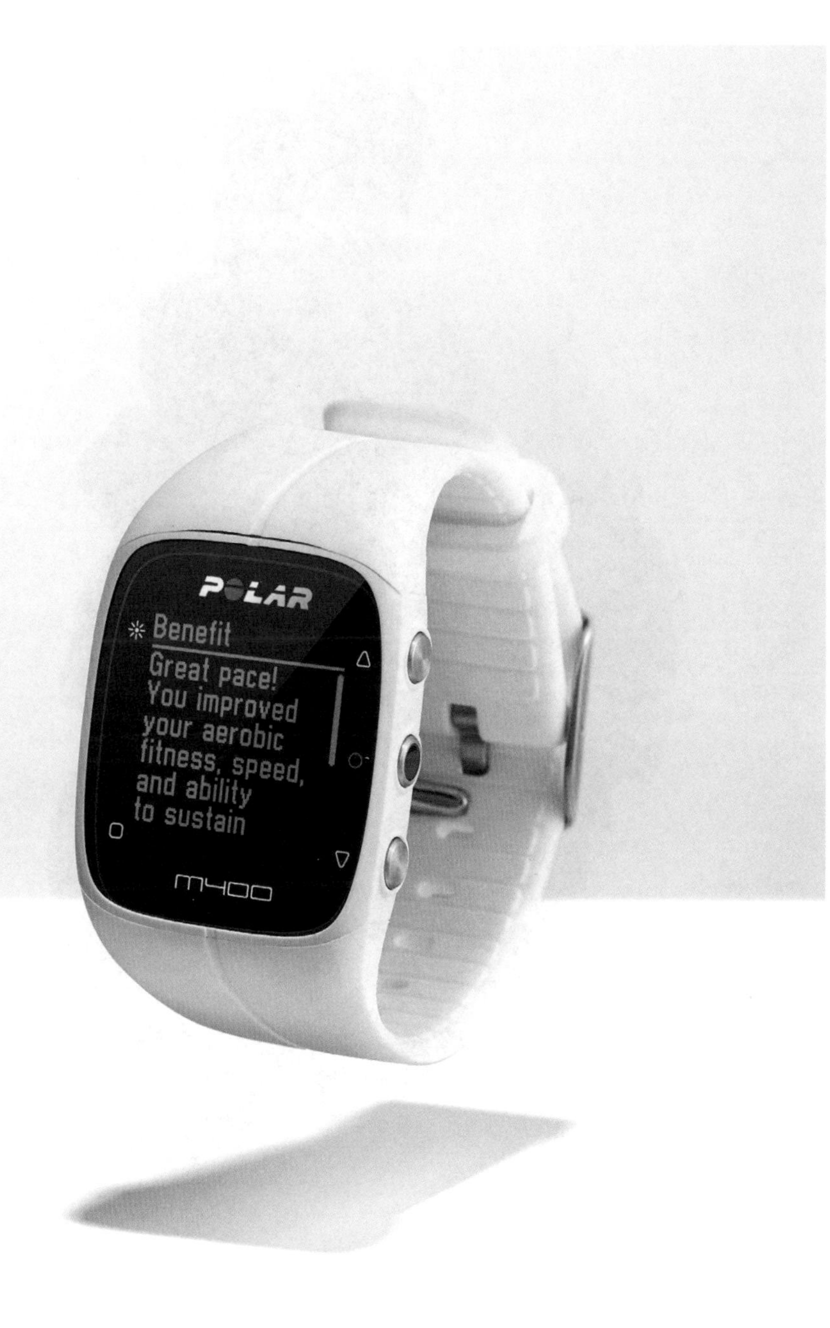

Pace and distance give you a clear measure of progress

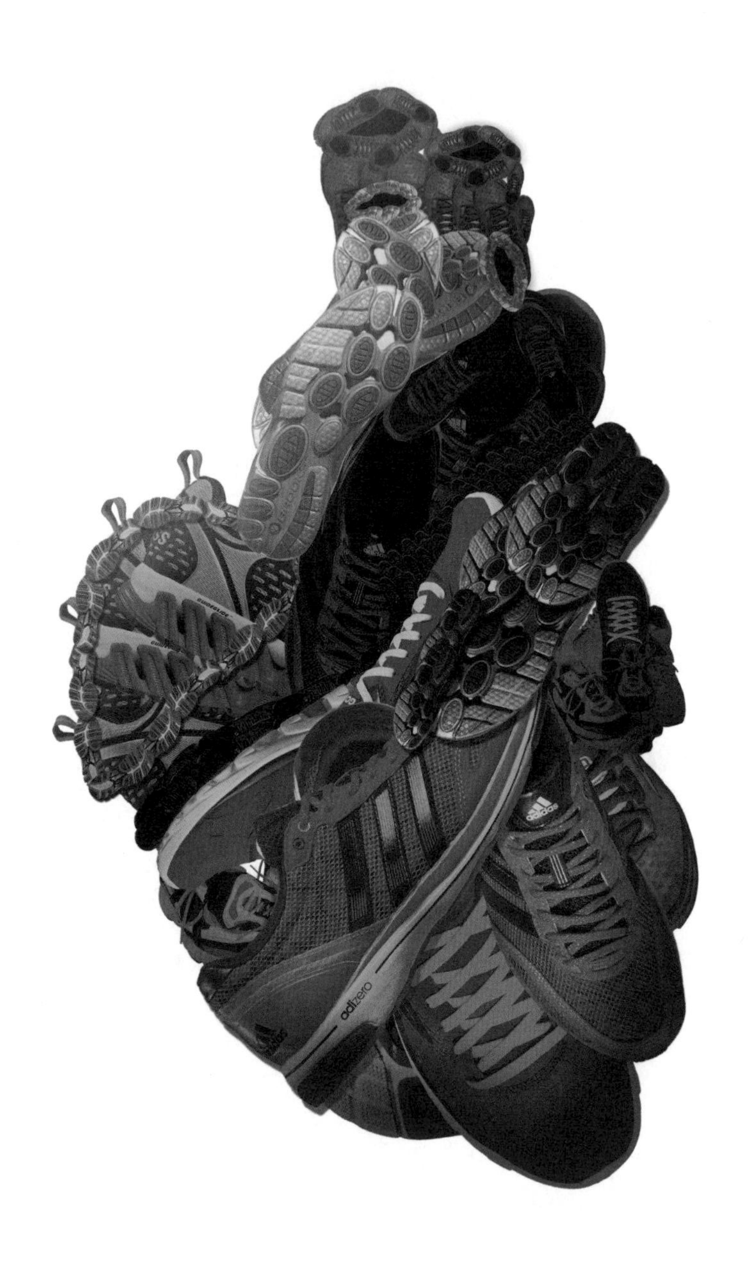

All that running will make for a healthier heart

What they leave out If your diet is still out of whack, it's not going to show up immediately in your 5K results. Because factors such as wind, heat and the hilliness of the course can all impinge on your race times, the number on the finish-line clock will not always be a direct reflection of your complete fitness profile or the dietary changes you're making.

Resting heart rate

Why it matters If your heart isn't healthy, it's likely that your running, weight-loss and overall health goals are going to remain out of reach. As you get fitter and build your aerobic power, your heart won't have to work as hard as it did before. Think about climbing the stairs. If you're unfit, you'll probably feel out of breath at the top of the stairs, with your heart pounding hard and fast in a panicky twitter. As you strengthen your heart through running, with each beat it can pump more blood. That means it'll take fewer beats to pump the blood you need to power your body up the stairs. So as you get fitter, your resting heart rate should go down.

When to measure First thing in the morning. Before you get out of bed, take your pulse for one minute and write it down.

How often Daily.

What it leaves out If the weather is hot, you're stressed, sick, sleep-deprived or in any other altered condition, your resting heart rate might be affected. It also doesn't measure your dietary improvements or any changes in your body composition.

How fast you're running

Why it matters The same thing we said about the scales applies here: if your goal is to get faster, it's important to track your pace to get a sense of how fast you're going.

When to measure On any run.

How often On every run.

What it leaves out If the weather is hot, humid, you're injured or you've fallen short on sleep, your pace is likely to slow and your level of effort is sure to spike. It also doesn't directly measure how you feel on each run (though if you feel awful, your average pace probably will reflect that – see Chapter 26 on measuring your running efforts). Your running pace also doesn't measure any dietary changes that could be either improving or derailing your running efforts, or lowering or raising your risk of chronic disease.

Body composition (body-fat percentage)

Why it matters Reducing your body fat and improving lean muscle mass can help you run faster, burn more calories even when you're not running and improve your overall health. By the same token, not enough fat can lead to injury and other health complications. For men, ideal body fat is 8-24%; for women; the ideal is 21-35%. For some athletes, it's going to be even lower. The most accurate measurements are by DEXA or Bod Pod scan, which are offered at some hospitals, research centres, doctors' surgeries, gyms and universities. You might have to pay for it. Other methods are easier and more accessible, but they're less accurate. Special scales offered at some gyms offer a body-fat measurement based on bioelectrical impedance analysis.

When to measure At the start of your workout or weight-loss efforts. At a gym, a personal trainer can use calipers to measure skinfold thickness in the chest, belly, triceps and thighs. These can be accurate if the trainer has experience, uses high-quality equipment and employs the right equation to translate those measurements into an estimate of body fat.

How often As your training progresses and as you make improvements, checking in on your body comp can be a great pat on the back. You might consider getting it checked as you move from one cycle of training to another – say, at the beginning of your marathon-training programme, then just before the race.

What it leaves out How you feel, any dietary changes and how fast you're running. And it won't indicate your risk of chronic diseases.

Your trousers

Why they matter These can offer an instant assessment of whether you're trimming your waistline and whittling away the belly fat that is linked to so many chronic diseases. They can also offer a big confidence boost, which counts for a lot. There's no better feeling than knowing you can fit into your 'skinny' jeans. And nothing can keep you more honest than how you feel in your trousers.

When to measure Before you've eaten; ideally first thing in the morning.

How often Once a week.

What they leave out Whether you're getting faster, your weight and your overall health.

Your macronutrients (carbs, fats, protein)

Why they matter Runners need all three macronutrients to run well. Diets that eliminate one group just can't give you the fuel you need to run your best, unleash your fitness potential and, ultimately, lose weight. For instance, if you try to completely cut out fats, which help the body absorb vitamins and minerals, among other important physiological functions, you set yourself up for nutrient deficiencies and injury. If you try to completely cut out carbs, you starve your body of its best energy source for running and set yourself up to run out of energy well before you're done with your runs. By counting macronutrients, you can ensure you're getting all the nutrients you need to run well.

When to measure At every meal.

How often Every day.

What they leave out The quality of the food you're consuming. As noted in Chapter 1, you can meet the recommended targets and still be consuming foods that aren't going to be any good for your waistline, your race times or your long-term health. Yes, with 20g protein, that protein bar can help you meet your daily protein target, but it's not going to satisfy you and offer you the nutrition or the sense of satiation that, say, the 20g in healthier foods such as egg whites, tuna or even Greek yogurt does.

Calories

Why they matter We should all be aware that weight loss is more than just calories in and calories out. But it *can* help to know how many calories you need to fuel your running and what your daily calorie limits should ideally be in order to lose weight. (Your best bet is to work with a registered dietitian to determine what your daily target should be. If that's not possible, use the formulas on pages 117-118 in Chapter 16 to get a general idea.) Even just the process of counting calories and looking up how many each food contains can be eye-opening. You might find that the fast-food breakfast you ate while barely thinking about it actually loads you up with a day's worth of calories before you even get to your morning meeting. And you may see that the bag of trail mix you don't even enjoy and could definitely do without is inflating your daily calorie intake unnecessarily. Studies have shown that people drastically underestimate the number of calories any food contains.[2] And the more calories a food contains, the more drastically they tend to underestimate those calories.

When to measure At first, try keeping a food log and tracking your calories for a week to get a sense of how many you're consuming at present. There are lots of free calorie-tracking websites and apps on the market. This may be an eye-opener, and give you a clue about where your weight-loss obstacles are.

How often Daily.

What they leave out Not all calories are created equal. Just counting how many you're taking in doesn't take into consideration the quality of those calories and the nutrition they provide. Some calories – say, those from sugar and processed foods – can rev up your appetite and set you up to hit the wall both in your races and at your afternoon staff meeting. Other calories – for example, those from whole grains, fruit and veg – offer a variety of nutrients and minerals, keep your GI system working efficiently, and keep you feeling full and satisfied until your next meal. The mere volume of calories you're consuming also doesn't say anything about the quality of your workouts, your body composition or your risk of chronic diseases.

Your healthy habits

Why they matter Each person has their own unique collection of practices that help them feel happy and keep them on track every day. (See Part V on 'Why We Eat'.) Scientists often call these 'process goals'. They're the steps in the process that help you achieve the results you're seeking. If you watch them accumulate, they keep you honest. If you don't see your weight or pace changing, you can examine these habits and see where you've either been diligent or lax. By the same token, you can draw confidence from all the healthy habits you're practising on a regular basis. Here are some examples: keeping a journal each day may help eliminate the stress that drives you to eat less healthy foods. Keeping track of the water you drink might help you stay hydrated and improve how you feel on your runs and how fast you go. If night-time eating is a problem, noting how many times over the course of a week you've managed *not* to sneak back into the kitchen after dinner might build your confidence.

When to measure As soon as possible.

How often As often as possible.

What they leave out Your healthy habits might not match up with how you feel about the numbers on the scales or the finish-line clock, but they will pay off in the long run. And if the other numbers aren't reflecting success, you can always draw confidence from seeing how long and how well you've reversed unhealthy habits. If you stick with healthy process goals, eventually your weight and your race times *will* cooperate.

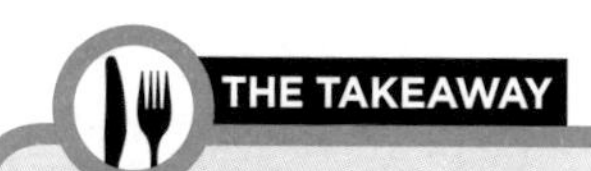

Find a good mix.
Use criteria you can measure on a daily, weekly and more long-term basis, and that are also affordable and easy to access. And think beyond the numbers. Remember, your overall health and happiness matter more than anything. If your heart, lungs, love life or job are breaking down, your running and weight-loss goals won't mean much.

Give it four weeks.
As running guru George Sheehan once said, you're an experiment of one. Try this mix for at least four weeks to see if it works for you. If after that you feel you're not getting the results you want, make some changes.

Make it personal.
Regardless of the science, or our advice, only *you* can decide what matters most to you.

Photography: Getty. **Sources:** 2. *BMJ*

A note on disordered eating

Reaching for your weight-loss and racing goals takes a tremendous amount of focus and effort – and making radical changes to what you eat, how you eat and how you exercise can feel all-consuming.

Before you consume a single mouthful as part of your new eating regime, you can spend a lot of time researching what you'll eat and where you'll buy it, deciding what you'll order at restaurants and standing in supermarket aisles scrutinising labels to assess whether a food's nutrient content earns it a place on your plate. It can be overwhelming, especially if you've never watched what you've eaten before.

'Your body will only perform optimally if you take care of it'

Rest assured it does get easier with practice. In this book, you'll find a lot of info to help you design your *Run Your Belly Off* diet, including the healthiest and most delicious foods that'll energise you and help you run your best. Soon that information will morph into knowledge; over time, knowledge will morph into understanding. And eventually, once you find the right mix of healthy foods that helps you feel and run your best, choosing healthy foods will become second nature.

However, if those around you don't watch what *they* eat, your new-found commitment to nutrition may seem difficult to understand. They might accuse you of being 'obsessed' or even of having an eating disorder. While over time they'll probably adjust to your new healthy habits just as you will, it's important to understand from the outset when a healthy commitment to weight-loss goals crosses the line into an unhealthy, disordered relationship with food and weight.

But where is that line? "It's not a simple answer," says Riley Nickols, clinical coordinator for a scheme that specialises in treating elite athletes with eating disorders.

Disordered eating isn't just about a new-found interest in monitoring calories and nutrients. Eating disorders – including anorexia, bulimia and binge eating – are serious problems that require urgent medical attention. "They're very similar to alcohol or substance abuse," says Nickols. "They affect your social life, work performance and start to filter over to other parts of life."

If you're concerned that you or a loved one has developed an eating disorder, there are certain warning signs – they include:

- Repeated injuries due to low fat, carb, and protein intake.
- Overwhelming guilt about taking days off from running or exercising.
- Overly rigid, abnormal eating patterns and behaviours.
- Lack of flexibility about what, when and how much to eat
- Isolation and avoidance of eating in social situations.
- Resistance to regaining weight in order to attain healthy weight.

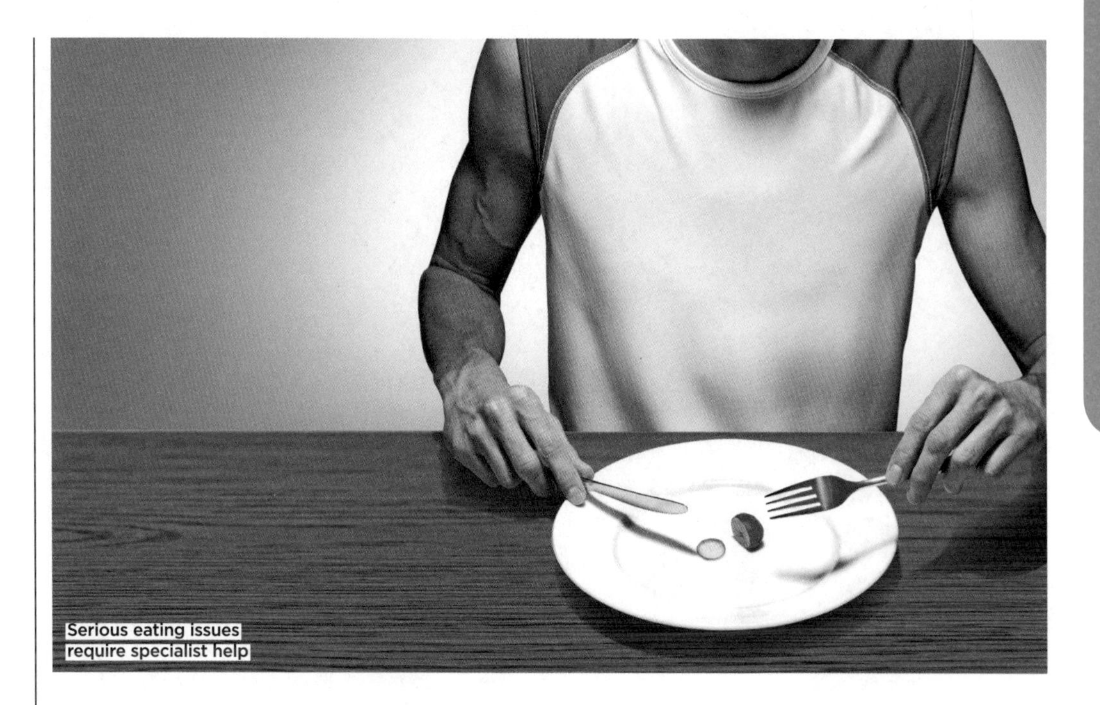
Serious eating issues require specialist help

- Poor body image; certain body parts feel intolerable.
- Body checking (repeatedly and obsessively grabbing or holding one part of the body).

"Normal eating incorporates a variety of foods, quantities and eating at different times of days," adds Nickols.

What's so difficult about disordered eating among athletes is that they tend to exhibit a lot of traits, such as commitment and discipline, that are admired in anyone who's working towards a goal. But, says Nickols, they "take the good traits to an absolute extreme".

While a runner with a new commitment to weight loss and racing might be willing to go out in any weather condition, someone with an eating disorder might actually run with a stress fracture. One prominent feature of an eating disorder can "involve a total denial of discomfort", Nickols says.

People with disordered eating patterns often struggle with anxiety and/or depression, and certain physical signs and symptoms can start to emerge. "Your body speaks to you all the time," says Nickols. "Whether you choose to listen to it is another question."

Following intense dieting and disordered eating, max VO_2 (aerobic power) plummets along with running performance. If you're severely restricting carbs and protein, it'll take longer to recover from workouts, and you risk injuries in bones, muscles and joints. While all runners can be susceptible to overuse injuries, the risk is "really heightened when you're not fuelling appropriately", says Nickols. "The body will only perform optimally if you take care of it and fuel it to meet your energy needs."

For anyone working on weight loss and racing, it's a good idea to consult a sports dietitian to understand how many calories and what nutrients you need to stay fit without becoming hurt or getting sick. Anyone struggling with disordered eating should seek treatment from a therapist who specialises in this area.

"Treating an eating disorder means transforming your relationship with your body and with food." says Nickols, "It's also about reshaping your relationship with exercise in order to be healthier and recover long term."

Part I

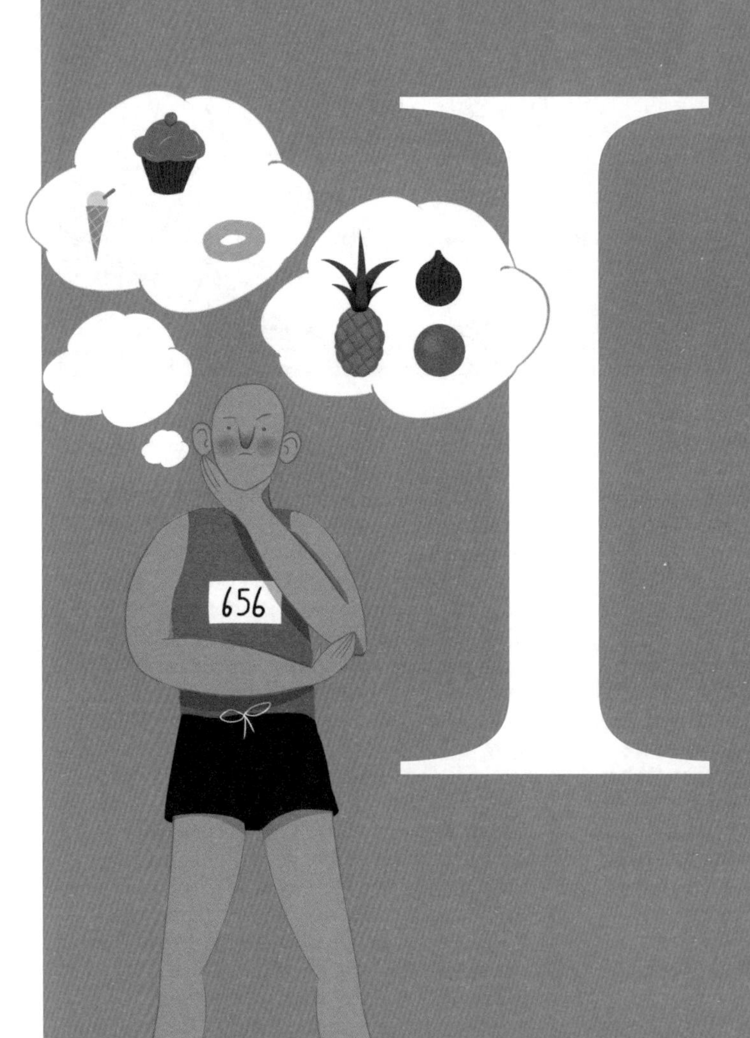

WHAT TO EAT

Confused by the constantly shifting advice we're given about what foods will aid weight loss? You're not alone, but you can be sure of one thing: if you run regularly, the rules aren't the same as those for non-running dieters. In this section you'll learn what you should be eating and drinking to shrink your waistline, improve your race times and boost your wellbeing. But *Run Your Belly Off* isn't about deprivation or saintly feats of restraint. In fact, chances are this section will make you realise you can indulge in a lot more of some truly delicious foods in order to reach your goals.

1.

ALL ABOUT CARBS

Since the 1970s, carbs have had a bad rap, thanks in large part to the popularity of certain diet plans. They've been demonised as the culprits behind everything from anxiety to dementia, not to mention chronic weight-control issues.

To some extent, this is justified. With over 520 calories, 74g carbs and 44g sugar, a large blueberry muffin[1] won't do you any favours. And yes, lots of runners tend to take the carb-loading too far (2,000-calorie plate of spaghetti the night before a 5K, anyone?).

But when it comes to carbs, quality counts for a lot. There is a huge chasm between that blueberry muffin, which contains lots of fats, calories and sugars with little nutritional benefit, and high-quality carbs such as a banana, an apple or a slice of wholemeal bread. These also contain fibre and nutrients that provide the fuel you need to run well and take your fitness to the next level, plus vital minerals that help protect you from chronic disease.

55-65% of your calories should be from high-quality carbs

As a runner, 55-65% of your daily calories should come from high-quality carbs. During times of heavy training and high mileage, aim for the high end of this range. If you're resting, or more focused on weight loss than high performance, aim for the lower end. Since carbohydrates are the fuel that the body can most quickly absorb and process for energy, you'll want to include them daily.

Why carbs are essential

Plenty of healthy carbs – fruits, vegetables and wholegrains – contain fibre, antioxidants, and a host of essential vitamins and minerals, so they deserve mainstay status in your daily diet, no

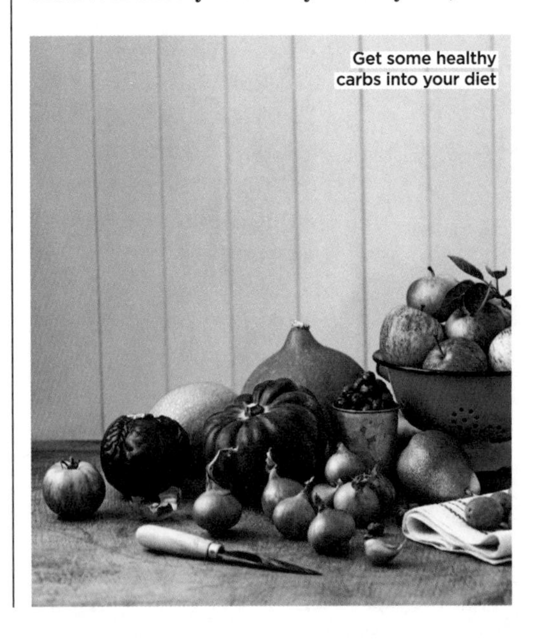
Get some healthy carbs into your diet

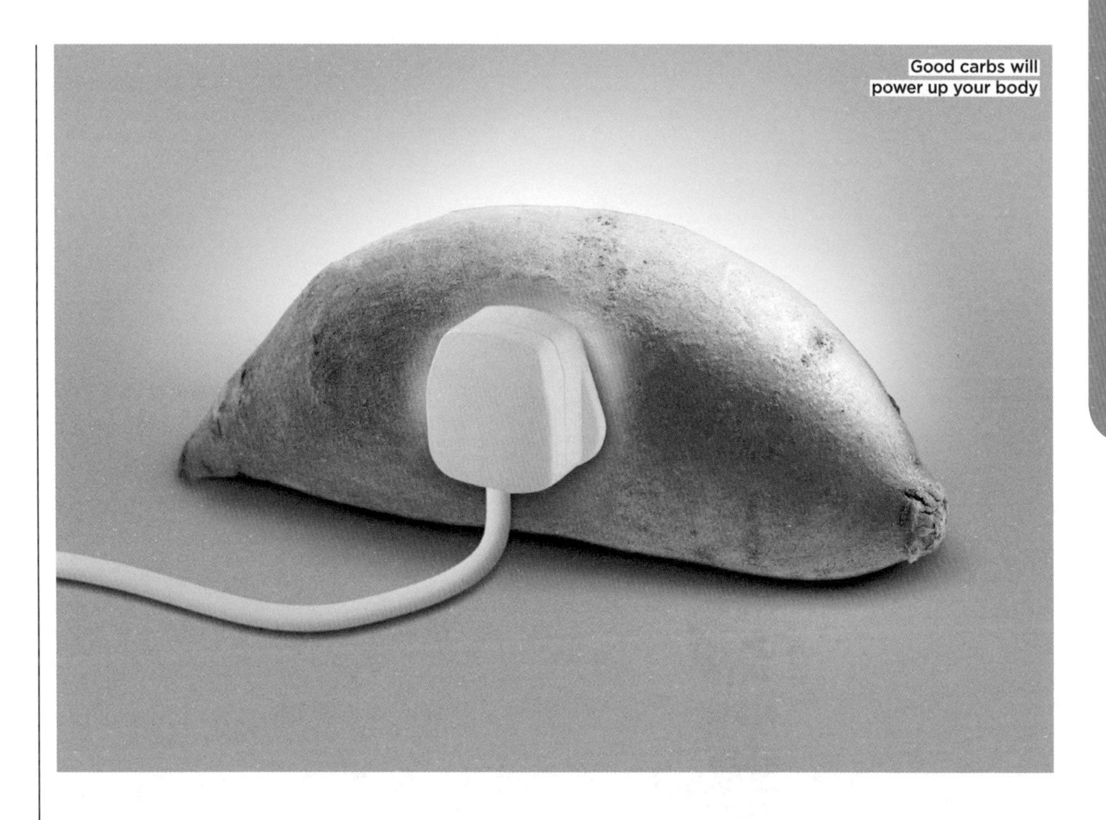

Good carbs will power up your body

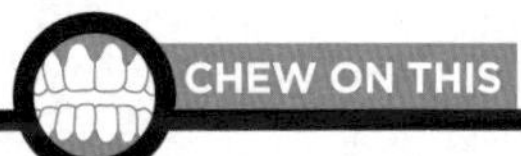

CHEW ON THIS

The pressure to eliminate carbs altogether can be tempting. But runners need carbs like cars need petrol. If you tried to go for a drive with an empty tank, you wouldn't get far. It's the same thing with running – heading off for a workout on a tank that's empty of carbs is a waste of time.

matter what your weight-loss or racing goals are. Without carbs in your diet, you have no fuel or glycogen stores in your muscles. And without any fuel in the tank, it's going to be very, very difficult to get the maximum calorie burn out of your workout – or even get through a long run without hitting the wall.

Carbohydrates are simply the easiest form of calories for your body to convert to energy. It's just like fuelling a car. If you're going on a long road trip – or trying to win the British Grand Prix – you want to fill up on the highest-octane fuel on the market. Approach running and carbs in the same way.

Yes, it's true that some athletes have found that if their pace isn't intense and if they've worked at it, they can run on fat stores, but for most runners carbohydrates are essential. It's simply impossible to meet the energy requirements for high-intensity workouts such as speed sessions or endurance workouts such as long, slow distance runs when your diet is depleted of carbs.

Not only that, but carbs help keep you hydrated. (It's called a carbo*hydrate* for a reason!) Water retention might not be music to your ears, but adequate hydration can help you run faster so that you burn more calories. And dehydration has been proven to make running at any pace feel harder.[2]

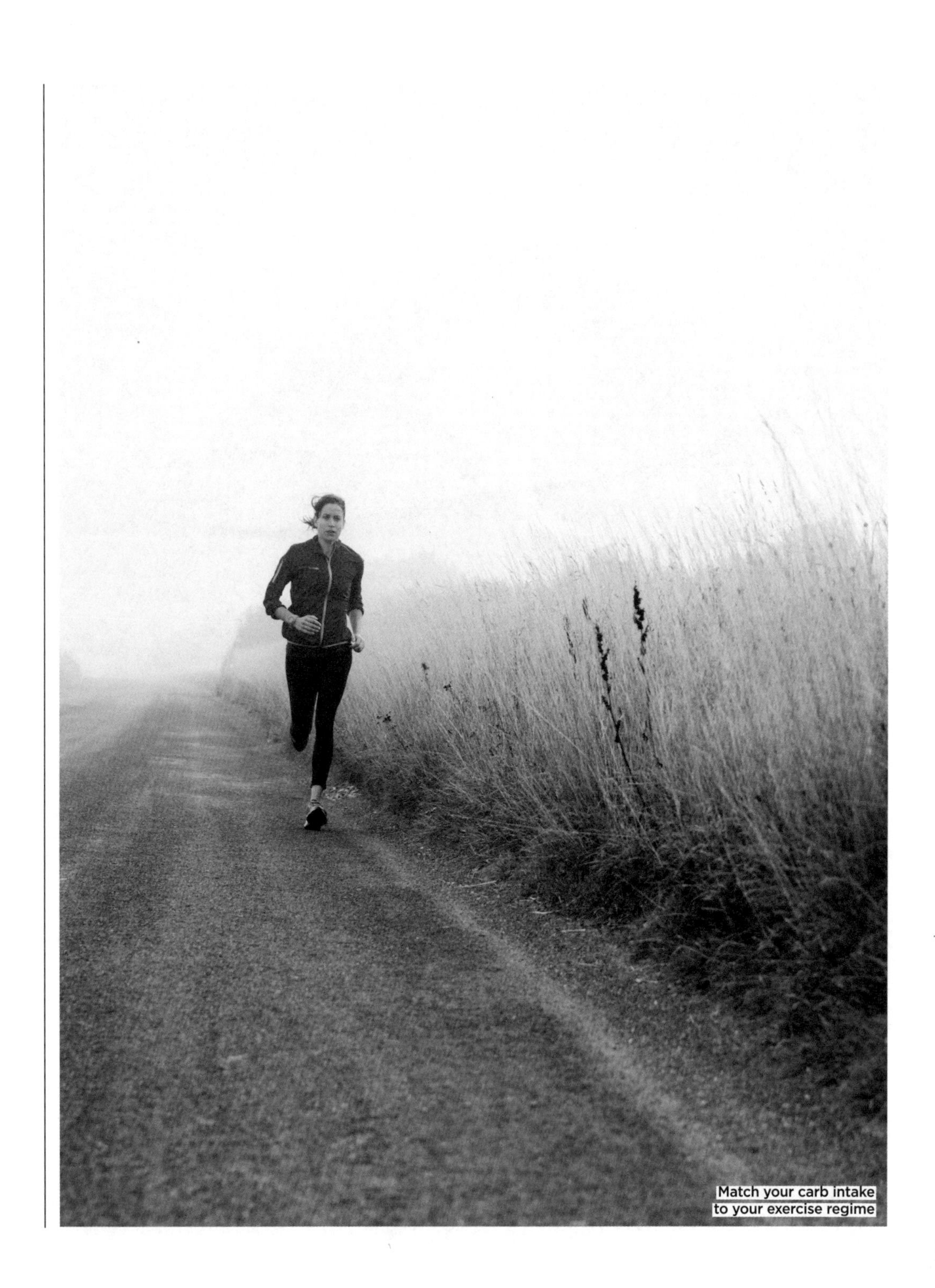

Match your carb intake to your exercise regime

Not all carbs are created equal

While you do need carbs, the type of carbs you eat and when you eat them can dramatically affect how you feel during a run and what you see on the bathroom scales.

You want to focus on getting the highest-quality carbs with the most nutrients and the fewest unhealthy additives. Look at the list below. Each serving contains approximately 25g carbs. To find the healthiest ones for you, see pages 49-50 for a list of whole grains, and 39-41 for a table of fruit and vegetables that can help you meet your carbohydrate needs.

- Grains (2 slices wholewheat bread, 80g porridge or 100g rice)
- Dairy products (500ml skimmed or semi-skimmed milk, or 125g fruit-flavoured yogurt)
- Beans and starchy vegetables (120g black beans, 240g green peas or 1 medium potato)
- Sports drinks, bars and gels (1 energy bar, 400ml sports drink or carbohydrate gel)
- Mixed dishes (150ml tomato soup, 1 slice thin-crust pizza or 1 small veggie burrito)
- Fruits and juices (1 medium apple, 300g fresh strawberries or 150ml orange juice)

How many carbs do you need each day?

This depends on how hard you're training and what stage of training you're in. Many runners fail to reach their weight-loss goals – or even gain weight – when they start running regularly because they're consuming more carbs than their level of activity demands. While it's fine to eat a large plate of pasta the night before a long run or a celebratory bagel after a long, hard workout, when you're trying to lose weight, there's probably no need for these types of food every day of the week. For weight-conscious runners, meeting your goals will come down to getting the carbs you need to avoid hitting the wall, but without stuffing yourself silly.

If you're not training for a race, aim for 2.2g of carbohydrates per lb of body weight per day. As you ramp up mileage and intensity, increase your intake to 3.2-4g per lb of body weight. If you're carb-loading a few days before a race (more on that in Chapter 17), aim for 4.5-5.5g carbs per lb of body weight per day. Here are two general rules to follow when it comes to carbs.

1. Tweak the formula

Remember, these are recommendations. If you're getting tired – during daily activities or your workouts – increase your intake a bit.

2. Time it right

Be sure to spread your intake over the course of the day to promote fuel availability before, during and after key training sessions. By consuming carbs before, sometimes during and after your workout (combined with protein) you'll feel energised during the run and ready to tackle future workouts without feeling overly fatigued and run-down. (See more on when to eat in Part III.)

THE TAKEAWAY

Count your daily carb needs.
Try tracking your intake of carbs – rather than calories – for a week and see how it matches up to our recommendations. You might need to add more carbs, or reduce your intake, to fuel your current running needs.

Add wholesome carbs to your diet.
If you've been eliminating *all* carbs in order to pursue a low-carb diet, try adding high-quality ones back for a week. Track how you feel on your runs and how quickly you recover for your next workout.

Time your carb intake right.
Plan your meals so that you have your most carb-heavy meals and snacks immediately before, during and right after hard workouts.

2.

FRUIT AND VEG: THE FORGOTTEN FUEL

For a good many of us, the word 'carb' is synonymous with pasta, potatoes and other starchy foods, along with tempting baked goodies such as bagels, doughnuts and croissants. But what many people – and many diets – overlook is the fact that fresh fruit and vegetables actually provide a lot of the carbohydrates any runner needs to rev up a workout, and without a lot of the additives and unsavoury side effects that can weigh runners down on the road and on the scales.

Just compare a banana and a bagel – which runners often choose between before a run or a race. From a cursory glance at the calorie count for each item, they seem roughly comparable. If anything, the bagel might seem like a slightly healthier choice. A small plain bagel has 180 calories, 36g carbs, 6g sugar and 7g protein,[1] while a medium banana has 105 calories with 27g carbs, 14g sugar and 1.3g protein.

Some fruit and veg are better than others for runners

But look a little closer. The banana has many other nutrients runners need – including vitamin B6 (which helps convert proteins and sugars into energy and is involved in cell building), magnesium (which assists in muscle contractions and energy metabolism, endurance and aerobic capacity), and potassium, which is critical for fending off electrolyte imbalances that can lead to muscle cramps on the run. The bagel has few, if any, of those special powers.

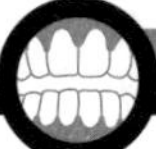

CHEW ON THIS

When it comes to the benefits of fruits and vegetables, your waistline and your workouts are just the tip of the iceberg. A 2012 study in the *European Journal of Nutrition* concluded there's convincing evidence that fruits and veg can reduce the risk of high blood pressure, heart disease and stroke, and may even lower risk of cancer, prevent weight gain associated with type-2 diabetes, *and* reduce the risk of eye diseases, dementia, osteoporosis, asthma, COPD and rheumatoid arthritis.[2]

What's more, in recent years researchers have discovered the degree to which fresh fruit and veg can protect you from some of the most prevalent and menacing chronic diseases, such as type 2 diabetes and cardiovascular disease.

That doesn't mean you have to become a vegetarian. But it does mean that getting plenty of whole fruits and vegetables into your diet can play a huge role in helping you have a long and healthy life, happily free of chronic diseases that have been accepted as part of ageing for most people. They can also provide a high-quality way to fuel up your runs.

Admittedly, bananas, apples and carrots may not have the sensual appeal of a freshly baked bagel smothered with cream cheese, or even the sweet memories or associations that go along with it. But the truth is that fruit and veg can fuel you just as well *and* provide important nutrients and minerals that will help you bounce back quickly from tough workouts, and prevent chronic diseases such as stroke, heart disease and high blood pressure. If you can fend off those ills, you're more likely to reach your goals at the finish line and on the bathroom scales.

That said, some fruits and vegetables are better than others for your running life. In general, those that you can consume with the peel attached (such as apples and potatoes), and most berries, will contain lots of fibre. Fibre is great, as it'll keep you feeling full and help ward off illness. But if you're heading out the door for a run in the next 60 minutes, avoid eating anything that has more than 7g fibre per serving.

Below you'll find a list of some of the highest-carb whole fruit and vegetables with extra nutrients that will support your running. Whenever possible, eat what's in season. When food is harvested before its peak to meet demand in a country thousands of miles away, it doesn't contain the full supply of nutrients it would have if it had been harvested when it was ready. Plus, when fruit or veg are being shipped long distances – eg, pears from Argentina; broccoli from Spain – nutrients can be lost on the journey, and preservatives are often added to protect it from spoilage during travel.

Fuelling up with fruit and vegetables

FRUIT/ VEG	CARBS (G)/ SERVING	FIBRE (G)/ SERVING	EXTRA NUTRIENTS FOR RUNNERS
Banana (1 large)	31	4	Bananas contain potassium, vitamin B6 and magnesium, which help maintain hydration on the run and fend off muscle cramps.
Figs, dried (1)	5	1	Figs are rich in carbs and potassium, and they're also easy to carry. Figs make a great mid-run snack.
Sweet potato (1 medium)	27	4 (with skin)	Sweet potatoes are tasty and loaded with vitamin A, which helps protect your eyesight.
Pear (1 medium)	27	5	Pears contain quercetin, a phytonutrient linked to preventing diseases such as cancer, as well as potentially improving athletic performance.
Cranberries, sweetened, dried (40g)	25	2	Cranberries contain compounds called proanthocyanidins, which have been shown to prevent stomach ulcers and urinary-tract infections, and improve cardiovascular health. Combine them with other dried berries and you'll have an antioxidant-rich blend that can prevent inflammation.

FRUIT/ VEG	CARBS (G)/ SERVING	FIBRE (G)/ SERVING	EXTRA NUTRIENTS FOR RUNNERS
Butternut squash (100g cooked cubes)	11	3	A superb source of vitamin A, just one serving offers men 64% and women 82% of the recommended daily intake of this vision-supporting nutrient.
Cauliflower (50g raw)	3	1	Cauliflower contains vitamin C, folate, and vitamin B6. Vitamin C boosts immunity and helps the body absorb iron and create collagen (a critical component of tendons, ligaments and connective tissue). Vitamin B6 plays a critical role in metabolism. If you're trying to cut calories, try mashed cauliflower, which has a look and texture similar to higher-calorie mashed potatoes.
Dates (1)	18	2	Like other dried fruits, dates are a portable source of energising carbs, so they're great for refuelling on the run. Dates are also rich in phosphorus, an electrolyte that plays a key role in maintaining fluid balance and is essential for healthy bones.
Raisins (40g)	34	2	Easily digestible, portable and energy dense, raisins are great for on-the-go fuelling. They're also quite high in potassium and other electrolytes such as magnesium, calcium and sodium.
Kiwi (1)	10	2	This fruit is rich in tissue-repairing vitamin C.
Navel orange (1 medium)	18	3	While an obvious choice for vitamin C to boost your immunity, an orange also contains carbs and fluids to help you stay energised and hydrated.
Strawberries, whole (150g)	11	3	Put more strawberries on your plate and you'll get more vitamin C in your body. They contain anthocyanins, which can help repair muscles and fight inflammation.
Baby carrots (10)	8	3	Eating carrots is one of the best ways to get your daily vitamin-A hit; they also contain vitamin B6 and carotene to give your immune system a boost.

Spaghetti squash (75g cooked)	5	1	**Compared with 'real' pasta, spaghetti squash offers more nutrients as well as filling fibre. If you're counting calories, spaghetti squash is ideal, as copious amounts contain just a handful of calories. Served with pasta sauce and cheese, it's a great alternative to pasta.**
Blackberries (75g)	7	4	**Low in calories and high in antioxidants, blackberries also contain fibre and vitamin C, plus vitamin K, which strengthens bones.**
Blueberries (75g)	10	2	**Blueberries contain powerful phytochemicals and antioxidants that may reduce risk of various cancers and heart disease. Research is now under way to understand how the phytochemicals in blueberries could improve brain function.**
Tomato (90g chopped)	4	1	**Tomatoes are a good source of vitamins C, K and A, as well as potassium, which can aid in recovery from tough workouts.**
Grapefruit (½ large)	13	2	**Grapefruit offers healthy doses of vitamin C, potassium and folate. Potassium can help keep your muscles from cramping. The red variety has the same amount of vitamin C as the white, plus extra vitamin A and pantothenic acid, which your body uses to transform proteins, fats and carbohydrates into energy.**
Cabbage (150g cooked)	8	3	**Cabbage is low in calories, has high concentrations of vitamins K and C, and is a good source of folate. Runners can protect the health of red blood cells by increasing their intake of folate.**
Yams (75g cooked cubes)	19	3	**Like sweet potatoes, yams can be mashed and taken on the run for a natural fuelling option. A sprinkle of salt combined with the 456mg of naturally present potassium makes it a great mid-run fuel option.**
Grapes (150g)	16	1	**Like the wine that's made from them, red and purple grapes contain the rare antioxidant resveratrol, which is linked to a healthier heart.**

Not all fruit and veg are created equal

Fruit has fallen out of favour in some circles in recent years, as low-carb diets have become more popular and researchers learn more about the dangers of sugar. But the 23g of naturally occurring sugar in an orange won't wreak the same havoc on your body as the same amount of added sugar in, say, a doughnut. Why? In addition to sugar, fruits contain important vitamins, minerals and phytonutrients to stave off chronic disease and keep you healthy, plus water to keep you hydrated. What's more, the fibre in the skins of fruit and veg means they're digested more gradually, so they don't cause the same kinds of energy spikes and crashes as table sugar. Plus the fibre boosts heart health and keeps your gastrointestinal (GI) system working efficiently. If you're looking to reduce the amount of sugar in your diet, cut out processed foods with added sugars; keep the fruit, which has so many other nutrients that are critical for good health.

That said, not all fruit and veg are created equal. Almost always, eating them in their raw form is your best bet. A 100g portion of dried apple pieces, for example, can have 49g sugar and 209 calories, and will probably leave you hungry. The same amount of raw apples will have just 52 calories and 11g sugar, plus water, fibre, and other essential vitamins and nutrients. Even dried veg can be full of added sugar and fat that you don't need. Packaged products such as kale chips, beet chips or freeze-dried sugar snap peas may seem like healthier alternatives, but check the nutrition breakdown and you'll see that many of these products rival potato crisps in terms of calories and fat. If you want something to satisfy a crunchy, salty craving, your best bet is to make your own.

The best of the best

So which fruit and veg are the healthiest? In 2014, researchers from the US Centers for Disease Control and Prevention attempted to rank them according to their nutrient density. This list of so-called produce powerhouses, created by Jennifer Di Noia, PhD, of William Paterson University in New Jersey, are found to reduce heart disease and some cancers. The list ranks 47 foods according to their density of 17 nutrients including iron, riboflavin, niacin, folate, and vitamins B6, B12, C and K.[3]

Topping the list is watercress, a leafy green packed full of antioxidants and vitamin K, followed by Chinese cabbage, chard, beetroot greens, spinach, chicory, leaf lettuce, parsley, romaine lettuce, collard greens, turnip greens, mustard greens, endive, chives, kale, dandelion greens, red pepper, arugula, broccoli, pumpkin, Brussels sprouts, spring onions, kohlrabi, cauliflower, cabbage and carrots.

Better together

Some foods can accentuate the nutrients in other foods. This is often referred to as food synergy. Here are some nutrients that bring out the best in one another.

Vitamin D + calcium Vitamin D helps the body absorb calcium, which you need to build strong bones and stave off stress fractures. The US Institute of Medicine recommends that the average adult gets 600IU (international units) vitamin D and 1,000mg calcium every day.
Serving suggestion Get calcium from dairy products such as milk, cheese and yogurt as well as from broccoli, kale, and Chinese cabbage. Some foods, such as porridge, orange juice and cereal, are fortified with calcium. Vitamin D can come from salmon, tuna, sardines, mackerel, prawns, mushrooms, egg yolks and fortified items such as selected orange juices and breads.

Iron + vitamin C In addition to boosting immunity so you don't get sidelined by coughs and colds, vitamin C helps the body absorb iron. That's especially important if you're a vegetarian and rely on plant-based sources of iron (which aren't absorbed as readily), such

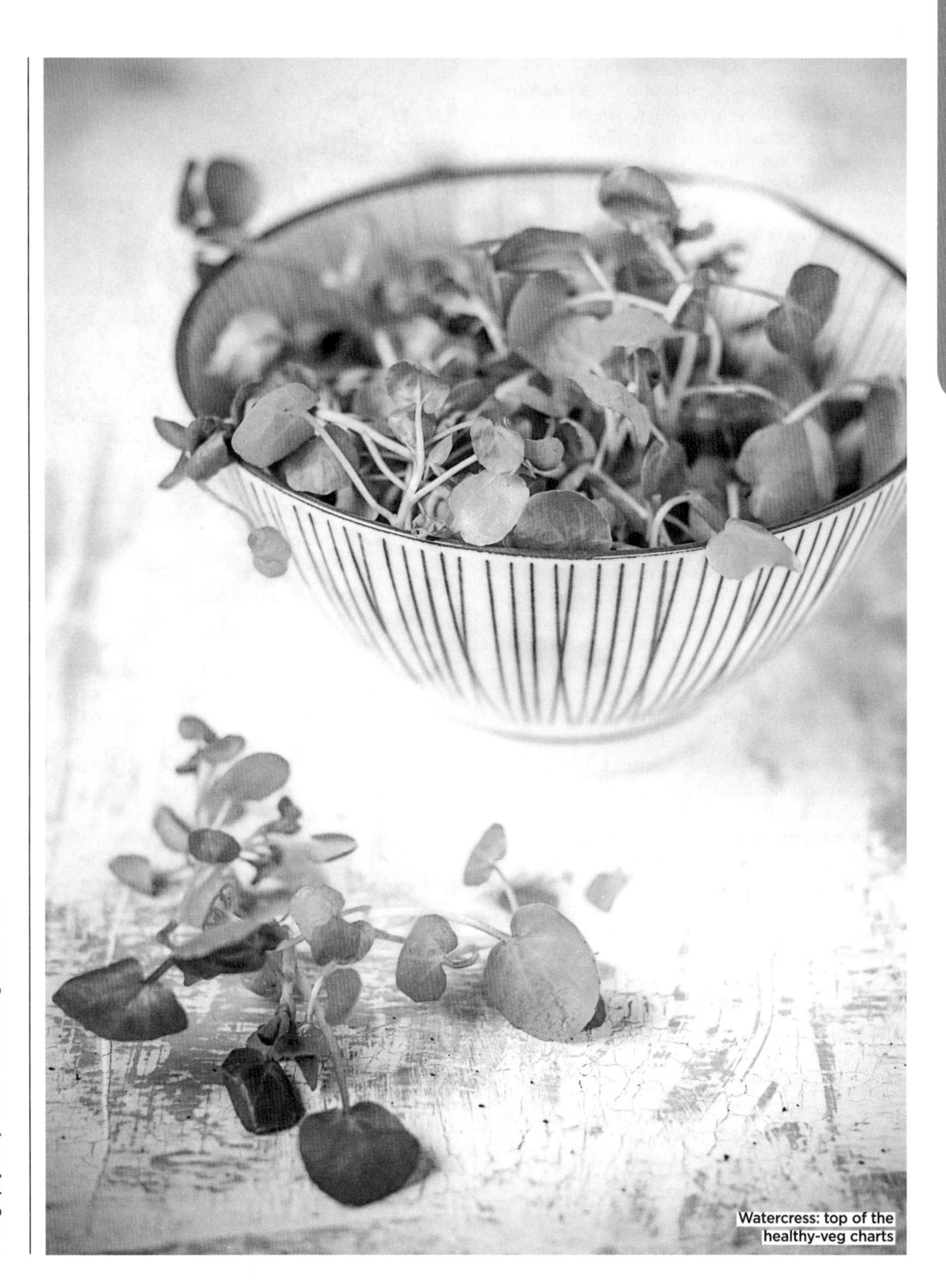
Watercress: top of the healthy-veg charts

Photography: Getty Sources: 3. *Preventing Chronic Disease*

as lentils, chickpeas and black beans.
Serving suggestion Good sources of vitamin C include tomatoes, broccoli, citrus fruits, leafy greens, strawberries and bell peppers. Iron can be found in beetroot leaves, kale, spinach, mustard seeds and fortified cereal.

Veg + healthy fats Monounsaturated fats – such as those in olive oil, avocado, walnuts and almonds – not only help lower cholesterol and reduce heart-disease risk, but also help your body absorb antioxidants and essential fat-soluble vitamins – such as A, D, E and K – from vegetables including carrots, broccoli, peas, spinach and sweet potatoes.
Serving suggestion Top your salad with a serving of full-fat dressing, walnuts, pistachios or grated cheese. Add olive oil to your favorite marinara pasta dish.

Protein + carbs Protein not only builds muscle and helps fill you up, but also slows the absorption of sugar from carbs into your body so you're less likely to have cravings. When you do eat healthy carbs from whole grains, fruit and vegetables, pair them with protein. This is especially important if you're refuelling post-run. Research has shown that having a protein-and-carb snack in the 30-60 minutes following a workout (see Chapter 20 on eating for recovery) can help you bounce back quickly for your next run.
Serving suggestion Cereal with milk, or digestive biscuits spread with peanut butter contain carbs and protein. Try apples with cashew butter or a pitta filled with hummus. Or tuna fish mixed with honey-mustard dressing on wholegrain bread.

Preserving the nutrients on the way to your plate

All those nutrient-packed fruits and veggies won't do you any good if, before they reach your plate, you kill all the nutrients in the cooking process. Many vitamins – including water-soluble ones such as C, thiamin (B1), riboflavin (B2), folate and B12 – are sensitive to heat, air and, in the case of riboflavin, even light exposure. In general, the longer you cook fruit and veg, the more water you use and the higher the temperature, the more nutrients (and taste) you'll lose. Here are some tips on how you can preserve the healing powers – and the flavour – of your ingredients.

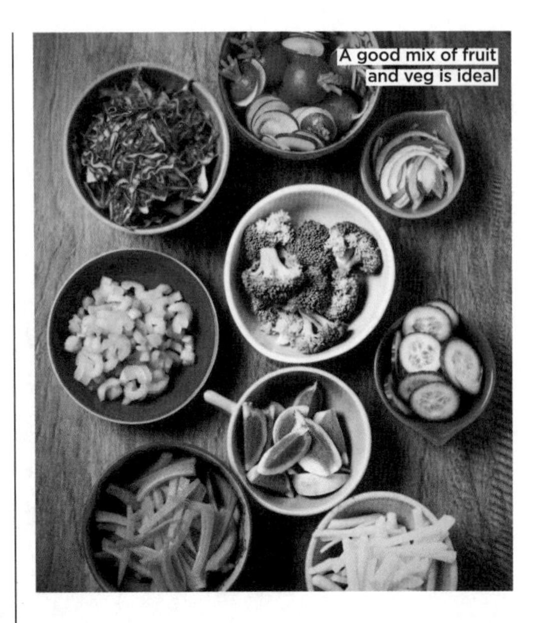
A good mix of fruit and veg is ideal

- **Go raw** In most cases, you can't go wrong consuming these foods in their natural state – in salads, smoothies or as a standalone snack.

- **Be a minimalist** Keep the cooking time, temperature and the amount of water needed to a minimum. Water leaches water-soluble vitamins from the food. Don't believe it? When you've finished cooking your veg, take a look at the water. If it's coloured, those are the water-soluble vitamins that have been washed away. If you want to save them, you could drink the water or use it as vegetable stock.

- **Steam it** Steaming is one of the best ways of cooking vegetables quickly so you can preserve valuable nutrients. It's particularly good for broccoli and courgettes as it helps retain the valuable antioxidants they contain.

Boil it Boiling water can wash away vitamins and minerals in certain veg. If you do cook them this way, keep the pan covered to minimise the cooking time. And use the leftover water – which will be packed with nutrients – in sauces and soups.

Zap it Microwaves were once associated with fears about 'nuking' your food and possible radiation. But scores of trials have established that they're perfectly safe. Cooks also know that that zap allows you to keep cooking time brief and use little water.

Stir-fry it Cooking your vegetables quickly over a high heat in a small amount of oil can minimise nutrient loss and is a tasty way to prepare julienned veg (as well as meat and rice).

Grill it This allows you to cook with minimal added fats, while preserving the flavour and the juiciness. While there's limited conclusive evidence, some research suggests regularly eating charred, well-done meat can increase your risk of some cancers. When you're barbecuing, stick with lean cuts and smaller portions that you won't have to cook for long. Also with lean cuts there's less fat to drip down and create flare-ups. And consider using a marinade; according to the American Institute for Cancer Research, studies have shown that by marinating your meat before grilling, you can potentially decrease the formation of carcinogenic compounds by up to 96%, possibly thanks to antioxidants in the marinade.[4]

Try baking or roasting This method helps some veg retain, and even boost, their nutrients. These include artichokes, broccoli, asparagus, green beans, aubergine, sweetcorn, Swiss chard, spinach and peppers. Other veg lose their antioxidant power when exposed to high heat, including Brussels sprouts, leeks, cauliflower, peas, courgettes, onions, beans, celery, beetroot and garlic. So either bake them quickly, blanch (don't boil) them, or consider eating them raw whenever possible.

Try juicing Juicing and making smoothies can be a great way to get raw fruit and veg into your diet, as long as you keep the drinks full of healthy things – sometimes they can be calorie bombs that rival the numbers you'd get with a milkshake. While juicing *can* have some health benefits – especially for those who weren't incorporating fruit and veg into their diets before – the juicing process that some juicers and extractors use removes the nutritious pulp and fibre, so you'll need to find sources of these elsewhere. If you're looking for a smoothie or shake that doesn't derail your daily calorie target, use whole fruit and veg (frozen varieties are fine). Avoid adding honey, fruit-juice concentrate, sweetened yogurt, whole milk, cream or ice cream. The most powerful smoothies should contain at least two servings of fruits and/or vegetables. If you're looking to make your smoothie into a recovery drink, be sure to include a source of protein such as 100% whey protein powder, skimmed milk or Greek yogurt. (For more on juicing diets, see page 104.)

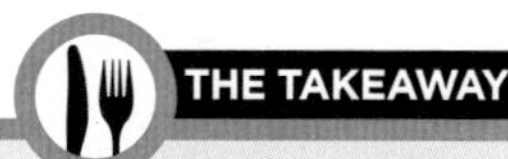

THE TAKEAWAY

Assess your fruit and veggie intake.
Think about your regular meals and snacks. How much fruit and veg are you getting on a regular basis? Be sure to get the timing right. If you're planning to go out for a run within the next 60 minutes, avoid eating or drinking anything that has more than 7g fibre per serving.

Add a serving of vegetables to one meal every day.
Not a great lover of veg? Chop them up finely and add them to a tomato sauce. Toss them in the blender with ice, yogurt, and milk for smoothies.

Add a serving of fruit as a snack.
Bananas, oranges, apples and other fruits make great portable, filling and satisfying snacks you can take with you when you're on the go.

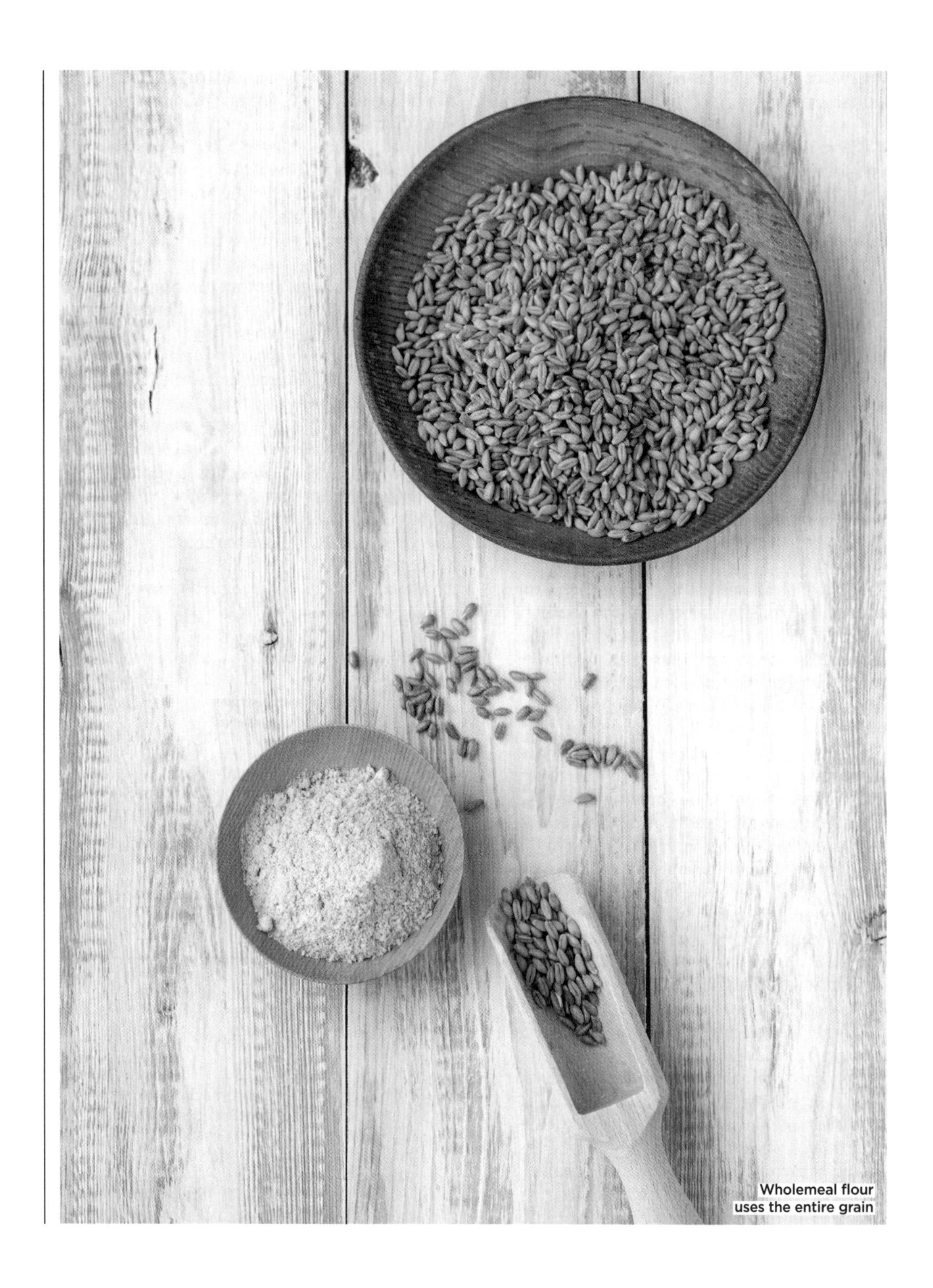

Wholemeal flour uses the entire grain

3.

GOOD GRAINS

With the uproar over carbs in recent years, grains have gained a bad name they don't deserve. They've been blamed for obesity problems, and many runners, dieters and celebrities advocate eliminating them.

But just as with sugars, there's a huge difference between the refined grains in products such as biscuits, cakes and doughnuts – which really are the culprits behind many people's weight problems – and the whole grains in foods such as oats, buckwheat, quinoa and wild rice, which have real health benefits.

While refined grains can be hazardous to your diet, whole grains are an essential part of it. Try to eliminate whole grains altogether, and you'll have a tough time reaching your weight-loss and racing goals. In this chapter, you'll learn why whole grains are such an important part of your diet and how to distinguish them from the more problematic refined versions that can derail your goals.

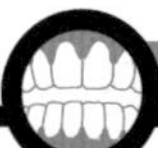

CHEW ON THIS

How do you tell if a product contains whole grains? If the first few ingredients listed contain the word 'whole' (for example, 'wholewheat' or 'wholemeal'). you can safely assume it's a whole grain. But other foods such as brown or wild rice, bulgur wheat, quinoa, oats, rye and Granary bread are also whole grains. Other terms, such as 'unbleached' and 'stone ground', may sound fancy but typically mean the grain is refined.

Whole vs refined

Whole grains include the endosperm, germ and bran, in the same proportions as when they were harvested from the earth. Rich in antioxidants and nutrients, they've been shown to lower blood pressure and cholesterol; reduce risk of cancer, heart disease, type 2 diabetes and obesity, and – thanks to their higher fibre content – even improve glucose and insulin response to a meal. A recent study in the *Journal of the American Medical Association* linked a diet rich in whole grains with a significantly lower risk of death from heart disease.[1]

And contrary to the widely held carbo-phobia that's taken hold in recent years, there's also evidence that whole grains can help you reach your weight-loss goals. A study published in 2008 in the *American Journal of Clinical Nutrition* found that individuals who consumed a diet rich in whole grains had less belly fat and a smaller waist circumference than those who predominantly ate white bread.[2] The high fibre content of whole grains helps you feel fuller for longer, which can help prevent overeating.

While refined grains – the kind found in white bread, traditional pastas, biscuits,

Photography: Getty Sources: 1. archinte.jamanetwork.com/article.aspx?articleid=2087877. 2. ncbi.nlm.nih.gov/pubmed/18175740

doughnuts and croissants – will energise you for your runs, they don't have the same long-term health benefits. They've been stripped of the nutrient-rich bran, germ and endosperm – often for the sake of taste, texture and a longer shelf life in the supermarket.

What's more, these items often have a lot of saturated fats, sugar, salt and empty calories, which can keep you from reaching your weight-loss goals. Plus, they can wreak havoc with your blood sugar. They tend to lack fibre and don't offer the same fullness benefits whole grains provide. Because they're digested so quickly, they cause the blood sugar to spike, then quickly plummet, leaving you feeling depleted. Since research links chronic illnesses such as diabetes and heart disease to diets that send your blood sugar on a roller-coaster ride, it's best to avoid refined, highly processed grains.

Whole grains, on the other hand, provide a steady, slow release of energy. Most score low on the glycaemic index (read more about that in Chapter 5). Whole-grain barley, for instance, has a GI score of 25, while a white baguette has a GI of 95.

How much whole grain do you need?

Because whole grains are a carbohydrate, the amount you should consume partly depends on your training regime and weight-loss goals. The more intense your workouts, the more you'll need. (For more on determining your daily carb count, see Chapter 1.) That said, most people need to up their whole-grain intake, no matter how hard they're training – it's recommended that most adults eat at least three to five servings of whole grains daily, making up at least half of all the grains you consume.

Timing it right

The key to working whole grains into your diet without derailing your racing and weight-loss goals is to make sure you're getting the right amounts at the right time.

Whole grains do pack a calorie punch, and because it's easy to overeat foods such as rice, porridge and cereal, it's important to measure out your portions. Here are some examples of single servings of popular whole-grain items.

- 100g cooked rice, bulgur, pasta or cereal
- 25g dry pasta, rice or other dry grain
- 1 slice bread
- 1 small muffin (weighing 25g)
- 40g cereal flakes

Due to the high-fibre nature of whole grains, it's important to time your intake right. Eating a piece of whole-grain bread immediately pre-run can lead to GI distress. To prevent a mid-run pit stop, whatever you eat up to an hour before you head out should have less than 7g fibre. It's best to save whole grains for a post-workout meal, when your body is primed to absorb the nutrients, repair muscle and restock spent glycogen stores. (Read more about eating for recovery in Chapter 20.)

Whole-grain foods also make an ideal post-run meal as they contain protein and amino acids, which can fire up the recovery process. Top a slice of wholemeal toast with scrambled egg; toss some wheat berries with spinach and grilled chicken breast; add some edamame to a bowl of brown rice, or enjoy a skimmed-milk latte with your morning whole-grain bagel.

Finding the best whole grains for you

With packaging employing 'natural' and 'earthy' colours, it can be difficult to tell a refined grain from a true whole grain. Not all brown or wheat breads have whole grains, and there are even some white whole-grain breads. A good indicator is to look for the word 'whole' before grains in the list of ingredients. See opposite for some of the best whole grains for runners and the extra health benefits they provide.

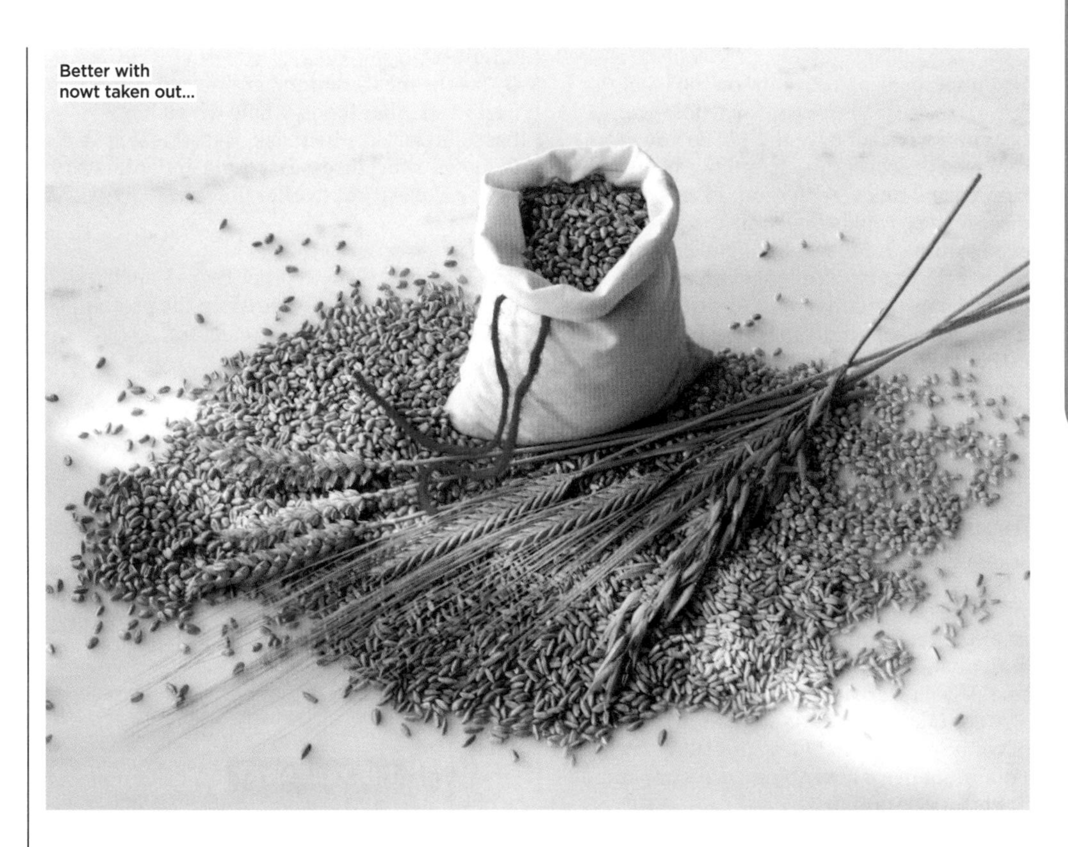
Better with nowt taken out...

Healthy whole grains

Amaranth
Amaranth – the seed of the plant also known as love-lies-bleeding – is rich in protein as well as minerals such as calcium, iron, magnesium and phosphorus. These nutrients promote strong bones and healthy blood but they're often limited in the average diet.

Barley
With 8g fibre in a 40g serving, barley offers more fibre than any other whole grain. It's also high in antioxidants, vitamins and minerals – such as magnesium and phosphorus – that are needed for bone health, plus iron and potassium, which are important for healthy blood and circulation. Be sure to buy whole-grain or hulled barley; pearl barley is missing at least some of the bran layer.

Buckwheat
A popular ingredient in pancake mixes, soba noodles, kasha and other foods, buckwheat contains relatively high levels of zinc, copper and manganese, essential nutrients that are needed in small amounts but can be hard to find in the average diet. Buckwheat also has a high level of muscle-boosting protein – about 6g in 170g cooked groats. It's also high in soluble fibre (which helps improve cholesterol levels) and resistant starch (to boost digestive health).

Corn
Corn provides more than 10 times as much vision-boosting vitamin A as other grains. It's is also high in antioxidants and carotenoids that are associated with eye health. And because it's gluten-free, corn is popular with those who have coeliac disease or follow a gluten-free diet.

Photography: Getty

Oats

If you see 'oats' or 'oat flour' on the label, you can be sure you're getting whole grain. Oats almost never have their bran and germ removed in processing. They have been widely studied and linked with reduced risk of heart disease, type 2 diabetes, some cancers and even asthma. And for the weight-conscious runner they're an excellent choice: 250g cooked oats contains about 6g protein (more if you make your morning porridge with milk rather than water) and roughly 2g heart-healthy unsaturated fat per serving – more than most other grains. That fat will help keep you feeling fuller for longer.

Quinoa

Because it's gluten-free and is one of the few grains that provide a complete protein, quinoa has undergone a surge in popularity in recent years. Easy to cook and ready in about 15 minutes, it's a popular choice for vegetarians, both on its own and as an ingredient in energy bars, shakes, cereals and other health foods. It also contains more potassium than other type of whole grain, with 159mg in a 180g serving. Potassium helps lower blood pressure and fights muscle cramps.

Rice (brown, black, red and others)

Easy to cook and easy to tolerate, rice is an excellent source of carbs for a post-run recovery meal. Most whole-grain varieties are high in fibre, and nutrients such as manganese and selenium, which is important for carbohydrate and fat metabolism.

Rye

Rye has a high amount of fibre in its endosperm – not just in its bran. Because of this, products made with rye generally have a lower glycaemic index than products made from other whole grains. Rye contains a unique type of dietary fibre, arabinoxylan, known for its high antioxidant activity, which helps fight inflammation and thus ease muscle soreness. Research has shown that rye boosts GI health and helps you stay feeling full for longer, which can help you manage your weight.

Whole wheat

By far the most common grain used in breads, pasta and other foods, whole wheat has been shown to reduce risk of stroke, type 2 diabetes, heart disease, asthma, inflammatory disease, obesity and other illnesses.

Wild rice

When compared with other types – such as brown rice – wild rice has twice the protein and fibre but less iron and calcium.

Gluten-free grains

Staying away from gluten? That doesn't mean you have to go grain-free. A variety of gluten-free grains are on the market.[3] They include:

■ Amaranth ■ Buckwheat ■ Corn ■ Millet ■ Montina ■ Oats ■ Quinoa ■ Rice ■ Sorghum ■ Teff ■ Wild rice

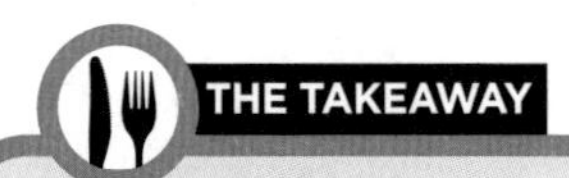

Make simple swaps.
To get your three to five servings of whole grains each day, cut back on refined-grain products such as white rolls and crackers, and increase your consumption of those made with whole wheat, whole-grain corn, brown rice, pinhead oats and quinoa.

Read the list of ingredients.
Look for the word 'whole' on the ingredients panel (not just 'wheat'). Remember, just because bread is brown in colour doesn't mean it contains whole grains.

Time your intake right.
Avoid eating whole grains just before a run, as they take longer to digest, and that could lead to GI distress. Make them a part of regular meals and have them just after a hard workout – like a long run or speedwork – when the body needs carbs to restock spent glycogen stores and repair muscles, so you can bounce back for the next workout.

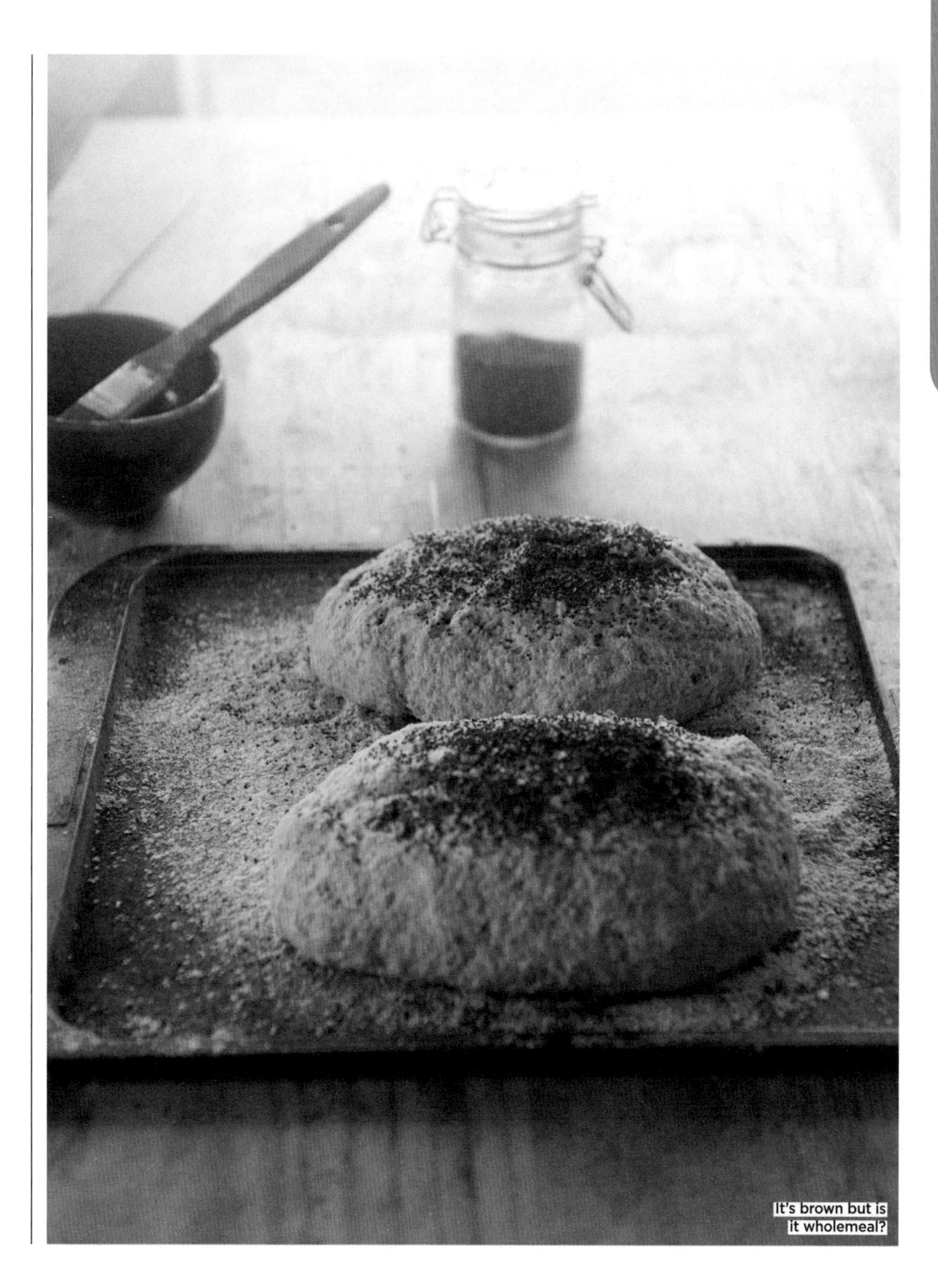

It's brown but is it wholemeal?

4.

GETTING SMART ABOUT SUGAR

Sugar is a diet demon that's earned its bad rap. Overloading on the sweet stuff can lead to weight gain and a wide range of health problems, including heart disease, diabetes and high blood pressure.

In the past few decades, the dangers of excessive sugar intake have been well documented. If you need motivation to steer clear, consider the following:

It can lead to diabetes

A constant intake of sugar forces your pancreas to work overtime, possibly leading to type 2 diabetes. It also lowers levels of HDL ('good') cholesterol while increasing triglycerides. Both factors increase the risk of heart disease.[1]

It can lead to other chronic diseases

In a study published in *Nature*, researchers pointed out that too much sugar leads to obesity, damages the liver and metabolism, impairs brain function, and increases the risk of heart disease and cancer.[2]

It makes you hungry

Overdosing on sugar sends your hunger hormones into overdrive. The satiety hormones that tell your brain, 'I'm full!' aren't properly triggered, which means you end up eating more than you need to.

It's as addictive as drugs

And since it's legal, maybe a bigger danger. In addition to having all these toxic effects on your health, sugar gives you a rush that makes you want more. If you've ever tried to eat just one square of milk chocolate, you've probably discovered there's no satisfying a sweet tooth. A study published in the journal *Current Opinion in Clinical Nutrition and Metabolic Care*[3] concluded, 'Evidence in humans shows that sugar and sweetness can induce reward

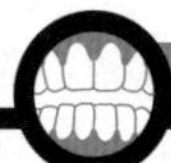

CHEW ON THIS

On packaged foods, the nutrition information label will show how many grams of sugar per serving the product contains. Although you can't always isolate the natural sugars from added sugars – normally 'sugars' are listed as part of the carbohydrate content – there *are* ways to tell whether a product might be high in dangerous added sugars. If the product has no fruit or milk products in the ingredients, all the sugars are from added sugars; if it does contain fruit or milk products, the total sugar per serving listed on the label will include both added and naturally occurring sugars.

Unless you're consuming a fruit or dairy product, in general it's best to aim for less than 10g sugar per serving. Keep in mind that 4g sugar equals about 1 tsp, or 16 calories. So a 330ml can of regular cola might have 35g or 8 tsp sugar. UK guidelines recommend a daily limit of around 30g added sugar – around 5% of your total energy intake – which equates to about 7 tsp.

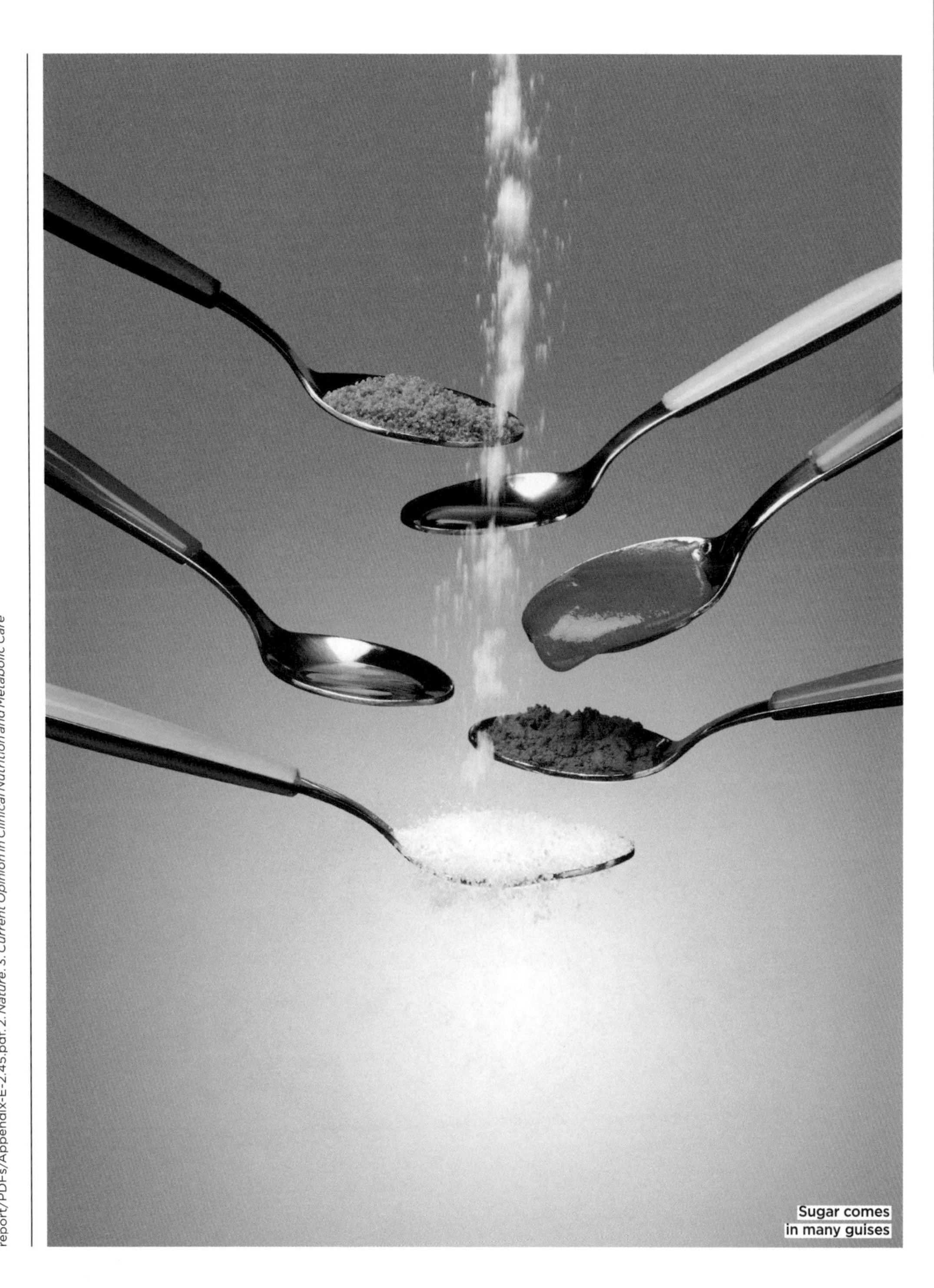

Sugar comes in many guises

report/PDFs/Appendix-E-2.45.pdf. 2. *Nature*. 3. *Current Opinion in Clinical Nutrition and Metabolic Care*

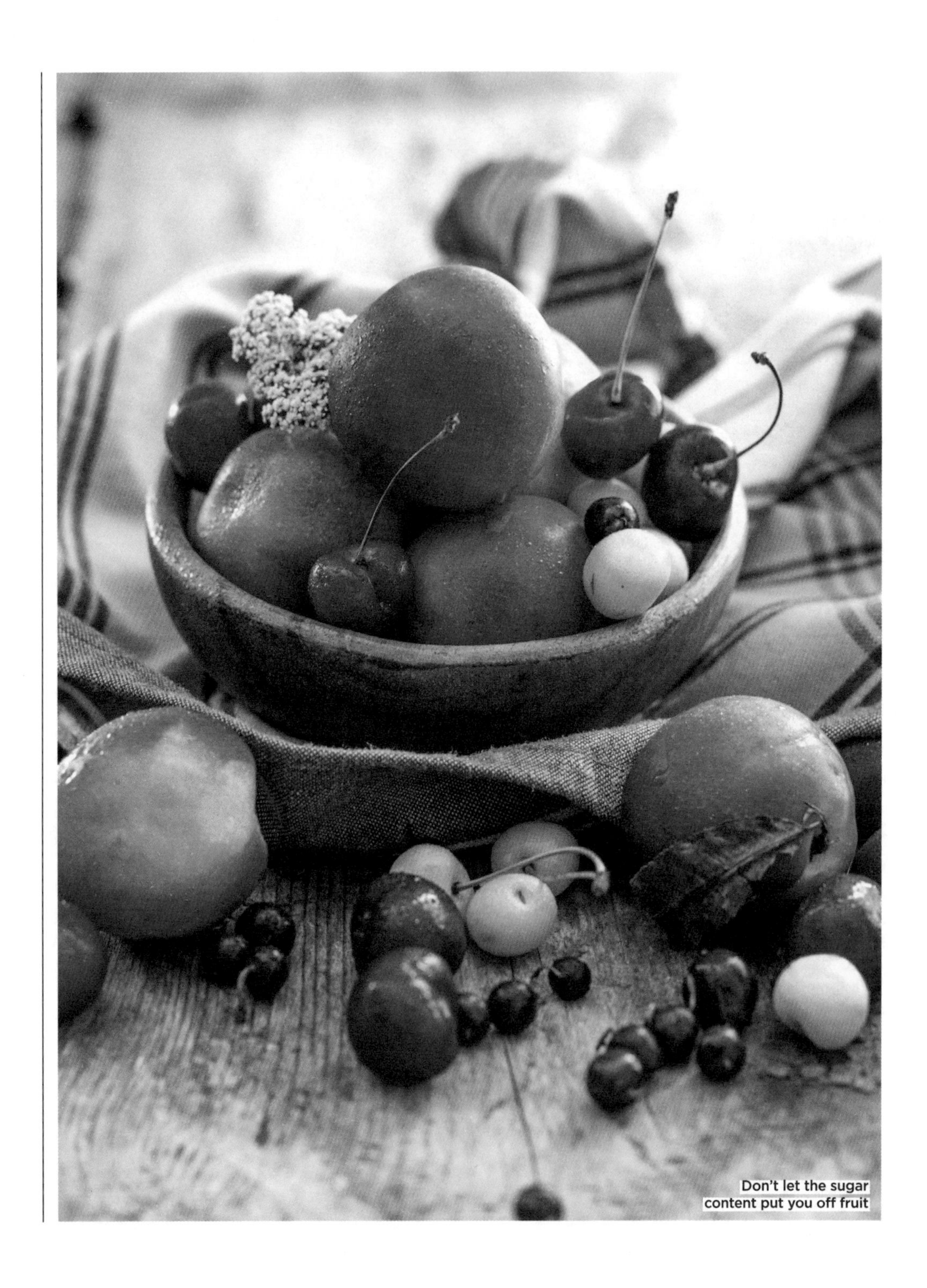

Don't let the sugar content put you off fruit

and craving that are comparable in magnitude to those induced by addictive drugs.' While it's difficult to compare the effects of a sugar high with what you might get from a drug like cocaine, in experiments on lab rats, the researchers showed that sugar and sweet rewards, 'can not only substitute to addictive drugs, like cocaine, but can even be more rewarding and attractive.'

With all these dire warnings about sugar, it's tempting to reach for calorie-free artificial sweeteners when you want a treat. But many people report that these sweeteners can drive up cravings for sweet stuff, too. (Read more in Chapter 11 on sugar substitutes.)

Why sugar from fruits and dairy is different

Many low-carb and high-protein diets discourage consumption of the natural sugars found in fruit, dairy products and some starchy vegetables (such as corn, peas, potatoes and baked beans). But cutting out fruit and veg for the sake of avoiding sugar would be a big mistake. The naturally occurring sugar in plain yogurt, vegetables, or a piece of fruit is much healthier than the added sugar in, say, a bar of chocolate, because it's packaged with the vitamins and minerals you need to run strong, lose weight and fend off chronic disease.

For instance, while bananas contain sugar, they also contain potassium, which helps prevent muscle cramping on the road. Raisins have fibre and iron; oranges, vitamin C to help ward off coughs and colds, while corn contains lutein, a vision-boosting nutrient that few other foods have. Carrots are high in vitamin A, which is also beneficial for eyesight, and while milk contains lactose – a naturally occurring sugar – it also has bone-building calcium and vitamin D to help you stay strong.

Take an apple and a chocolate bar, for example, notes Dee McCaffrey, author of *The Science of Skinny*. The apple has, "the perfect package of vitamins, fibre, enzymes and phytonutrients", says McCaffrey, a chemist who lost more than 7st by eliminating processed foods and starting a regular exercise regime.

"When you eat an apple, it actually cleanses your body, and your liver, the body's main fat-burning organ and its main filter. It actually supports your whole metabolism, and the detoxification pathways and fat burning," she explains. "It's a very efficient form of calories that your body will use up and not store."

> 'Eating an apple cleanses your body and your liver'

In contrast, when you eat 100 calories-worth of a bar of chocolate, you'll get fast energy, but you'll also be consuming a lot of sugar and you'll miss out on the cleansing, fat-burning and general health benefits that you'd get from the apple. What's more, the refined sugar is inflammatory to the body: "Even though you might get a burst of energy from having that sugar, the chocolate bar could leave undetected chronic inflammation in your body and the arteries," says McCaffrey. "So the calories it contains could be causing a long-term health issue, while the apple will give you long-term health benefits."

Regardless of your daily calorie target, it's important to make room in your diet for whole, unprocessed fruits and starchy vegetables. Because fruit and veg contain fibre, and dairy products contain fat and protein, they won't make your blood-sugar levels soar then crash, the way the sugars in processed foods will. And the health benefits they provide vastly outweigh the fact that they also contain sugars.

How much sugar should you have?

The short answer is that you should consume as little added sugar as possible. According to NHS guidelines, it shouldn't make up any more than 5% of the energy you get from food and drink – which for adults means your limit is about 30g a day. That said, it's nearly impossible to determine how much sugar in a packaged product is 'added sugar' (from unhealthy additives) and how much of the sugar comes from natural sources such as fruits and dairy.

To make it simple, try to keep under 10g sugar per serving and don't stress about the sugar content in raw fruit or milk. To stabilise your energy levels, try to spread your sugar consumption throughout the day.

How to avoid sugar

Even if you steer clear of obvious sugar shocks, you may still be consuming a lot that you don't need in your meals and snacks. Here's how to avoid sneaky sources of sugar:

Avoid added sugar

Look for packaged products that clearly state on the label that there's 'no added sugar'. Often sugar is added to sauces and dressings to bolster taste when other substances such as fat are taken out.

Check the ingredients

Ingredients are listed by weight, so those listed first make up a larger percentage of the product. If sugar (including any of the forms included in the list on this page) is one of the first three ingredients, put it back.

Check the claims

Packaged-food manufacturers make a variety of claims about sugar content. Some of those claims have set definitions; others do not:

- ***Reduced sugar:***
  At least 30% less sugar per serving compared with a standard serving size of the traditional product.
- ***No added sugar:***
  This does not necessarily mean that the product is sugar-free: it simply means that no sugar has been added to it as an ingredient; any sugars in the product occur naturally.
- ***Low sugar:***
  No more than 5g total sugars per 100g
- ***High sugar:***
  22.5g or more total sugars per 100g

(To find out more on decoding food labels, turn to Chapter 12.)

Be aware of sugar's other names

Sugar is added to products in many different forms, but all of them offer calories and the same ill effects of sugar without any nutritional benefit. The following is a list of other forms of sugar you should look out for.

- brown sugar ■ cane sugar ■ corn sugar ■ fructose ■ glucose ■ dextrose ■ fruit juice concentrate ■ corn syrup ■ honey ■ maltodextrin ■ invert sugar ■ maltose ■ molasses ■ raw sugar ■ sucrose ■ turbinado sugar ■ hydrolysed starch

THE TAKEAWAY

Take stock of your daily sugar habits.
Look at your average daily intake and calculate how much sugar you take in on a regular basis. Where can you cut out sugar? Try a three-day detox from added sugars. Before you start, stock up on three different pieces of raw fruit that you enjoy. During the detox, anytime you crave a sweet, rather than trying to strain your willpower have a piece of fruit. At the end of three days, reassess how you feel and whether you miss anything you've taken out of your diet.

Don't drink it.
Avoid all drinks with sugar, including sports drinks (unless you're actually running) and dressed-up coffee drinks. These won't fill you up the way foods do, or offer any nutrition.

Set a standard for yourself.
Avoid packaged foods with more than 10g sugar per serving, or foods that list sugar (in any form) in the first three ingredients.

5.

THE GLYCAEMIC INDEX

If you've been searching for weight-loss guidance in recent years, it's likely you've heard about the glycaemic index (GI). The index, which ranks foods according to how they affect your blood sugar, is designed to help you avoid foods that cause big swings in blood sugar, which in turn can lead to cravings, energy crashes and even chronic diseases such as type 2 diabetes. By the same token, the index can help you identify foods that will help you feel fuller for longer.

The index assigns scores to different foods based on how quickly they're digested and enter the bloodstream, and how much they make your blood sugar spike.

High-glycaemic foods, such as bagels, pasta and white bread, are ranked at 70 or higher, as they cause blood sugar to rise quickly. Lower-GI options – such as fruit or traditional porridge oats – tend to be higher in fibre, protein and fat, are slower to digest and absorb, and produce more gradual rises in blood-sugar and insulin levels.

When using the glycaemic index, timing is everything

For the purpose of managing your weight, timing is everything when using the glycaemic index. High-GI foods might be ideal for giving you the burst of energy to power through that speed workout, for example. But if you're constantly loading up on high-GI foods while engaged in sedentary activities such as a day at the office, it can be a problem. Why? Because once your blood sugar rises, your body produces insulin to shuttle it back into the organs that need it. Too much of that over time can lead to chronic disease. And once your blood sugar falls, your energy level plummets, which leaves you feeling tired and hungry.

Like so many other factors, the glycaemic index isn't a magic bullet that's going to catapult you to the PB of your dreams or get you to your feel-great weight. But used with all the other nutrition data you're gathering, it can help you tailor your diet to your racing and weight-loss goals.

How to use GI to reduce finish times *and* your waistline

While there is a fair amount of research looking at performance when fuelling with a low- or high-GI diet, there is no solid answer as to how runners or dieters can best use the GI.

Some research shows that runners benefit from low-GI foods, as they provide a slow, steady supply of energy rather than cause you to crash and burn. In other words, you'll burn fat while saving the fuel that's in muscles, and be able to run a bit longer before needing to pause for a snack. A study published in the journal *Metabolism* in 2001 concluded that when a moderate-GI carb (in this case, rolled

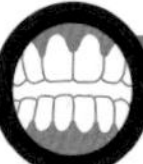

CHEW ON THIS

Agave nectar has been touted as a healthy alternative to sugar, because it has a low glycaemic index relative to other forms of sugar. But agave nectar contains more fructose than the widely demonised high fructose corn syrup (HFCS). Why does that matter? Fructose, unlike other sugars, is metabolised directly by the liver, and that can lead to fatty liver deposits, which has been linked to weight gain, insulin resistance and heart-disease risk in studies of animals. What's more, as with other forms of sugar, the more you consume, the more you'll crave it. (The fructose in agave nectar should not be confused with the fructose found in, for example, apples and bananas. Because of their fibre content and the other nutrients they contain, the fruits are not digested in the same way and therefore don't cause the same kinds of problems as agave nectar and HFCS.)

oats) was given to cyclists 45 minutes before exercise, they had more long-lasting energy than with higher-glycaemic food (puffed rice).[1]

On the other hand, a study published in 2007 in the *Journal of Strength and Conditioning Research*[2] found that there was no significant difference in performance or endurance between athletes who consumed raisins (a moderate-glycaemic food) and those who had a sports gel (a high-glycaemic food.)

One word of warning with low-GI foods: because they tend to be higher in fibre and fat, they will take longer to digest. So you'll want to leave plenty of time between your meal and your run. Also, if your blood sugar is low and you're feeling too tired to run, a low-GI food isn't going to give you the energy surge you need to get out the door. In this case, a high-GI food might be a better choice.

And remember, just because a food has a low GI number doesn't mean it's healthy. A chocolate bar, for instance – which no one would list as health food – has a low GI number of around 51, in part because its high fat content takes a long time to digest. But that fat is all saturated, which isn't going to help your heart or your long-term health.

During a race or a long endurance event such as a marathon, when you need a quick burst of energy to boost you and avoid hitting the wall, foods that are higher on the glycaemic index are going to be your best bet. They're also ideal straight after a hard workout, such as a speed session or a long run, when your muscles need a quick boost of carbs to repair torn muscle fibre and replenish spent glycogen stores. But on an everyday basis, sticking with foods that rank low on the glycaemic index is the best way to avoid blood-sugar spikes. Because they take more time to digest, they'll help you feel fuller for longer.

The GI index

The GI is not listed on nutrition labels, but you can find a complete list in the international GI database at the University of Sydney in Australia (glycemicindex.com).[3]

Remember that foods are ranked according to 50g servings, and a single serving of many foods will be either more or less than that. Also, the GI only ranks foods with carbs, so it doesn't include meat, fish or poultry. The following lists, adapted from the 'international tables of glycaemic index and glycaemic load values', published in *Diabetes Care*,[4] show where foods rank on the glycaemic index:

Low-GI foods (under 55) make great meals and snacks any time of day

- Chickpeas (10)
- Grapefruit (25)
- Fat-free milk (32)
- Low-fat yogurt (33)
- Pear (38)
- Apple (39)
- Baked beans (40)
- Orange (40)
- Peach (42)
- Dried dates (42)
- Brown rice (50)
- Orange juice (unsweetened) (50)

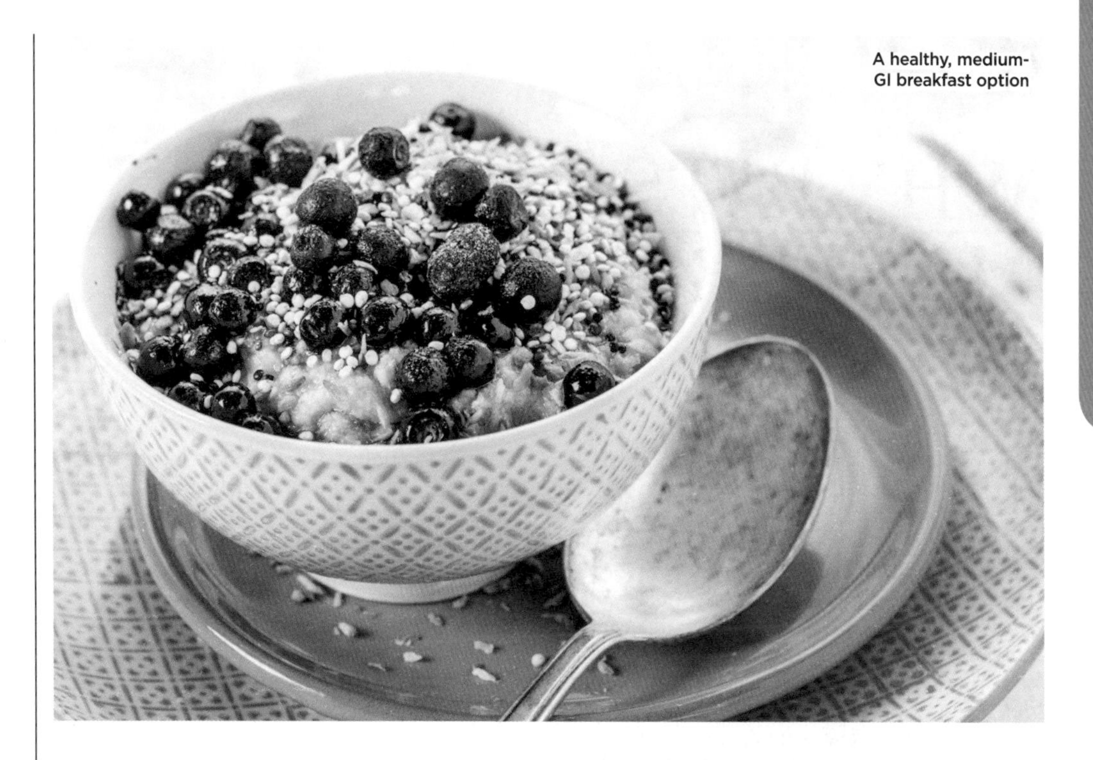

A healthy, medium-GI breakfast option

- Quinoa (53)
- Yam (54)

Medium-GI foods (between 55 and 70) can be consumed in moderation

- Traditional porridge oats (55)
- Grapes (59)
- Corn on the cob (60)
- Banana (62)
- Raisins (64)
- Couscous (65)
- Special K cereal (69)
- Plain white bagel (72)
- Instant oatmeal (78)

Save high-GI foods (over 70) for mid-run energy boosts or post-workout refuelling

- Rice cakes (82)
- White rice (89)
- Corn flakes (93)
- Baked potato (111)

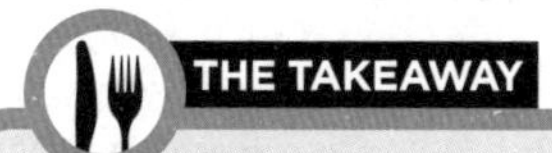

THE TAKEAWAY

Make smart swaps.
Look at the GI index and work out where you can exchange high-GI foods for low-GI alternatives in your regular meals and snacks.

Make room for high GI in your diet.
Don't eliminate high-GI foods from your diet; just eat them strategically so you don't feel deprived. And an all-out ban usually leads to a disastrous binge. Pick a high-GI food and reserve it for a pre-workout boost or a post-workout treat, when you need fuel fast to bounce back quickly for the next session. (See Part III for more on when to eat.)

Know the combinations.
You can slow down the absorption of high-GI foods by combining them with foods that contain fibre, protein and fat, which take longer to digest – eg, peanut butter on toast, or a baked potato with veggie chilli.

6.

WHY FATS MATTER

Fats have been another casualty of the dieting mania of the past four decades. The fat-free craze of the 1980s – which opened the door to a huge number of products for the weight-conscious – left us only more overweight decades later. Like so many other food fads that look to eliminate one group of nutrients altogether, it was a case of a good idea taken to an extreme, creating a problem.

Not that cutting back on fat was such a bad idea. Saturated and trans fats have been linked to higher levels of cholesterol and increased risk of heart disease and stroke. And fats do pack a calorie punch, so it's important not to go overboard (fat contains 9 calories per gram, compared to carbs and protein, which each have 4 calories per gram).

> Fats play an important part in every runner's diet

But in the rush to extract fat from popular foods while preserving taste, texture and shelf life, many manufacturers added sugars and the likes of high-fructose corn syrup, which only fuelled overconsumption. Many fat-free yogurts are good examples of this. Check out the sugar quantities in some popular fat-free yogurts, and you'll see that they violate a lot of the best practices for sugar that we recommended in chapter 4. So it's no wonder that – in the US at least – more than two decades since the tidal wave of fat-free products flooded the supermarket shelves, over half the population wants to lose weight, and one-third of people report being overweight, according to a Gallup poll.[1]

Fats play an important role in every runner's diet– especially if you're trying to lose weight and stay injury-free. Much like carbs, in order to use the properties of fats to get the results you want, it's important to focus on eating the right kinds and the right amounts.

How fats keep you healthy

Dietary fat helps the body absorb the fat-soluble nutrients it needs to log a peak performance, including vitamins D and K – both of which are vital for bone health – and

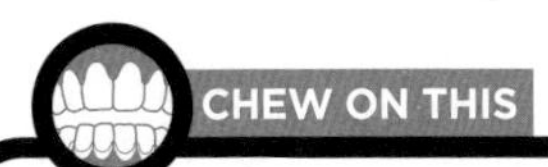

Try to consume as few trans fats as possible. Look for foods that have zero trans fat per serving. But beware: even if a product claims to be 'trans fat-free,' it may still have up to 0.5g trans fat per serving. To make sure it's truly free of trans fat, check the ingredients list: if it includes any partially hydrogenated oil, it has a small amount of trans fat. But if one serving is one biscuit and you have more than one, the trans fats can add up.

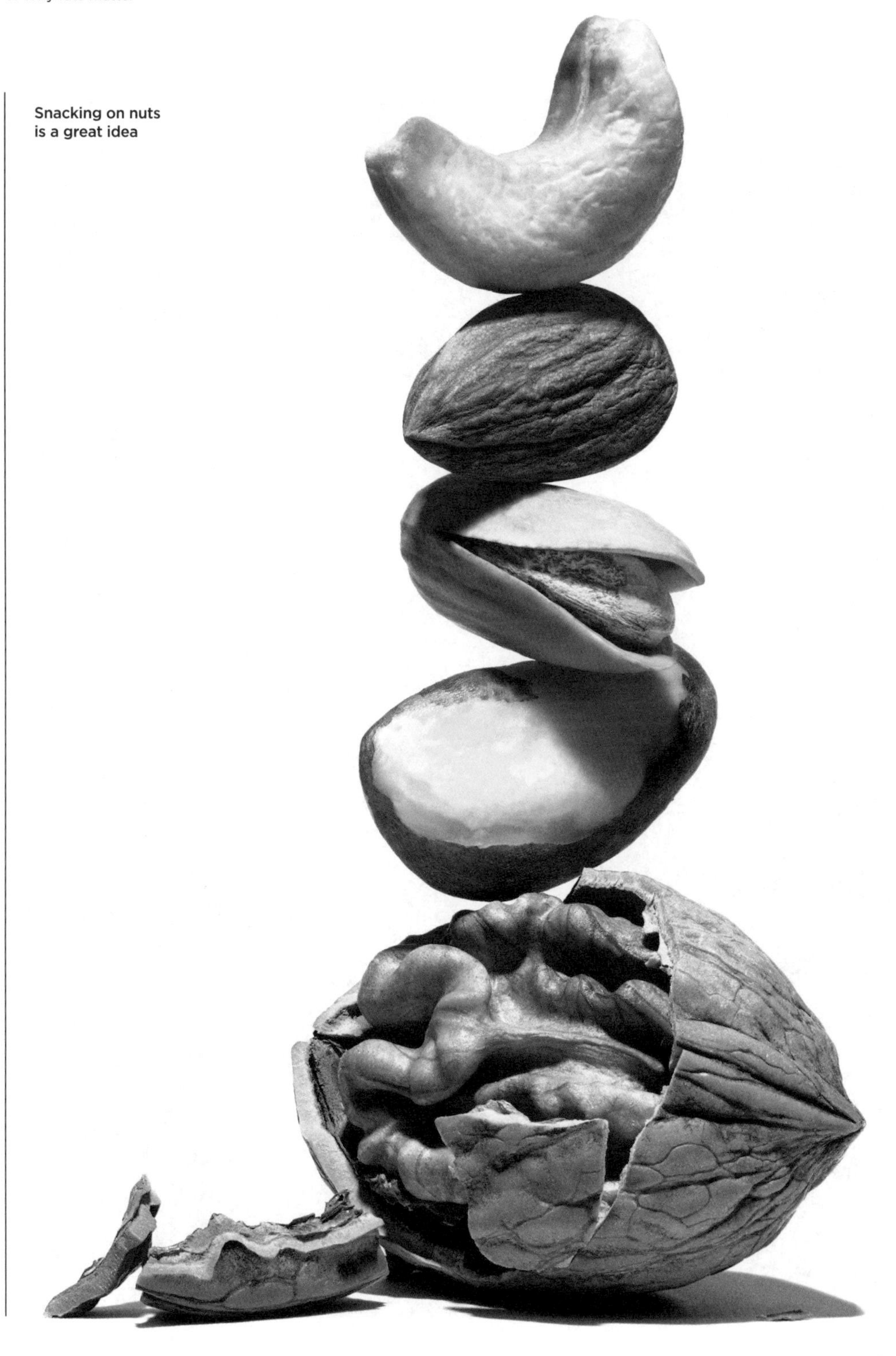

Snacking on nuts is a great idea

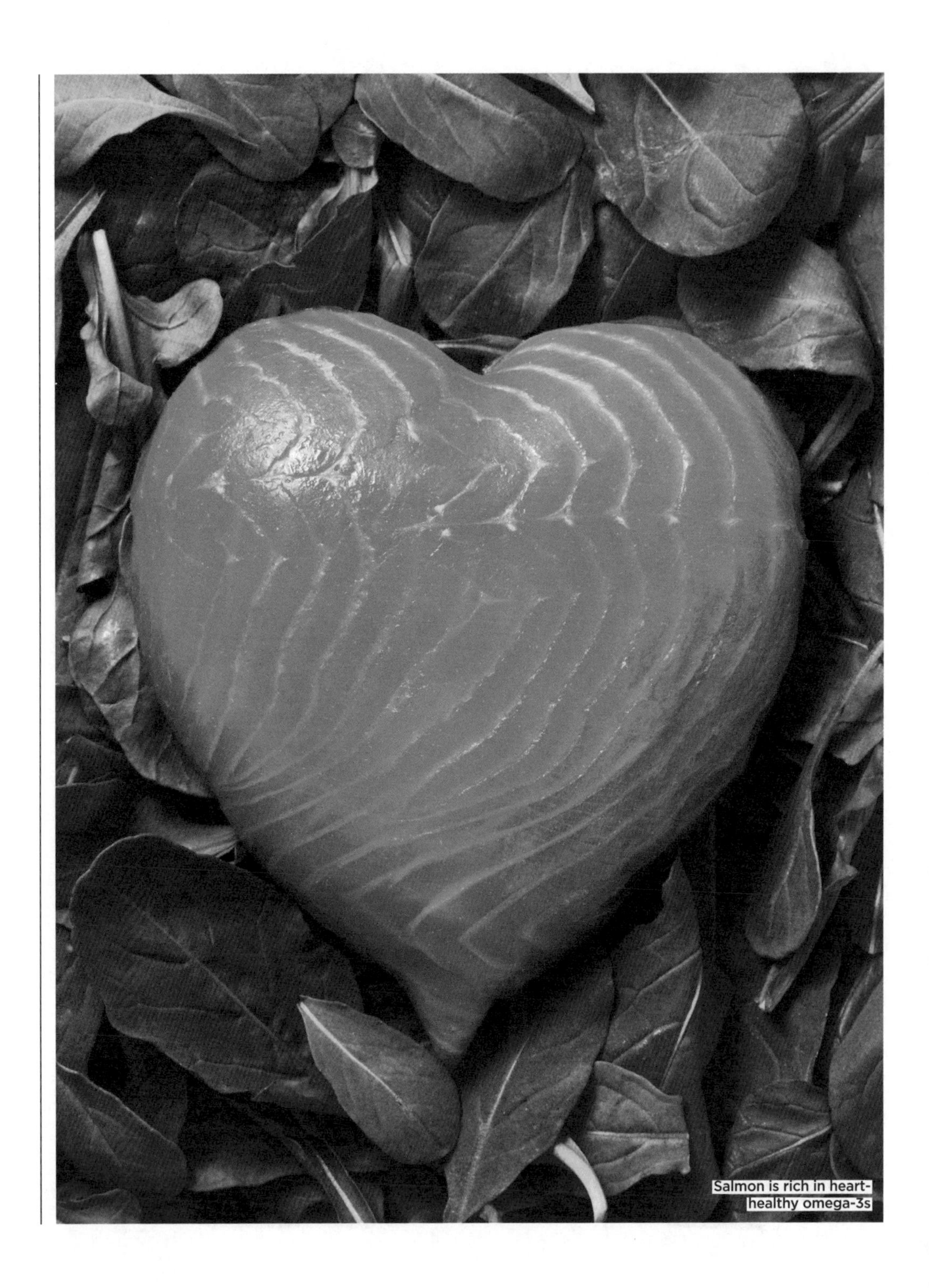

Salmon is rich in heart-healthy omega-3s

vitamin E, which acts as an antioxidant and helps keep the body from breaking down. Omega-3 fatty acids – the kind found in salmon, walnuts and ground flaxseed – help fight inflammation and soothe aches and pains. Polyunsaturated fats (PUFAs) – such as those found in avocados, nuts, seeds and olive oil – have anti-inflammatory properties, so they may help repair the microscopic muscle tears and bone breakdown cause by a hard workout. And because fats promote the feeling of fullness, they're good for runners who want to shed weight. They also help prevent blood-sugar spikes and crashes, as well as the cycle of craving and overeating that can trip up your training. The right kind of fats – unsaturated – are allies, and that's why you shouldn't fear fat. Instead, aim for an intake of fat within the suggested range of 25-35% of your daily calories and make sure the vast majority of that is from healthy, unsaturated fats.

Still not convinced? There's evidence that a low fat intake is associated with injury risk in female runners. A study in the 2008 *Journal of the International Society of Sports Nutrition* found that injured runners had significantly lower intakes of total fat (63 ± 20 versus 80 ± 50 g/d) and lower percentages of calories sourced from fat (27 ± 5% versus 30 ± 8%) compared with non-injured runners. In addition, the runners who consumed lower amounts of dietary fat – 27% rather than 30% of their daily calories – experienced cases of tendonitis, iliotibial band (ITB) problems, and more stress fractures than those who consumed the recommended amount.[2]

Know your (fat) type

The type of fat you consume makes all the difference in the world. While unsaturated fats can improve your cholesterol and heart health, saturated and trans fats have been found to raise your levels of bad cholesterol (LDL). Trans fats are especially bad because they actually lower your levels of good cholesterol (HDL). So unfortunately the 11g fat in that honey-glazed doughnut is not going to bestow

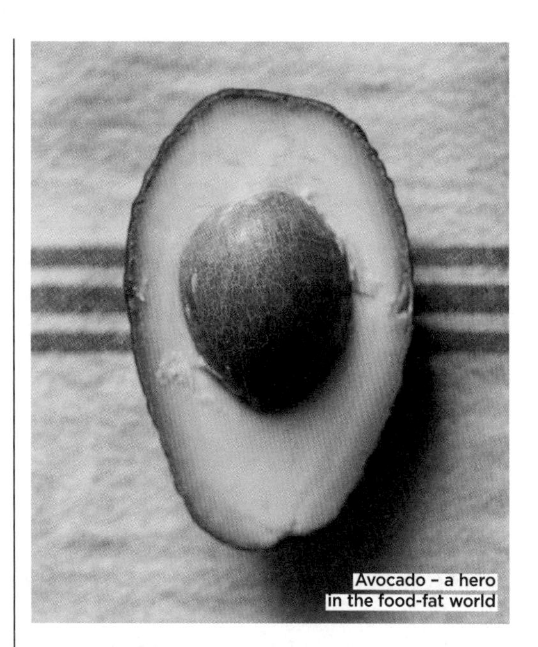

Avocado – a hero in the food-fat world

the same benefits as a tablespoon of avocado – and could indeed be hazardous to your health.

As a runner, there's no reason to be afraid of fat, but you do need to focus on the kinds of fat you're consuming. Unsaturated fats, such as those from plants, nuts and seeds – including avocados and olive oil – lower bad cholesterol and help reduce your risk of heart disease.

Unsaturated fats

These fats lower total cholesterol and LDL cholesterol, and so can help safeguard you against heart disease. Find them in vegetable and nut oils, including almond, avocado, rapeseed, olive and peanut.

There are two types of unsaturated fat. Monounsaturated fats (sometimes referred to as MUFAs) lower your total cholesterol as well as your LDL cholesterol, and have been proven to help reduce belly fat.[3]

Polyunsaturated fats, referred to as PUFAs, have anti-inflammatory properties, so they may help repair muscle tears and bone breakdown after a hard workout. They promote heart health by lowering LDL cholesterol levels. Some PUFAs – omega-3 and omega-6 fatty acids – are called essential fatty acids. That means the body doesn't make them, but it needs them for maintaining brain and nerve function, so they must be derived from foods. They also lower the risk of heart disease and protect against type 2 diabetes, Alzheimer's and age-related brain decline.

The American Heart Association recommends that at least 5-10% of food calories come from omega-6 fatty acids, such as those found in certain oils (eg, corn and sunflower); nuts and seeds, and certain fish (such as tilapia).

When it comes to omega-3s, two types – eicosapentaenoic acid (EPA) and docosahexaenoic acid (DHA) – have been found to promote healthy and flexible joints, improve cognition, fight off inflammation, promote a healthy immune system and bestow a raft of other health benefits. If you're feeling run-down, sore or just want to ensure good health, you might consider increasing your intake of fatty fish, which naturally contain omega-3 – good sources include sardines, salmon and tuna. If you're not keen on fish, try walnuts, flaxseeds or chia seeds. Or you could opt for fish-oil supplements. These come in various sizes and dosage levels – look for pills that contain 1-2g EPA and DHA. This means the fish oil might contain more than just 1,000-2,000mg in total; it's the level of EPA and DHA that's most important.

Where the healthy fats are

Best sources of healthy fats for runners

FOOD	FAT CONTENT PER SERVING LISTED	EXTRA NUTRIENTS FOR RUNNERS
Avocado, 25g (about ⅕ medium)	5g	Avocados are an excellent source of monounsaturated fats, which lower levels of bad (LDL) cholesterol and boost heart health. Like most sources of fat, avocados are dense in calories, so limit your intake to a serving or two a day. Substitute avocado for fatty products such as butter, cream cheese or mayonnaise.
Mackerel, salmon, sardines, trout or tuna, 75g cooked	Mackerel = 15g Salmon = 6g Sardines = 10g Trout = 5g Tuna = 5g	Oily fish such as mackerel, salmon, sardines, trout and tuna contain a healthy dose of omega-3 fatty acids – known to fend off heart disease and fight inflammation. NHS guidelines recommend eating around 2 x 75g portions of oily fish per week. Canned varieties can be a smart choice, especially where the bones are included, which means you'll boost your calcium intake along with your protein and omega-3 intake.
Olive oil, 1 tbsp	14g	Olive-oil intake has been linked to reduced risk of stroke and heart disease, as well as improved blood pressure. Olive oil burns more quickly than some other oils, so be careful. Choose extra-virgin olive oil when you can, since it contains health-boosting antioxidant polyphenols.

FOOD	FAT CONTENT PER SERVING LISTED	EXTRA NUTRIENTS FOR RUNNERS
Rapeseed oil, 1 tbsp	14g	Rapeseed oil is high in the omega-3 fatty acid ALA (alpha-linolenic acid), which has been shown to reduce inflammation and improve heart health. It's also easy to cook with, as it has a high smoke point.
Hemp-seed oil, 1 tbsp	14g	Best used cold due to a low smoke point, hemp-seed oil is an excellent source of omega-3s and polyunsaturated fat. It should be stored in the fridge.
Flaxseed, 1 tbsp	Flaxseed oil = 13.6g Ground seeds = 4.3g	Ground flaxseed is a great source of heart-healthy fats. Buy ground seeds or cold-pressed oil.
Wheat germ, 2 tbsp	1.5g	In addition to healthy fats and fibre, wheat germ provides thiamin, an essential B vitamin that converts carbs into usable energy and helps the heart, muscles and nervous system to function properly. It also contains zinc, a nutrient that aids immune function and healing.
Nut butter, 2 tbsp	Almond = 18g Cashew = 16g Peanut = 16g	Though high in calories, nut butters are a great source of unsaturated fats, fibre and protein. While peanut butter is certainly the most common variety, almond and cashew butters offer tasty options for those with peanut allergies. Avoid nut butters that contain palm oil or other substitute oils. Look for all-natural nut butters with the fewest ingredients.
Almonds (25g or 23 kernels)	14g	Almonds contain heart-healthy monounsaturated fats, plus they provide vitamin E, an antioxidant that boosts circulation. Studies have shown that eating nuts several times per week lowers levels of LDL cholesterol.
Pistachios (25g or 49 kernels)	13g	Like almonds, pistachios contain vitamin E and heart-healthy fats. They also contain lutein and zeaxanthin, both important for eye health, and offer 3g fibre per serving. Because you have to work to extract pistachios from the shell, you don't have to worry about getting carried away with snacking.
Walnuts (25g or 14 halves)	18.5g	Walnuts are one of the few plant-based sources of omega-3 fatty acids. While high in calories compared with other nuts, walnuts are still a good choice. Research shows nut eaters are generally slimmer, less likely to develop type 2 diabetes and have a reduced risk of heart disease.
Egg (1 whole)	5g (1.5g saturated fats)	Whole eggs are a good source of choline, an important B vitamin that helps regulate the brain, nervous system and cardiovascular system. Choose omega-3-enhanced eggs to further increase your intake of healthy fats.

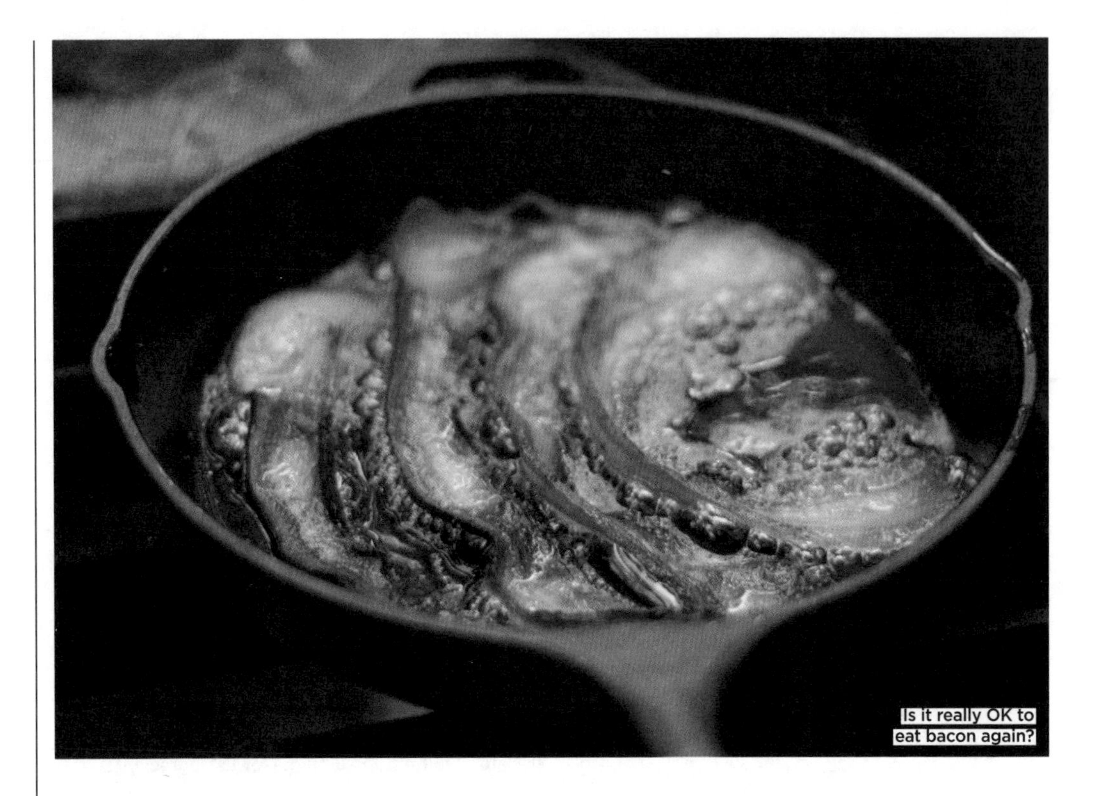

Is it really OK to eat bacon again?

Saturated fats

These fats, often found in animal products such as butter, lard, bacon, beef, lamb, poultry with skin, and dairy (both full-fat and low-fat products) can lead to high cholesterol. Some tropical oils, such as palm oil and cocoa butter, also have saturated fats. The Department of Health recommends limiting intake of saturated fat to no more than 11% of total energy intake from food. In other words, if you consume 2,000 calories per day, your intake should be around 25g per day – about the amount found in 50g butter.

New questions

For years, health and nutrition experts have urged people to avoid saturated fats as much as possible and recommended that we replace them with the heart-healthy monounsaturated and polyunsaturated fats. But recently that advice has come into question.

A review of more than 70 research studies published in the US journal *Annals of Internal Medicine*[4] did not find that people who ate higher levels of saturated fat had more heart disease than those who ate less. Nor did it find fewer instances of disease in those eating more unsaturated fats, including monounsaturated fats such as avocados and olive oil and polyunsaturated fats – for example, soybean and rapeseed oil.

Needless to say, the study provoked a good deal of controversy and left many people wondering whether they now had the green light to fill their dinner plates with bacon, butter and sausages.

Not so fast. Decades of research still support the theory that you'll lower your risk of heart disease by replacing saturated fats with heart-healthy ones found in nuts, seeds, avocados, fish, plant oils and vegetable-oil-based soft spreads.

In addition, there are no health benefits to saturated fats. But this doesn't mean eliminating them from your diet will make you bulletproof to a heart attack, especially if you replace them with products that have high amounts of sugar. The same holds true for unsaturated fats. While guacamole has plenty of heart-healthy avocado, if you're using it to dress up a bowl of high-fat tortilla chips, you're not doing your body much good.

Trans fats

While saturated fats have been engulfed in controversy in recent years, on trans fats, sometimes called trans fatty acids, experts universally agree: they're hazardous to your health and you should eliminate them from your diet or consume as little as possible.

Trans fats became widely used by food makers in the 20th century because the compound, created when hydrogen is added to liquid vegetable oils, offered a cheap and easy way to extend shelf life and preserve flavour in packaged foods.

We now know how harmful trans fats are to our health. They increase risk of stroke, heart disease and type 2 diabetes. Not only do they raise LDL ('bad') cholesterol like saturated fat does, but they also actually lower HDL ('good') cholesterol levels.

In the UK there is no specific requirement for the level of trans fats to be included on food packaging (unlike in the US, where this has been in place since 2006), although some manufacturers do so voluntarily. But the presence of 'partially hydrogenated' fat or vegetable oil in the ingredients list indicates the presence of trans fats – and the higher up the list it appears, the more there'll be.

There have been calls from health bodies in the UK for a total ban, following similar moves in other countries, including Denmark, Switzerland and the US (effective from 2018). In response to the backlash, many fast-food chains, food manufacturers and supermarkets have taken trans fats out of their products – and heavily advertised that fact.

But what about the foods that don't come in a package? Unless they specifically say 'trans fat-free' or free of 'partially hydrogenated oils', certain foods are highly likely to contain trans fats. These include:

- Biscuits
- Crackers
- Doughnuts
- Muffins
- Pies
- Fried foods
- Cake icing
- Pancake mixes
- Solid vegetable fat
- Spreadable butter and margarine
- Buttered popcorn
- Pie crusts
- Hamburgers
- Beef sausages, hotdogs and beef mince
- Ready-to-bake cookie dough
- Biscuits
- Ready-to-eat noodles
- Ice cream

THE TAKEAWAY

Replace bad fats with good fats.
If you're taking in saturated or trans fats, substitute healthy forms of unsaturated fat.

Make sure you're getting enough healthy fat.
Make sure your diet includes at least some healthy fats. At least 15-20% of your daily calories should come from unsaturated fats. Add avocados to your tuna sandwich, cook with olive oil or have a 100-calorie pack of nuts as an afternoon snack.

Consider omega-3 supplements.
If your family has a history of heart disease or you're concerned that you're not consuming enough fatty acids from foods, talk to your doctor about whether you should take supplements.

Photography: Getty Sources: 4. Annals of Internal Medicine

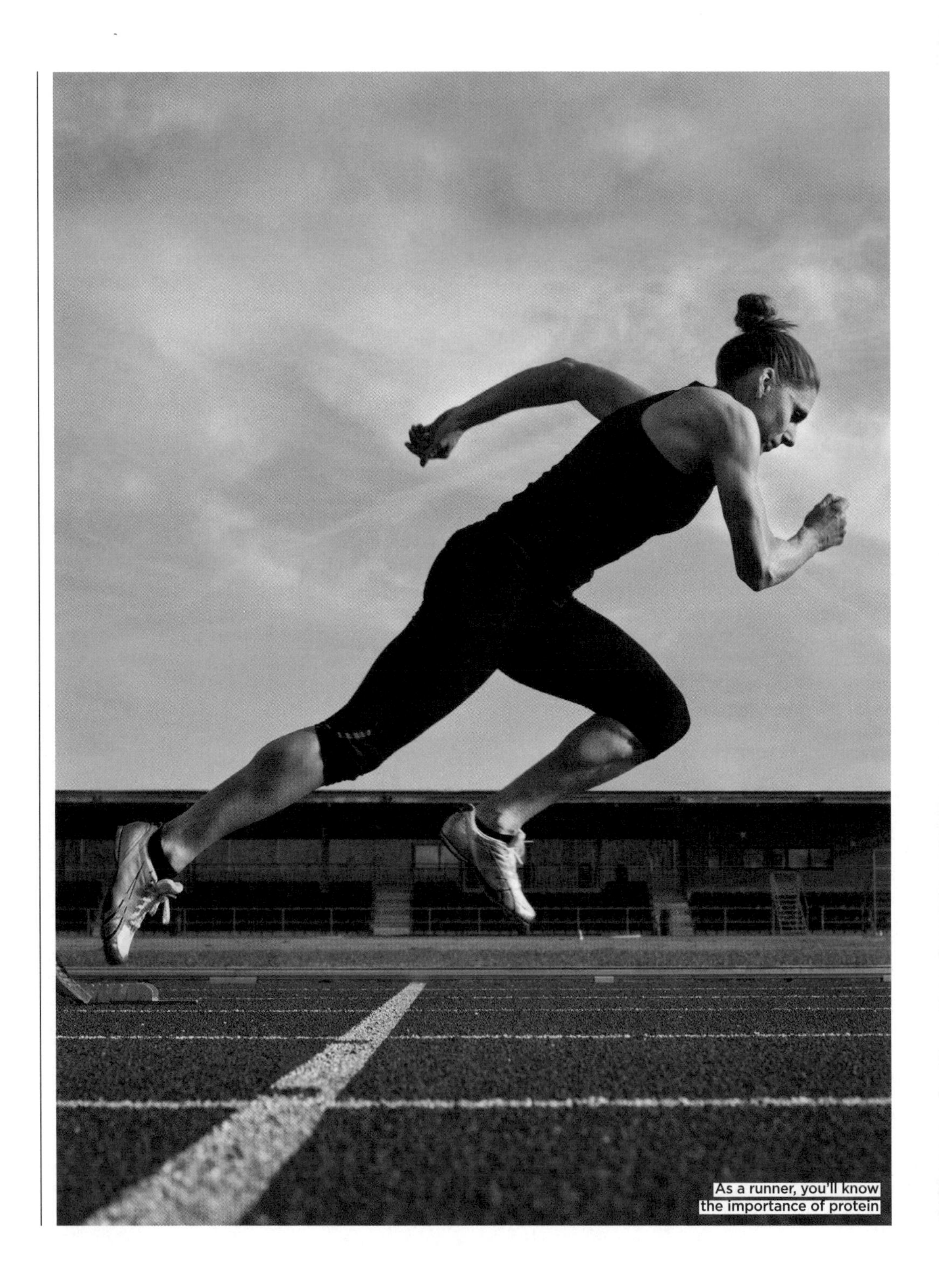

As a runner, you'll know the importance of protein

7.

PROTEIN

Scientists have long known protein builds lean muscle mass and provides a feeling of fullness that can aid weight loss. A raft of studies linking protein-rich diets to shedding weight have kept that idea in the spotlight.

One such study, in the *FASEB* [Federation of American Societies for Experimental Biology] *Journal* in 2013, reported that people who ate twice the (US) recommended dietary allowance (RDA) of protein, while cutting calories and exercising, lost more fat and kept more lean muscle than those who stuck with the RDA.[1]

Another, published in 2014 in the same journal[2], showed that eating a high-protein breakfast (with 35g protein) curbed appetites later in the day and reduced cravings for high-fat, high-sugar snacks in the evening; it also helped stabilise levels of blood sugar and insulin, thereby reducing risk of diabetes.

Manufacturers have rushed to add protein to some foods

Yes, protein is important for weight loss. And as a runner, you need more than what's recommended for sedentary people, because as you log miles, you need to replace the protein you break down during intense and long workouts in order to build lean muscle tissue.

That said, as with fat and carbs, protein's importance has become distorted in the dieting hysteria. Enticed by the link to its proven weight-loss benefits and buoyed by the popularity of low-carb diets, food makers have rushed to add protein to some foods, such as cereal and granola bars, and promote the naturally high protein content of others such as nuts, beef jerky and Greek yogurt. There's been a 54% increase in the number of new products with a high-protein or vegan claim since 2008, according to research company Mintel.

But not all high-protein products are healthy. Often protein is added to processed foods along with artificial additives sugar, fat and salt to make them taste good. So always check the nutrition panel. A 50g serving of a certain cereal with added protein, for instance, has 7g protein[3] – compared with 4g in the original variety. But it also has about 100 more calories and 16g more sugar per serving. Another high-protein chocolate bar has 20g protein, but it also has other chocolate-bar-like attributes: 290 calories, 9g fat and 22g sugar.

It's a confusing time to be a consumer. As is true with other nutrients, if you want to lose weight, it's important to get the right kinds of protein at the right time and not overdo it.

Why you need protein

You need plenty of protein every day. It builds muscle and runners need it to bounce back quickly from tough workouts. In the 30 minutes after a hard speed session or long run, the body is particularly receptive to protein and carbs to repair muscle tissue and restock

Photography: Getty. Sources: 1. FASEB Journal; 2. Ibid; 3. marathonbars.com/products.php

glycogen stores. That's why experts advise runners to have a snack with a 2:1 ratio of carbs to protein in the 30-60 minutes following such a workout. (To learn more, see Chapter 20.)

Protein is also crucial to the regulation and maintenance of the body and plays a role in blood clotting, fluid balance (so you stay hydrated), hormone and enzyme production, and cell repair. If your protein intake is low, you may start to feel fatigued, lose muscle mass, become run-down and increase your risk of illness and injury.

Your daily protein target

Protein may be good for you, but it does have calories. So as with carbs and fats, if you consume more protein than you need, it's going to get stored as fat.

Most runners should aim for 0.55-0.9g protein per lb of body weight per day to recover from workouts and continue to build fitness. And if you're logging more miles or are incorporating lots of strength training into your routine, you're likely to need more protein. So if you weigh 9st 4lbs, aim for 72-100g per day, while a 14st runner will need to take in approximately 107-123g per day.

It's best to spread your protein intake evenly at meals throughout the day, aiming for 30g at most meals and the remainder from snacks. Protein at each meal and snack will help quiet your appetite, and the 30g at mealtimes will make sure you're eating enough muscle-repairing amino acids at each sitting.

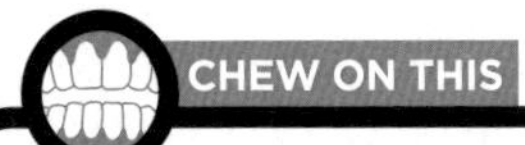

For any food labelled as a 'source of protein', protein must provide at least 12% of the food's calories, according to European Commission regulations on nutrition claims. If it's labelled 'high protein', it must account for at least 20% of the calories.

The best protein sources

Some types of protein are better than others, while some are more readily absorbed by the body. Here are some considerations when choosing your sources of protein:

Go for high quality

Aim for protein-rich foods with the most vitamins and minerals, and the least saturated fats and other ingredients you don't need. For example, while a burger made of 90%-lean mince, with 23g protein in a 75g serving, will help you reach your daily target, but 50% of those calories come from saturated or trans fats. So it's best not to make it a part of your everyday diet. A 75g yellow fin tuna steak, however, has 25g protein and just 0.5g unsaturated fat – and no saturated or trans fats. So tuna is the healthier choice. Remember, just because a food is high in protein doesn't mean it should become a staple of every meal.

Variety matters

Some protein sources are naturally 'complete', ie, they contain all nine essential amino acids your body needs but can't make on its own. You can find complete proteins in animal-based foods such as meat, fish and dairy, as well as some vegetable-based proteins such as soy and quinoa. Other protein sources are 'incomplete' because they don't contain all nine of the essential amino acids; these must be combined with other foods to provide them.

Take red beans and rice: eaten alone, the red beans are incomplete, but eaten with rice, the dish provides the amino acids you need to repair tissue and stave off injury. But you don't have to worry about getting these so-called complementary proteins in the same meal; the body can pool nutrients throughout the day. So if one food is low in an essential amino acid, another can make up for it. As long as you amass a variety of complete and incomplete proteins throughout the day, you'll be good to go.

Pick wholesome sources first

Proteins in some foods are easier for the body to use (or more 'bioavailable') than others. In

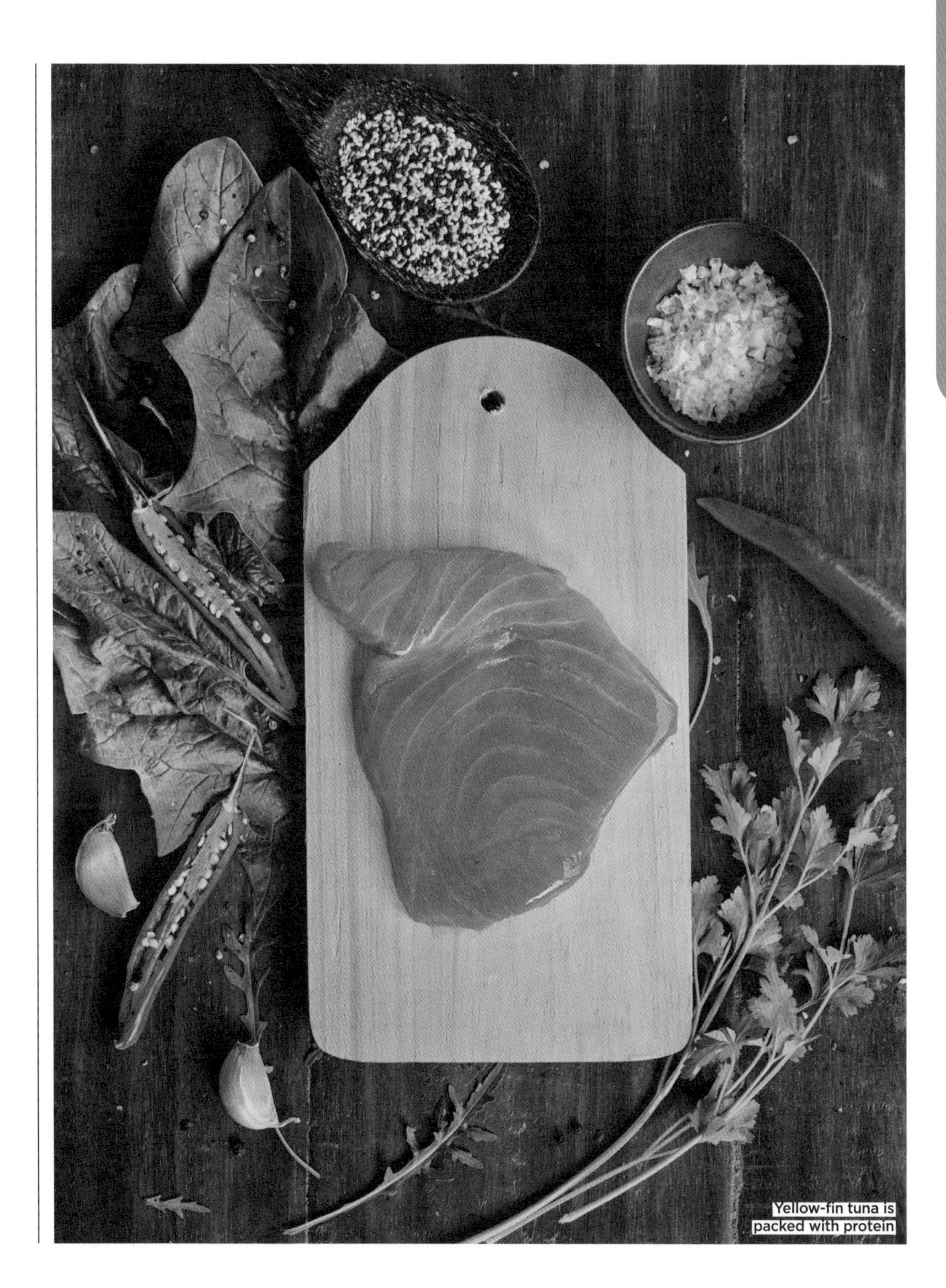

Yellow-fin tuna is packed with protein

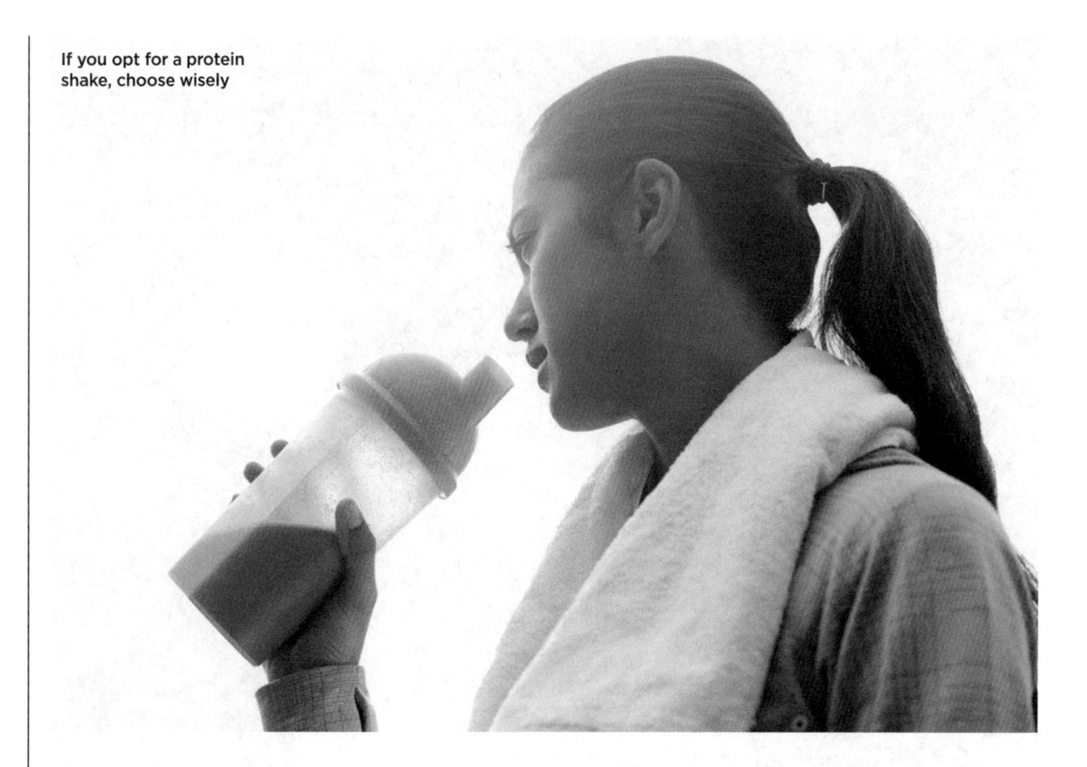
If you opt for a protein shake, choose wisely

general, it's best to get most of your protein from unprocessed whole foods, as these also contain other nutrients your body needs. If you're too pressed for time or don't have access to a refrigerator or cooker immediately after a run, you can find high-quality, bioavailable protein in certain protein bars and powders. Because protein is so critical to muscle repair and appetite regulation, it's better to grab a protein shake than have nothing at all.

When it comes to supplements, be cautious
Protein powders, available as shakes, bars and capsules, are marketed as helping you attain peak physical performance. But they should be used in moderation, given that the Department of Health advises against consuming more than twice the recommended daily intake of protein (which is 55.5g for men and 45g for women). A single (28g) scoop of whey protein power has 20g protein.

In addition, according to a spokesperson from the British Dietetic Association, "You could get the same benefits from introducing high-protein foods to your diet as snacks, or adding them to your normal meals."

If you do decide to use a supplement, opt for one that derives protein from a high-quality source such as whey, casein or soy – or a blend of all three. Whey, which is derived from milk, is digested quickly and rapidly assists muscle repair and recovery. Casein, also derived from milk, is digested more slowly, so it keeps you feeling full and assists with muscle repair and maintenance for a few hours after you consume it. Soy is digested a little faster than casein, but a little slower than whey and is ideal if you're seeking a vegetarian source of protein. If you're a vegetarian, you could also try pea protein. (Other types of vegetarian protein are widely available.) Pea protein is nearly 'complete', so it provides nearly all the amino acids you need for muscle repair. It's also not a risk for anyone with food allergies, generally less expensive than sources of animal protein and high in arginine, which assists with blood flow.

Best sources of protein for runners

FOOD	PROTEIN CONTENT (G)	EXTRA NUTRIENTS FOR RUNNERS
Chicken breast (75g boneless, skinless white meat)	25	Contains the mineral selenium, which helps protect muscles from free-radical damage that can occur during running, and niacin (vitamin B3), which helps regulate fat burn during a run.
Lean beef (75g, 90% lean)	24	Beef boosts iron and zinc to keep your immune system healthy. Choose cuts labelled 'loin', 'round', or '90% lean'.
Pork (75g)	22	Pork has iron levels similar to beef, but with less fat, plus thiamin (vitamin B1) and riboflavin (B2). Look for lean cuts such as tenderloin or loin.
Turkey breast (75g boneless, skinless white meat)	22	With only 125 calories, one serving offers more than 50% of your daily niacin and B6 intake.
Salmon (75g)	22	Choose canned for additional calcium. Any variety will give you a healthy dose of vitamin B12.
Tofu, firm (125g)	20	A vegetarian- and vegan-approved source of complete protein. A serving of firm tofu set with calcium contains nearly 100% of your daily calcium needs and can help lower cholesterol.
Lentils (200g)	18	High in iron, which is vital for transporting oxygen to muscles and organs. Lentils also offer 16g fibre per 200g serving.
Greek yogurt (150ml)	12–17	This style of yogurt packs more protein, calcium and vitamin D than traditional yogurts. Aim for low-fat or fat-free varieties.
Chickpeas (150g)	12–15	Chickpeas are a good source of the mineral manganese, which promotes bone health and also helps regulate blood sugar.
Kidney beans (170g)	13	Rich in iron, kidney beans are also a useful source of fibre, providing 11g per cup.
Black beans (180g)	15	Black beans provide fibre and folate, a B vitamin that plays a key role in heart health and circulation.
Quinoa (180g cooked)	8	One of the few vegetarian-friendly foods that provide all the essential amino acids – the building blocks for your body to make more proteins and build muscle. Quinoa also contains fibre and complex carbohydrates.

FOOD	PROTEIN CONTENT (G)	EXTRA NUTRIENTS FOR RUNNERS
Milk (250ml)	8	Contains calcium to build bone health. It's also one of the few dietary sources of vitamin D. To avoid extra calories and saturated fat, opt for skimmed (aim for 1% or less) varieties.
Almonds (35g)	8	They provide vitamin E, an antioxidant that boosts circulation; many runners fall short on this because there are so few good food sources. Almonds also contain heart-healthy monounsaturated fatty acids. Studies have shown that eating nuts several times per week lowers levels of LDL ('bad') cholesterol.
Pistachios (25g or 49 kernels)	6	Like almonds, pistachios contain vitamin E and heart-healthy fats. They also provide 3g fibre per serving. Another benefit of eating pistachios from the shell is that you have to work to eat them, and the shells left behind provide a reminder of how much you've consumed, so you won't get carried away with snacking.
Egg, whole (1 large)	6	Eggs are rich in protein and choline – a nutrient that's vital for brain health. Choose omega-3-enhanced eggs to increase your intake of healthy fats. And don't lose sleep over the cholesterol found in whole eggs; experts now say we should worry less about cholesterol from foods and more about saturated fat (eggs contain only 1.5g of this).
Egg, white (1 large)	3.6	For runners looking to shed lbs but still boost protein intake, 1 egg white offers a lot of protein for very few calories.

Vegetarians

Switching to a plant-based diet can improve your health and won't take anything away from your running. Because vegetarians aren't eating meat – which can be high in saturated fat and cholesterol – and are eating fruits, veggies and beans, which are usually higher in fibre, minerals and nutrients, they tend to have lower risks of heart disease, high blood pressure, type 2 diabetes, and cancer. If you're a vegetarian, you don't necessarily need more protein than meat-eating runners. But you do need to be diligent about meeting your needs. Certain nutrients are harder to get, including omega-3 fatty acids, vitamin B12, zinc and iron.

You can get the protein you need from a variety of soy products, as well as beans, nuts and whole grains. If you consume a diet that's rich in these items and other fortified foods, you'll be more likely to meet your needs for optimal health as well as performance.

Almonds are a good source of vitamin E

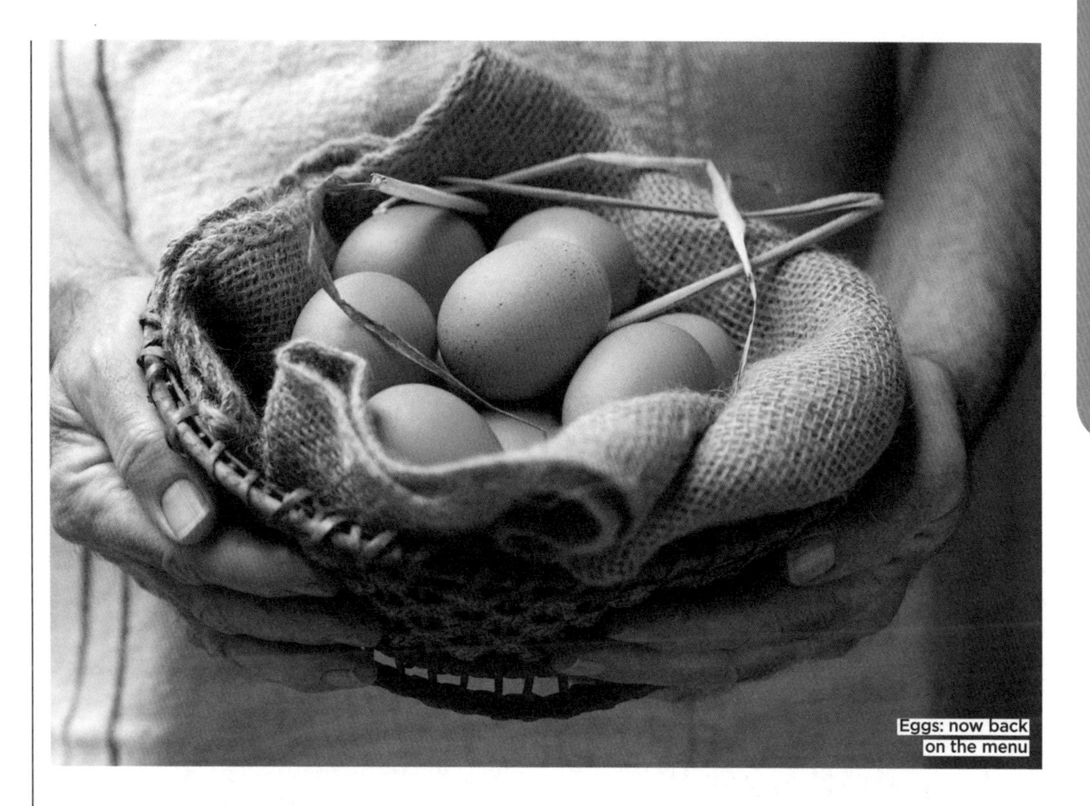

Eggs: now back on the menu

Where to get it

To boost your protein without upping your fat intake, increase the amount of lean proteins you already enjoy. Choose lean minced beef (90% lean or higher); substitute beans for potatoes as a side dish, or use plain, fat-free yogurt as a condiment. And incorporate some protein into breakfast, too. When making pancakes or muffins, substitute a scoop of protein powder for a scoop of flour, or substitute egg whites for whole eggs to double the protein (4 whites equals 2 whole eggs). And replace your regular yogurt with Greek yogurt, which provides up to four times as much protein as standard varieties.

Protein will help repair torn muscle tissue and keep you feeling fuller for longer. For the best sources of lean protein, and the extra benefits they provide for runners, see the chart on the preceding pages.[4]

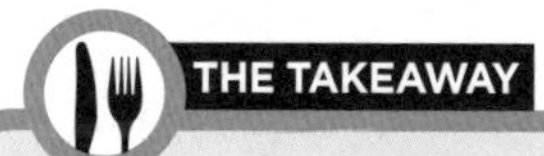

THE TAKEAWAY

Figure out how much you need.
Aim to consume around 0.55-0.9g protein per lb of body weight each day.

Spread your protein intake throughout the day.
Protein helps your belly feel full, so make sure it's a part of each meal and snack to stave off bouts of hunger and cravings.

Focus on natural forms of protein.
Avoid products with added protein that are high in other ingredients you don't need (eg, sugar, saturated fat). A good source of protein will have 5-9.5g per serving. A food that is high in protein will have at least 10g per serving.

8.

WHAT TO DRINK

If you want to unleash your potential on the road *and* reach your weight-loss goals, proper hydration is essential. But that doesn't mean you have to start buying water bottles in bulk. Nor does it mean you lugging around a two-litre container and force-hydrating yourself. As with food, proper hydration involves getting the right amounts of fluids at the right time.

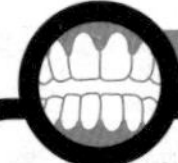

CHEW ON THIS

If you're looking to replace the electrolytes you lose through sweat, choose a calorie-free sports drink, or one with less than 50 calories in a 500ml serving.

Why it matters

Water supports all the major body processes, from regulating temperature to flushing waste products out of your system. All the organs and cells in the body need water to properly function. Studies have shown that you can't hit the same paces – and, by extension, incinerate the maximum number of calories – when you're dehydrated.[1] And because the sweating you do through your regular workouts depletes the water in your system, you need to replenish your stores by making an effort to hydrate throughout the day, particularly around your workouts. If you start the next workout dehydrated, it'll be slower and feel harder than it needs to be.

Water also has an impact on weight loss. Often the fatigue and drain that feel like hunger are actually being caused by thirst. So in a fit of thirst, you may be consuming unneeded calories when what you really need is a drink. What's more, when you're dehydrated, you retain water. This is because your body is working to protect you; when it senses it's not getting the fluids it needs to function properly, an antidiuretic hormone is released, which spurs the kidneys (the body's filtering system) to conserve water.[2]

The result? Dehydration could drive up the numbers on the scales – and drive you crazy – unnecessarily. Plus, because water helps you feel fuller, you'll be less likely to overconsume empty calories that pack on the pounds.

How much do you need to drink?

No blanket formula applies for all people all the time. In recent years, hydration experts have concluded that during exercise and the activities of everyday life, simply drinking when you're thirsty will help you stay adequately hydrated.[3] That said, many people want more concrete directions than simply 'drinking to thirst'. And because so many people try to satisfy thirst with food instead of water, many nutritionists recommend you drink half the number in ounces of your body weight in lbs each day. So if you weigh 160lbs (11st 6lb), aim for 80 fl oz (2.3ltr) per day. Drink more when it's hotter or if, when you're done with a run, you have salt streaks on your skin.

Staying hydrated throughout the day is the best way to avoid a last-minute need to quaff fluids before a workout, a sloshy or nauseous feeling while you're on the road, and unwanted pit stops on your run. So sip regular small amounts of water or calorie-free drinks.

If you're well hydrated, your urine will be the colour of pale lemonade or straw. If it's clear, you're drinking too much; if it's the colour of apple juice, drink more.

Want a formula for staying hydrated on the run? Do the sweat test: weigh yourself naked before heading out, and again when you return. Note how much fluid you consume during the run and add it to the amount of weight you lose. For every pound of body weight you lose, aim to drink an additional 500ml fluid. Perform the sweat test in different weather conditions, as you'll lose – and need to replenish – a lot more fluid after a hot and humid run than after a perfect, 13°C day. Record the results and refer to them before you head out on runs.

What drinks hydrate you best?

Boring as this may sound, water is the best source of hydration for most circumstances. If you're not keen, any calorie-free variety of flavoured water or soda water is an acceptable alternative. Or you can flavour your own with a slice of lemon, orange, cucumber or mint.

Store shelves are filled with sports drinks that promise to help you go longer, get stronger, run faster and recover better. Many of them are loaded with calories, sugar and artificial additives that won't benefit your running and can drag down your weight-loss

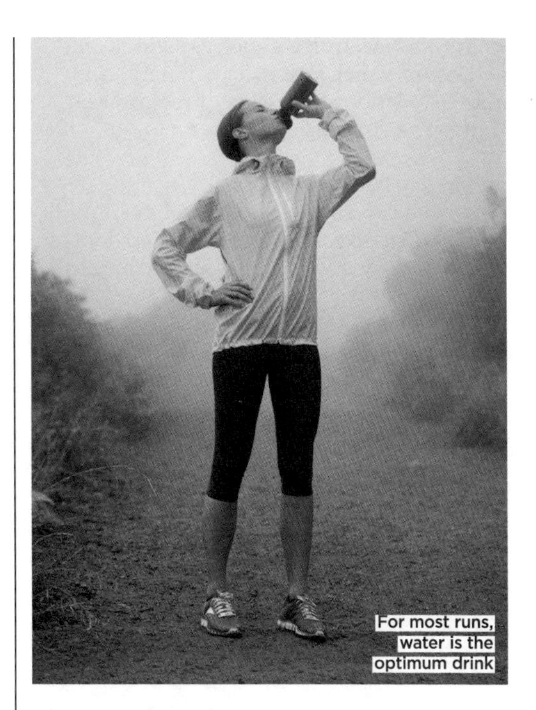

For most runs, water is the optimum drink

progress. Whether you need a sports drink is going to depend on heat and humidity, and the length and intensity of your workout.

Many people start hitting the fluorescent-coloured sports drinks as soon as they begin exercising on a regular basis, because they associate them with being a serious athlete. But the reality is that most of the time, you just don't need them. It's just way too easy to swallow a meal's worth of calories in just a few swigs, and they don't come with the satisfaction and nutrition of a real meal. You certainly don't need a sports drink to hydrate you when you spend eight hours at the office, and unless you're running in the Sahara or an extremely humid environment, you also don't need it after that easy 5K.

When mere water isn't enough

There are some cases where you need the nutrients that sports drinks provide: carbs for

comments/dehydrationandaging.pdf?sfvrsn=6. 3. *Clinical Journal of Sports Medicine*

energy and electrolytes such as sodium and potassium, which are critical for nerve and muscle function and are lost through sweat. Here's when to consider using one:

It's hot and humid outside
When you sweat, you lose electrolytes. Sports drinks will help you restore them and hold on to fluids, so you can keep running strong.

You're running for more than an hour
On any run of an hour or more, you need to refuel on the road with 30-60g carbs per hour. If eating on the road gives you GI distress, sports drinks can offer an easy alternative.

You're a salty sweater
If there are white streaks on your skin post-run, it means you've lost quite a bit of salt through sweating. You've probably also lost other electrolytes such as potassium, magnesium and even calcium. Sports drinks can help you replenish these electrolytes.

You're doing two runs close together
If you're doing two workouts a day, or running in the afternoon and again the next morning, rehydration is critical to helping you through the next workout. Complete rehydration involves replacement of both fluid and electrolyte losses. After your run, drink 700ml fluid for every lb of weight lost during activity. Water will suffice if you're also eating salty, solid foods. A protein shake with electrolytes will also offer protein, carbs and fluids for rehydration and recovery. If you can only tolerate fluids and don't have time to digest a protein shake before your next workout, rehydrate by grabbing a sports drink.

Best sources of electrolytes

If you want to replenish your electrolytes without the added calories, your best bet is to reach for a low-sugar and low-calorie electrolyte formula. Examine the nutrition label and steer clear of drinks with extra calories, sugars and artificial sweeteners; look for electrolyte drinks with fewer than 50 calories per serving. If you want a zero-calorie formula, there are many sugar-free drinks, as well as low-calorie electrolyte tablets, which dissolve quickly in water.

When you've finished a run and are looking for a quick, easy-to-digest drink that will rehydrate you and help your muscles recover, a protein shake can be a great choice. You can make your own, blending some fruit and vegetables (spinach or kale leaves are good choices) with a protein powder and 250-500ml water or milk, plus ice. This combination has water and electrolytes to rehydrate you, and protein and carbs to help you recover. If you don't have immediate access to a blender, ready-to-drink protein shakes are the next best choice. (For more, see Chapter 20 on post-run eating.) If you're a salty sweater, add high-sodium veg such as celery to your shake, or try vegetable juice, which is a good source of sodium.

> After a run, a protein shake can be a great choice

Benefits of caffeine

One of the most persistent myths is that caffeine causes dehydration. But unless you're consuming large quantities, it's OK to drink coffee or caffeinated tea before a workout. (Large quantities – 2.7mg caffeine per lb of body weight per day, or 400mg per day for a 10st 10lbs person – can lead to unwanted side effects for some people. A 250ml cup of coffee has about 85mg caffeine; a 330ml can of cola typically contains 30-40mg caffeine, while an ordinary cup of tea has about 40mg.)

A 2014 study published in *PLOS ONE* concluded that coffee can hydrate you just as well as water.[4] The study didn't involve runners, but the American College of Sports Medicine says that while caffeine can have a modest diuretic effect in some people, for most

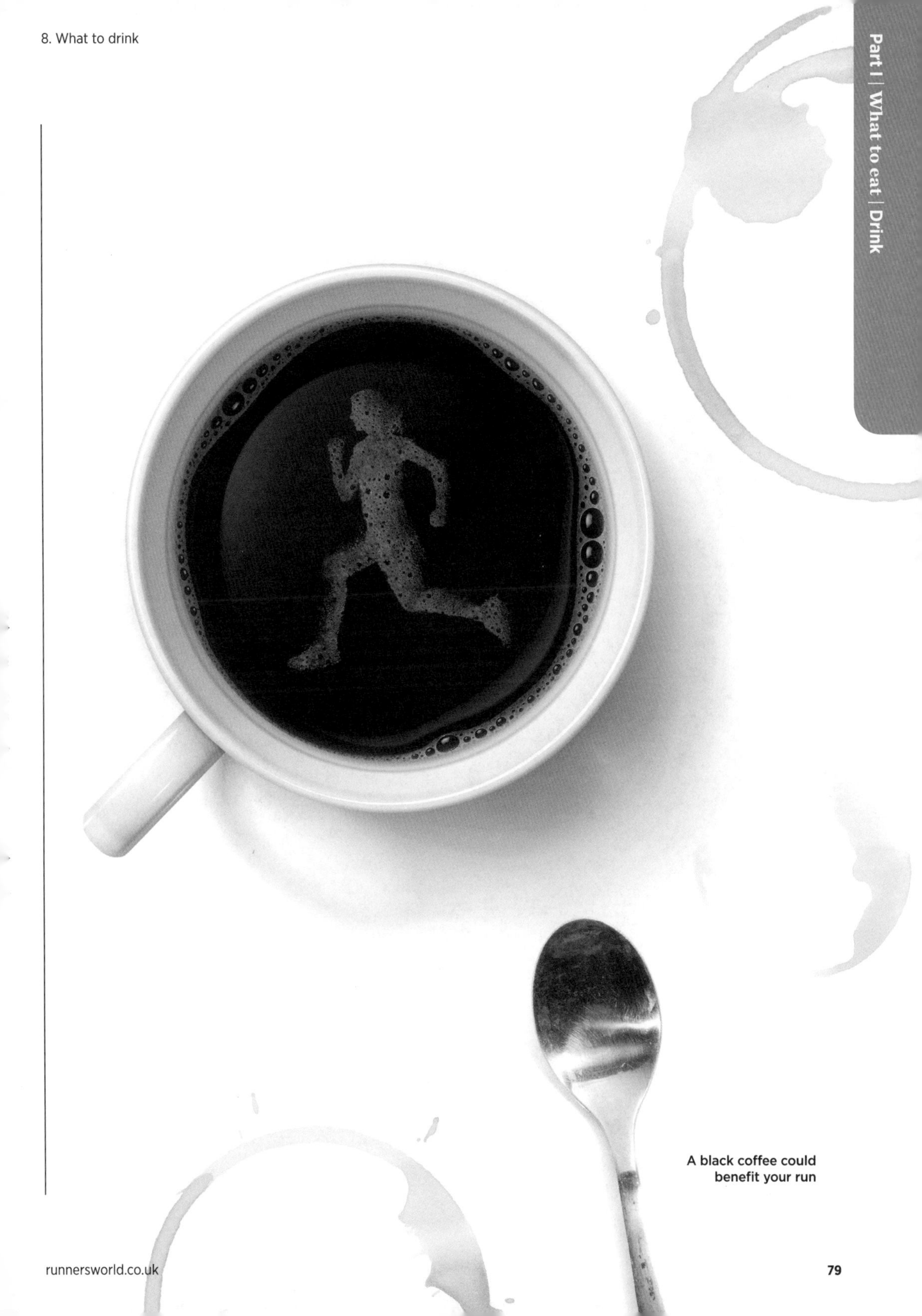

A black coffee could benefit your run

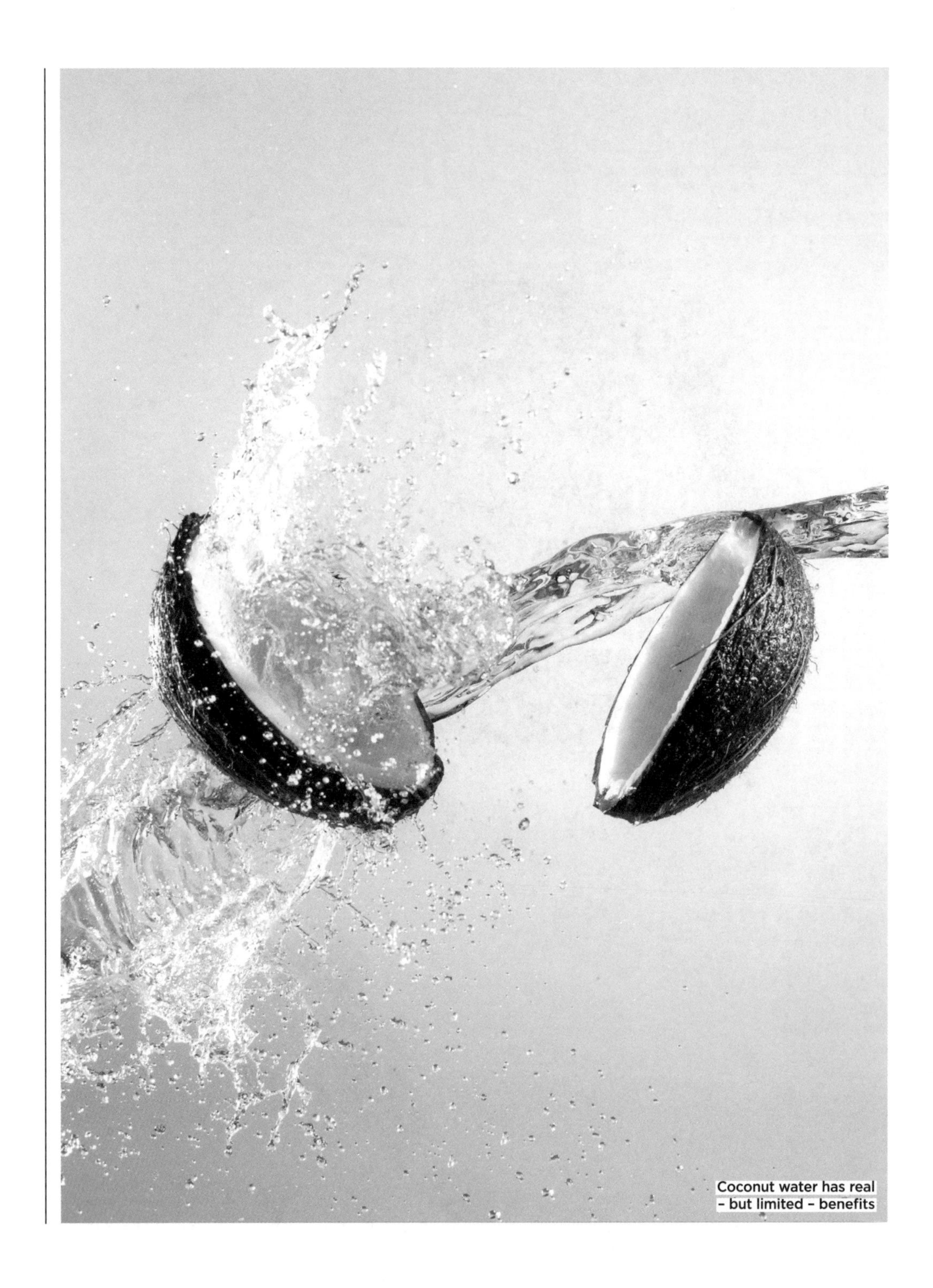

Coconut water has real – but limited – benefits

people who drink it regularly, it's fine.[5] Other studies have shown caffeine boosts performance; staves off depression;[6] may reduce risk of heart disease[7] and type 2 diabetes,[8] and lessens pain during exercise.[9]

Just steer clear of certain speciality coffee drinks, or treat them as 'sometimes treats'. That large white chocolate mocha has more than 400 calories – a meal's worth of calories for some – without providing the nutrition or satisfaction of a meal.

And be sure to leave enough time between your java and your run to hit the bathroom. Hot fluids stimulate the bowels (clearing out the system is part of why so many runners rely on pre-run coffee), and you don't want to have to make an unwanted stop on the run.

Coconut water

Coconut water has become the thirst quencher *du jour*. It's now a permanent fixture in supermarket fridges and health-food shops, alongside traditional sports drinks.

But a closer look at the product offers an enduring lesson in how certain foods and drinks acquire a 'health halo', where certain nutrition information is swept up in marketing hysteria. It also reminds us why we should look beyond the claims on food labels before we make any 'healthy' processed food part of our regular diet.

Coconut water does offer some benefits. It's a natural way to replenish certain electrolytes after hard workouts. Unsweetened varieties are free of the sugar, artificial sweeteners and dyes contained in many conventional sports drinks. And it's high in potassium and magnesium, two nutrients the body needs for general health and good performance. Coconut water contains approximately (depending on brand) 600mg potassium per 250ml serving, getting you one step closer to the daily reference intake (RI) of 3,500mg, which few of us meet.

Coconut water also provides a handful of other electrolytes, such as calcium and magnesium. With 60mg magnesium, a 250ml serving will give you approximately 20% of your daily needs. However, compared with conventional sports drinks, coconut water is way too low in two key things your system needs after a tough workout: sodium, the main electrolyte you lose through sweat, and carbohydrates, which help restock the body's spent energy stores. So if you're looking for electrolytes to rehydrate during or after a long run, a speed session or a tough workout in hot weather, a traditional sports drink is still going to be the best bet to rehydrate and replenish your energy.

While coconut water will replace the small amount of potassium you lose during a workout, it won't replace your sodium losses. But if you're not in the middle of a taxing workout and are simply looking to cut calories and keep your fluids au naturel, coconut water can be a fine choice. Just be sure to choose unsweetened varieties. For more on how to look beyond food labels, go to Chapter 12.

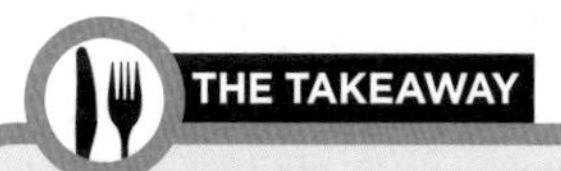

Drink water.
Sip calorie-free fluids throughout the day. Aim for half the number (in ounces) of your body weight (in pounds). So if you weigh 120lb (8st 8lb), aim for 60oz (1.7ltr) a day; if you weigh 180lbs (12st 12lb), aim for 90oz (2.5ltr).

Watch the colour.
To determine your hydration levels, do the pee test. If you're well hydrated, your urine will be pale yellow or the colour of straw. If you're dehydrated, it'll be the colour of apple juice. If you're overdoing the fluids, it will be clear.

Reserve sports drinks for special occasions.
You only need them for workouts in hot and humid conditions, in which you're losing lots of fluids through sweat or could use the energy boost from carbs that sports drinks contain. Those occasions include speed sessions, runs in hot weather or runs that last more than an hour. When you're having a sports drink, opt for a low-calorie formula with the least amounts of sugar, artificial sweeteners, flavours and colours, and fewer than 50 calories per serving.

8. *Diabetologia*. 9. *International Journal of Sport Nutrition and Exercise Metabolism*

9.

ALCOHOL

You've probably heard the maxim, 'Don't drink your calories.' But if you're like most runners, you probably also enjoy the reward of a post-run beer or glass of wine. And, in fact, it's widely believed that moderate consumption of alcohol *can* fit into a healthy-eating and training regime if you get the timing – and the amount – right.

That said, recent guidelines from the UK chief medical officers have cut the recommended level of alcohol consumption for men from 21 to 14 units a week (for women it's still 14), ideally spread over three or more days. (A unit equates to a measure of spirits, a third of a pint of beer (5-6%ABV) and ½ x 175ml glass of wine.) Their advice is now that there is no 'safe' level of alcohol, due to a review linking it with increased risk of cancer. Also, a Canadian study[1] has cast doubt on earlier research linking moderate drinking with health benefits – including the theory that a glass of red wine can cut the risk of heart disease.

The UK does now have one of the lowest recommended levels of alcohol intake (in Spain the limit for men is 35 units per week; for women it's 21), although it's unlikely that many people will be persuaded to give up as a result. Besides which, there is still evidence that sensible consumption of alcohol can be compatible with both your running life and your weight-loss goals.

So our advice is to read on, decide what's right for you and don't beat yourself up over the odd glass of Pinot...

Can alcohol be 'healthy'?

A variety of health benefits have been linked to moderate consumption of alcohol, including a lower incidence of gallstones, decreased risk of type 2 diabetes, greater bone-mineral density, and improved cognitive function in older adults. *Moderate* consumption of alcohol has also been shown to lower levels 'bad' LDL cholesterol and increase 'good' HDL cholesterol.

Beer has been associated with a lowered risk of kidney stones in men. It's also a source of multiple B vitamins, such as folate, niacin, riboflavin, vitamin B6 and pantothenic acid, which help keep the body functioning as a well-oiled machine. In general, the more malt in the brew, the higher the level of B vitamins.

As for red wine, the news is less positive. It's long been believed that the resveratrol it contains gives it anti-inflammatory properties that could reduce the risk of heart disease and even cancer. But a study published in *JAMA Internal Medicine* in 2014 showed resveratrol may not be the miracle cure it was touted as.[2] Red wine does have catechins, though, which could help improve HDL cholesterol.

What alcohol means to your waistline

If you're watching your weight, it's best to stick with beer or wine, as the calorie counts in mixed drinks and cocktails can be sky-high. Treat alcohol like you would a dessert – as a "sometimes treat," advises dietitian Karen Ansel, author of *The Calendar Diet*. If you can

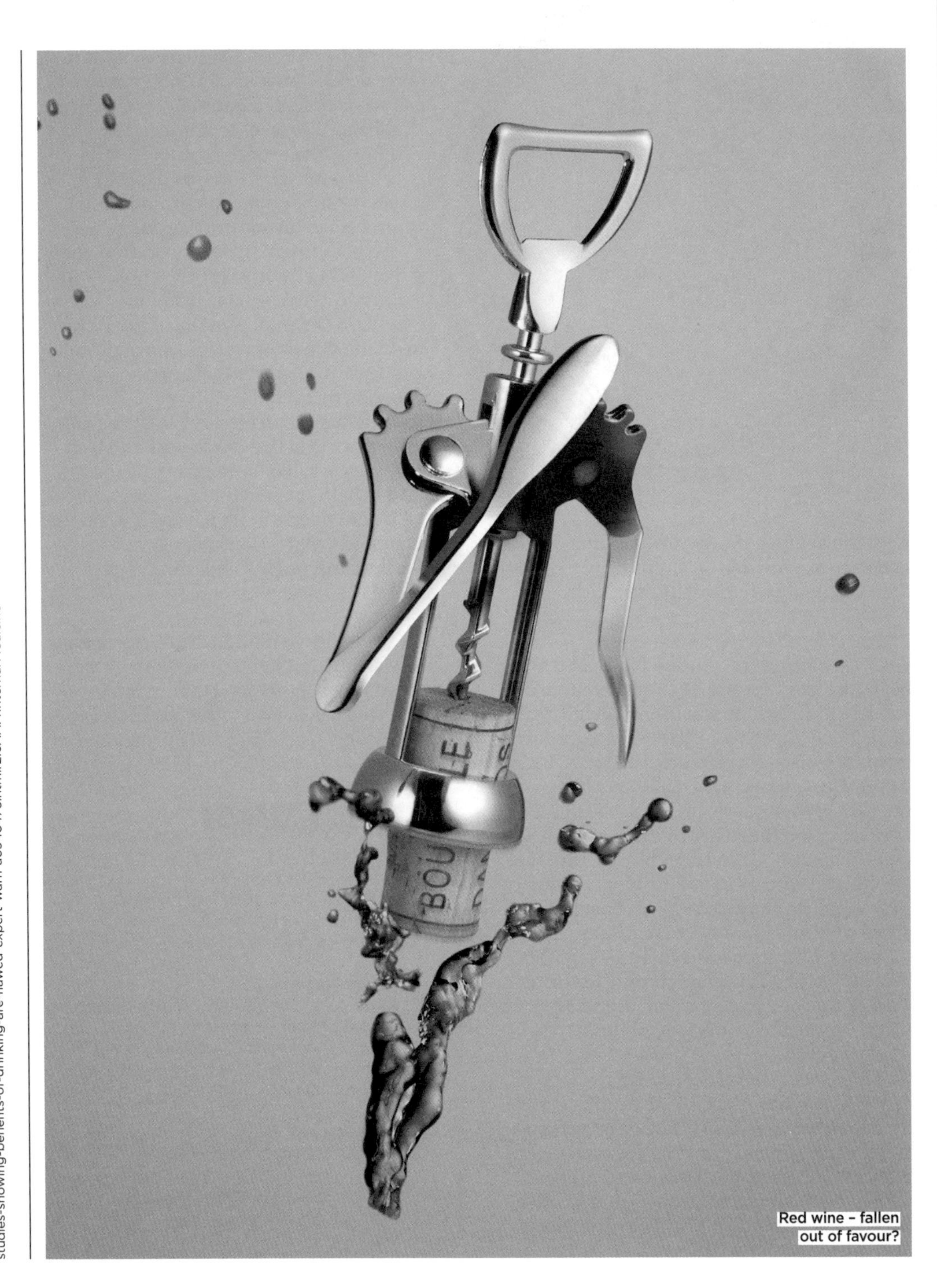

Red wine – fallen out of favour?

Photography: Hearst Studios. **Sources:** 1. independent.co.uk/life-style/health-and-families/health-news/alcohol-studies-showing-benefits-of-drinking-are-flawed-expert-warn-a6945476.html. 2. *JAMA Internal Medicine*

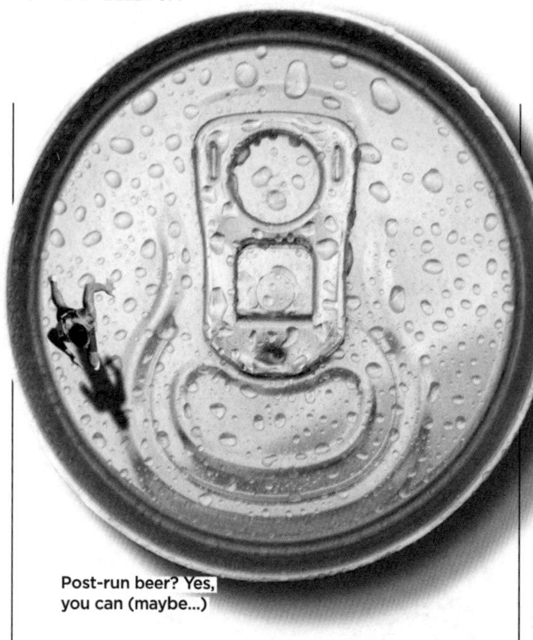

Post-run beer? Yes, you can (maybe...)

limit the number of days you have that drink – and keep to one drink on any day – you can cut down without feeling totally deprived.

Another thing to note

Once alcohol lowers your inhibitions, you may be more likely to reach for the nachos and dip and less likely to stop when you feel full. "All of a sudden that extra pizza slice or handful of crisps doesn't seem like such a bad idea," says Ansel. This is especially true if you've been restricting your calories at regular meals. To avoid going off the rails, avoid drinking on an empty stomach. "If you sip while you eat, the alcohol will enter your system more gradually, so you'll make more clear-headed decisions about what and how much to eat," she says.

Delay dehydration by having a glass of water before your first drink and chasing the drink with at least one glass of water afterward. That will also promote a feeling of fullness.

How alcohol affects your training

Downing a few beers as you're heading out the door for a run is obviously not a wise move. While some runners swear by a few beers the night before a race, the American College of Sports Medicine (ACSM) warns that alcohol affects aerobic power and impairs the body's ability to regulate its temperature, particularly in cold weather. The ACSM advises runners to skip alcohol for at least 48 hours before a marathon or half marathon.

Alcohol also leads to dehydration, reduces uptake of glucose and amino acids by muscles, inhibits the body's energy supply and impairs metabolic processes during exercise. But when it comes to post-race rehydration, the benefits or otherwise of alcohol are still open to question. One study, published in *PLOS ONE*, showed that it interferes with the signals that would normally tell your body to adapt and get stronger, thus hampering recovery.[4]

However, Australian research by Dr Ben Desbrow has found that a cold post-run beer (with a pinch of salt or accompanying salty snack) will help you rehydrate, as long as it's 3.5% ABV or under. But try pairing it with water and/or a sports drink, along with a recovery meal of protein and carbs.

Bottom line

It's OK to indulge in the odd drink. If you want to lose weight, limit it to a 'sometimes treat', as you would any other food that adds 'empty' calories. And if you want to get faster, steer clear of alcohol just before and during runs.

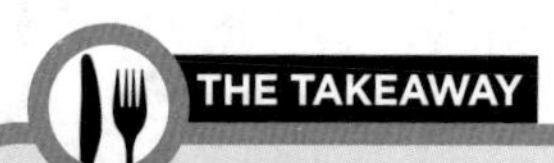

Remember moderation.
Stick with the official guidelines and limit your intake to 14 units a week – spreading that out over three or more days.

Get the timing right.
Drinking alcohol immediately before a run or race can hamper your performance, and it could lead to injury. But moderate alcohol consumption at other times of day won't hurt and can arguably offer some health benefits.

Wash it down with water.
Drinking water before and after you have alcohol can promote a feeling of fullness and help prevent the dehydration that alcohol consumption can cause.

10.

SPORTS FOODS

Engineered bars, sports drinks and energy gels are convenient, tasty ways to help you power through a workout or recover afterwards. But with so many on the market – some with nutrient profiles that rival chocolate bars – how do you find products that are compatible with your weight-loss goals?

Many novice runners are tempted to overdo the sports foods. And just like any other excess calories, they can negatively affect both your waistline and your race times. After all, an energy bar that packs 250 calories, 43g carbs, 21g sugar and 10g protein, is designed to get you through a three-hour distance run without hitting the wall. Grabbing one to get through a gentle 5K is definitely overkill.

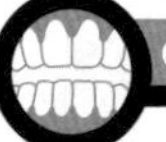

CHEW ON THIS

Sports bars, gels and drinks can have a place in your diet, even if you're watching your weight. As with so many foods, it's a matter of choosing a product that meets your needs for a particular workout without providing calories and additives you don't need.

Smart choices

If you're going to incorporate engineered foods into your diet, become a label detective. Make sure you know you're getting the amount of calories, fat, carbs, fibre and sugar you need for a specific workout. You'll also probably need to try a few products to discover what gives you a boost without upsetting your stomach. Here's what to look for in different situations.

Pre-run snack

Choose products high in the muscle-fuelling carbs you need to energise your workout but low in the fat and fibre that could lead to GI distress on the road. For an easy run of a hour or less, limit it to 200 calories or fewer, with less than 10g fat, 10g protein and 7g fibre.

Mid-run refuelling

Choose products high in the carbs you need to sustain energy over a long period and, again, low in fat and fibre that could upset your stomach. If you'll be running for one to three hours, aim for a product that provides 30-60g carbs for every hour you're on the road.

Post-run refuelling

In the 30-60 minutes after a long run or a tough speed session, your body is extra-primed to absorb carbs and protein to rebuild muscle tissue so you can bounce back strong. A sports bar with a 2:1 ratio of carbs to protein will help you do just that. For more, see Chapter 20.

Meal replacement

At mealtimes it's best to have, well, a meal. But if you're in a rush and need something quick to keep your appetite at bay, it's OK to reach for a

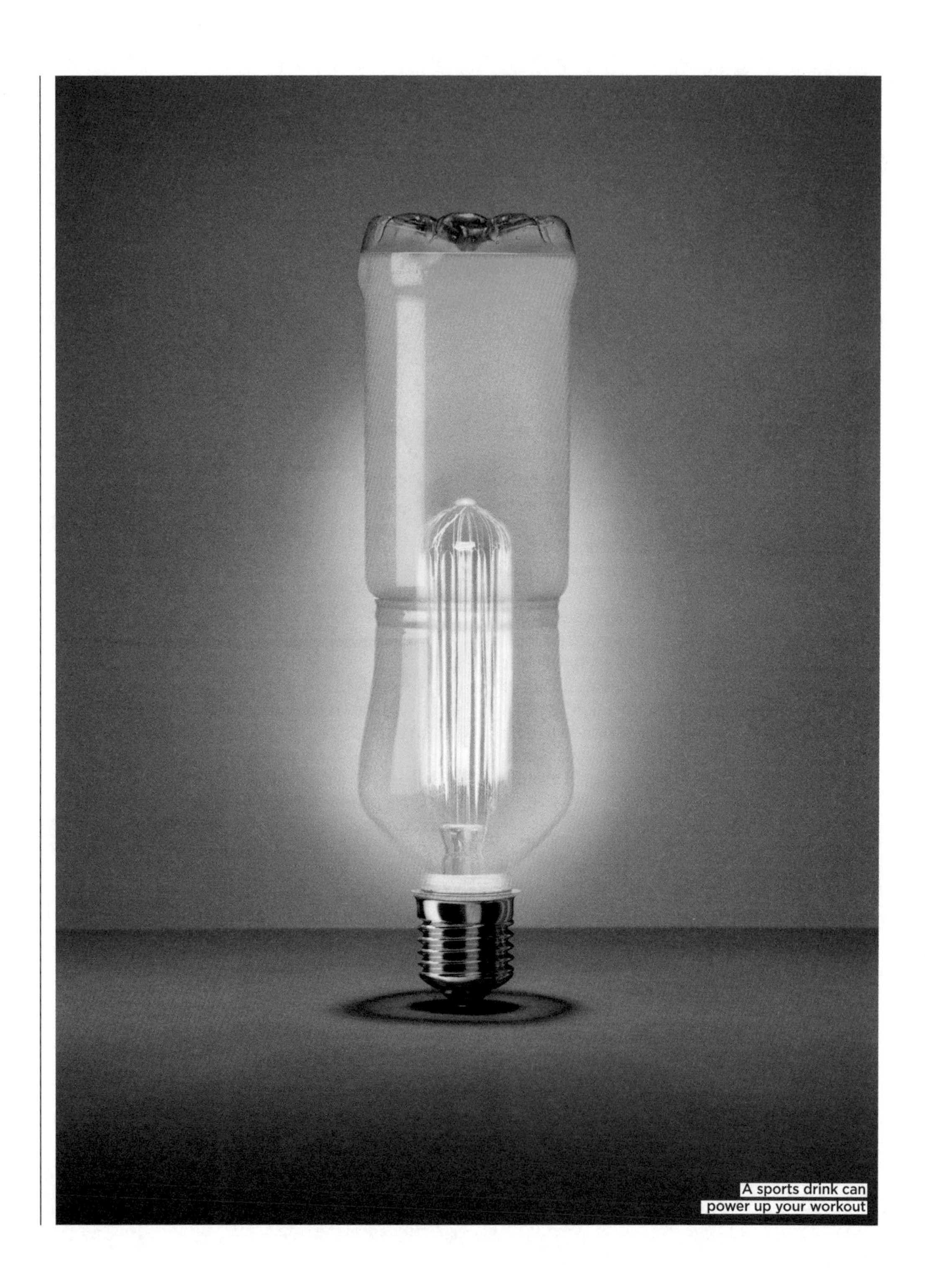

A sports drink can power up your workout

sports bar. Just make sure it doesn't contain more calories than you'd have in a regular meal. Check the serving size, and go for one with a balance of carbs, protein, fat and fibre; at least 10g protein and 5+g fibre is ideal, as that's what you'd get from whole foods.

Strength-training session

A strength-based workout requires fuelling up beforehand so you feel energised and strong; otherwise you might be tempted to skip reps or use momentum instead of muscle to go through the motions. While some strength athletes consume protein during workouts, it's unnecessary for most runners if you simply want to get stronger, tone up, trim your waistline and prevent injuries. During your workout, sip water to prevent dehydration. If you do start feeling dehydrated and develop muscle cramps, add a low-calorie or calorie-free electrolyte drink. Just like you would after a tough run, once you've finished your strength session, have a recovery meal or shake within 30-60 minutes of completing the workout. Aim for an intake of 15-25g protein with two to four times as much carbohydrate.

Even when you're looking for a convenient pre-run or pre-workout snack, good, portable whole-food options such as apples, oranges or bananas will give you the vitamins and minerals you need, along with your energy boost – and no worrying about additives you don't need or that might upset your stomach. Discover more pre-run snacks on page 127.

Read the ingredients

Baffled by the content of many sports foods? Here's a guide, compiled by *Runner's World* contributor Kelly Bastone.[1]

Maltodextrin

This processed carb is more quickly absorbed than other carbs, so it delivers a fast hit of fuel. Easier on the stomach than the concentrated glucose found in some sports drinks, it's also relatively tasteless, so a useful choice if overly sweet gels and chews don't sit well with you.

Protein (whey and soy) isolates

Whey and soy proteins are first extracted from a food and then added to bars to boost protein content. Hydrolysed proteins undergo further processing that removes vitamins but makes the protein more digestible.

Glucose syrup

AKA corn syrup, used because it bonds easily with dry or solid ingredients. Its short, simple sugar chains are rapidly absorbed, so it offers instant fuel that's ideal for pre-run energy.

Sugar alcohols

Eg, sorbitol, xylitol, maltitol, mannitol and isomalt, these are reduced-calorie sweeteners often found in sugar-free and no-sugar-added products, and have less of an effect on blood glucose (blood sugar) than other carbs. Treat with care, though: sugar alcohols can lead to GI distress, and can have a laxative effect.[2]

Brown rice syrup

This sweetener is a bit higher in nutrients and is slower-burning than corn syrup. But organic versions can contain traces of arsenic, which is naturally present in the water, air and soil. Its health threats haven't been confirmed, but some companies might stop using it.

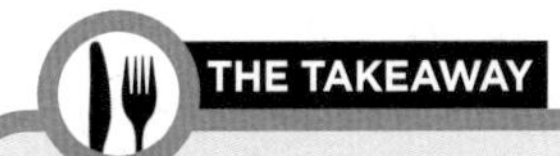

Shop around.
Try different brands and flavours to find out which products give you a boost without upsetting your stomach.

Use 'em, don't abuse 'em.
Think about when you eat engineered sports foods. Are you using them to fuel your workouts and recover afterwards? Or are you using them as snacks and pick-me-ups when you don't really need them?

Find whole-food alternatives.
By sticking with wholesome sources of energy, you get more of the vitamins and minerals you do need and less of the additives and calories you don't.

11.

ARTIFICIAL SWEETENERS

For anyone watching their weight, diet soft drinks, low-calorie foods and sugar-free treats seem like gifts from the gods. They give you the green light to enjoy your favourite sweets without getting weighed down by the guilt or the calories associated with their regular counterparts.

Or do they? While zero-calorie versions of foods can make it easier to meet daily calorie goals, new doubts have emerged about whether, over the long term, such products really will help weight-loss efforts.

Safety concerns

But the first point to establish is that, after decades of research, health authorities in the UK and the US have deemed that all the popular sweeteners on the market – from saccharin to aspartame — are safe. Studies in the early 1970s linked saccharin to bladder cancer in lab animals, but since then numerous further studies have disproved any link.[1]

Can they really aid weight loss?

So artificial sweeteners won't kill you and they can help you meet your daily calorie targets. But are they the best bet for long-term weight loss? Well, sugar-free doesn't always mean healthy, points out dietitian Jenna Bell, director of food and wellness at New York-based consulting firm Pollock Communications. If you're limiting your calorie intake but really, really want a biscuit or some hot chocolate, the sugar-free version *is* going to save you calories, but it isn't necessarily good for you. Sugar-free baked goods, ice-cream treats and sweets seldom offer any nutritional benefits, and they still have calories. So if you go overboard, you're going to see the effects on the scales.

And there's plenty of evidence that consumers *do* tend to go overboard when eating diet foods. A study published in the *Journal of Marketing Research* in 2006 found that people ate up to 50% more of products that were deemed 'low-fat'.[2]

Diet drinks

Health authorities such as the US Academy of Nutrition and Dietetics have concluded that diet drinks are associated with weight loss and don't affect appetite for food. And certainly, if you want to shed a lot of weight and you drink a lot of fizzy soft drinks, swapping your full-calorie variety for a diet version will have an impact. Consider this: if you drink three regular fizzy drinks per day, you're consuming more than 400 calories, which adds up to

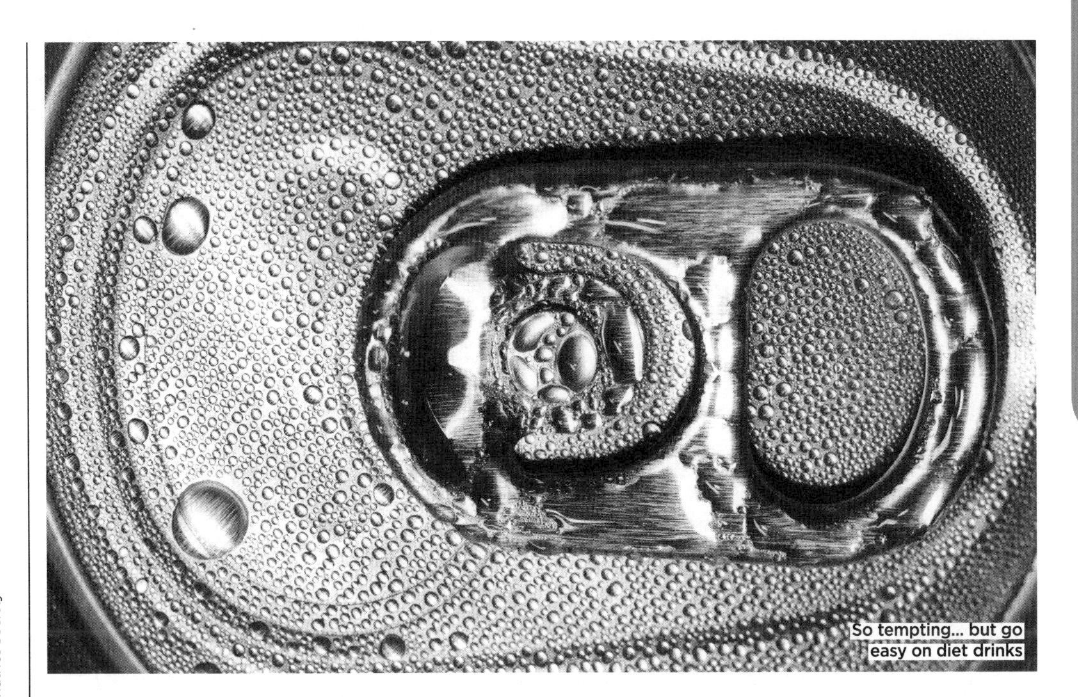

So tempting... but go easy on diet drinks

about 3.5lbs over the course of a month. If you simply switched to diet soft drinks and made no other changes, you'd be likely to lose those 3.5lbs instead of gaining them.

That said, research has emerged in recent years that actually links carbonated diet drinks to higher risks of belly fat, weight gain and chronic diseases.

A study published in the *Yale Journal of Biology and Medicine* in 2010 concluded that, 'Artificial sweeteners, precisely because they are sweet, encourage sugar craving and sugar dependence.'[3] Another study, published in 2015 in the *Journal of the American Geriatric Society,*[4] found that diet fizzy drink users had 70% bigger waist sizes than non-users; those who drank two or more diet fizzy drinks a day over 10 years saw an average increase in waist size five times that of non-users. And we hear plenty of anecdotes from runners who report that giving up diet drinks gave their weight-loss efforts and running a lift.

"I felt sluggish when I would drink fizzy drinks, but I was hooked on them," says Amy White, a runner and mother of two who lost 7st 4lbs. "It wasn't until I stopped drinking them altogether that I felt I could go faster, longer, and harder. I have the occasional fizzy drink, and I always regret it afterwards because I can feel it messing with my body."

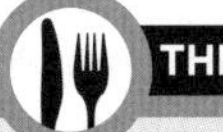

THE TAKEAWAY

Make your calories count.
Foods should provide nutrients that keep your body in its best shape. Before indulging in products sweetened with sugar substitutes, ask how nutritious it is. Low-calorie doesn't always mean 'good for you'.

A 'diet' label isn't a licence to go overboard.
It's easy to overdo it on foods labelled as low in fat. Remember, extra calories are extra calories, even when they're from diet foods.

When in doubt, cut it out.
Wondering if diet foods are stopping you feeling your best? Cut them out for a week. You may be surprised by the difference.

2. *Journal of Marketing Research*. 3. *Yale Journal of Biology and Medicine*. 4. *Journal of the American Geriatrics Society*

12.

DECODING FOOD LABELS

One of the most powerful tools you can use to reach your feel-great weight and your dream time on the finish line is hidden in plain sight: it's on the nutrition label of your favourite packaged foods.

Studies have shown that people who read food labels are more likely to lose weight than those who don't.[1] When we take the time to study the nutrition information, we're often shocked to find out just how many calories a small snack contains, or to realise we're consuming half a day's calories on the way home from work. Evidence suggests that, when left to our own devices, we vastly underestimate calorie counts.[2]

But deciphering those labels – and identifying what foods will help you reach your goals – isn't always easy. From gluten-free to no high fructose corn syrup to non-GM, there's been a barrage of so-called health halos, some of which have no legal definition and many of which can be pretty misleading.

Here are some tips on how to reads labels so you find the products that will help you meet your goals.

Watch your portions

Even if a health claim is legitimate, it's not a licence to go overboard. Excess calories can lead to weight gain even if they come from 'healthy' foods. A study in the *Journal of Marketing Research* found that people who were given a food labelled 'low fat' ate 50% more than those who ate the normal version.[3] And some foods that look like just one serving are actually two – or more. So check the 'serving size' before you eat.

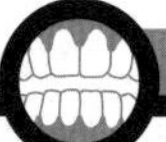

CHEW ON THIS

Don't get derailed by a health halo. While terms such as gluten-free may be important for people with coeliac disease, and non-GM may be important for those worried about genetically modified ingredients, those terms do not necessarily mean the foods are going to help you achieve your weight-loss goals. Read the food label with your personal weight-loss priorities in mind.

Prioritise

What to look for depends a lot on your unique health concerns. If you have high blood pressure, you may want to target products labelled 'salt- or sodium-free', which have less than 0.01g salt per serving.

Don't forget the ingredients

Ingredients are listed in descending order of weight. And don't forget, if you're trying to avoid sugar, it also goes by a lot of other names. If a product says 'no added sugar', it means there is no table sugar or any other sugar-containing ingredient added, but it may include naturally occurring sugars such as fructose or lactose. So while yogurt may have no sugar added, the lactose in the milk

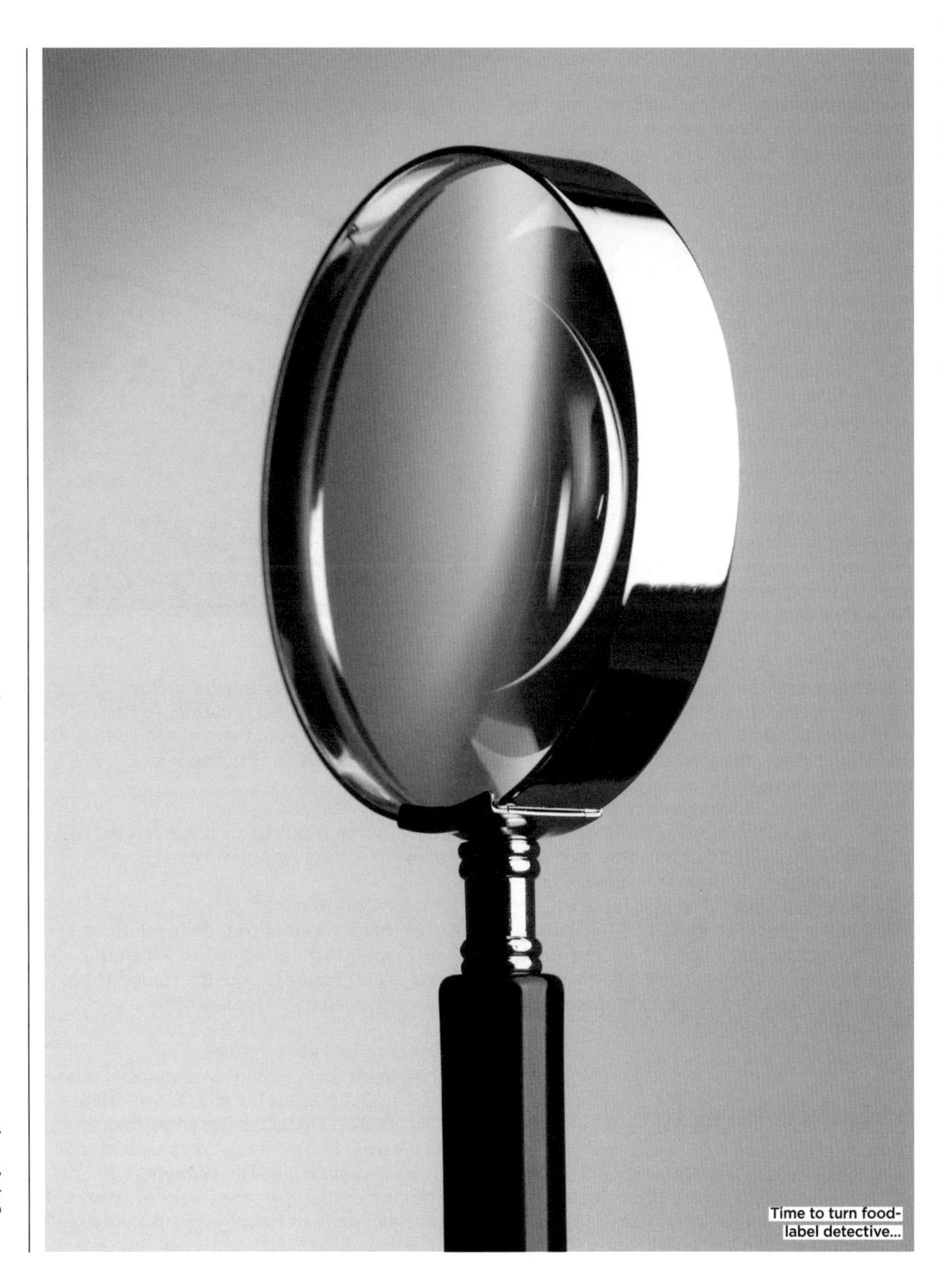

Time to turn food-label detective...

Photography: Getty. Sources: 1. Journal of Consumer Affairs. 2. BMJ. 3. Journal of Marketing Research

naturally provides low amounts of sugar. Foods labelled as being free from high-fructose corn syrup may sound healthier, but they're not if they're higher in other sugars such as evaporated cane juice, agave syrup, brown rice syrup, or even apple or grape juice concentrate.

Gluten-free does not necessarily mean good

The term gluten-free is critical for anyone with coeliac disease – a digestive condition in which gluten damages the small intestine and causes other health problems. But lots of people buy gluten-free foods on the assumption that they're automatically healthier. That's just not necessarily true. Indeed, scores of crisps, biscuits and chocolate bars sport the 'gluten-free' label. And many gluten-free foods have refined carbs and added fats. So check out the other vital stats on the package to make sure the calories, fats, sugars and other ingredients are going to help you achieve your weight-loss goals. (See Chapter 1 for more on carbs.)

Eco-friendly isn't always diet-friendly

The 'organic' label means the food is grown without pesticides, antibiotics or growth hormones. But now that many cakes, biscuits and other not-so-diet-friendly items are organic, you should still closely examine the nutrition info and ingredients. Likewise with foods labelled 'non-GM' (containing no genetically modified organisms); this is meant to distinguish them from foods that have been genetically altered to increase resistance to pests and disease. While labels such as 'organic' and 'non-GM' may be good for the farmer or the environment, if you're concerned about your weight, they're not the most important variable.

What to look for

When you're examining the nutrition panel and ingredients list on your favourite foods, here's your 12-step guide to what you should look for to help you lose weight and get faster.

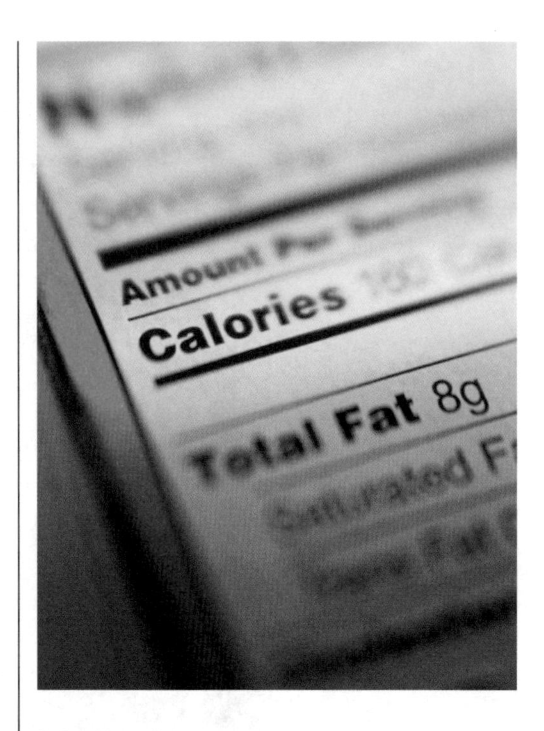

1. Serving size

Many serving sizes are much smaller than people are accustomed to eating. To stay on track, you may want to break out your measuring spoons and kitchen scales.

2. Number of servings

Some foods that look like a single serving are actually two servings or even more.

3. Calories per serving

Assess this in terms of your daily calorie target (see Chapter 16 for more on this.) If your target is 1,600 calories and that smoothie has 600, you'll need to cut back in other places.

4. Saturated fat per serving

Eating foods that contain saturated fats raises the level of cholesterol in your blood. High levels of saturated fat increase your risk of heart disease and stroke, so keep your intake as low as possible. The Department of Health recommends limiting your intake of saturated fat to no more than 11% of your total energy intake from food. So if you aim for 1,600 calories a day, you shouldn't consume more than about 20g saturated fat per day.

5. Trans fats per serving: avoid altogether

Found in processed foods such as biscuits and cakes, and usually listed as hydrogenated or partially hydrogenated vegetable oil, trans fats have virtually no nutritional value. Official advice is that they should make up no more than 2% of your energy intake (about 5g a day).

6. Sugar per serving

Aim as low as possible – no more than 10g sugar per serving. To keep your energy levels stable, try to consume this at even intervals throughout the day. If you're craving an item with more sugar, have it just before a workout, when your body can use it for energy, or within 30 minutes of finishing, when your body needs carbs to restock your glycogen stores so you can bounce back for your next exercise session. (Adding protein to that sugary snack will speed up this process. To read more, turn to Part III on when to eat.) And if you're eating raw fruit or a dairy product, don't stress about sugars.

7. Protein per serving

Aim for as high as possible, while still maintaining your calorie target. Protein helps repair and rebuild torn muscle tissue so you can recover well for your next workout. And it promotes a feeling of fullness, so you won't feel hungry. That's why it's important to spread protein intake throughout the day. Be careful with special 'high-protein' foods: some bars have a meal's worth of protein, but also a meal's worth of calories.

8. Cholesterol

Because cholesterol has been linked to a higher risk of heart disease, keep intake as low as possible. Focus on cutting down saturated and trans fats, as these drive up levels of LDL or 'bad' cholesterol in the blood.

9. Fibre per serving

Like protein, fibre makes you feel full. It also keeps your GI tract healthy and, because it can reduce your cholesterol levels, fibre promotes heart health. The Government recommends aiming for 30g a day. But to avoid GI distress on the run, your pre-workout snack or meal should have less than 7g fibre.

10. Vitamins and minerals

The best foods are nutrient dense, which means that in addition to having a good blend of carbs, fats, and protein, they contain a smattering of the vitamins and minerals you need to stay healthy, such as calcium, vitamin C, iron and B vitamins. Look at the "recommended daily allowance" column to see how high the product is in these essentials.

11. Ingredients list

Remember, ingredients are listed in descending order of weight. If you see sugar in any of its other forms (see Chapter 4 for more details) listed in the first three ingredients, choose another food. But even if it's not in the first three, if you see lots of other forms of sugar throughout the list, it can add up.

12. Salt

Most adults should limit their intake to no more than 6g salt per day (and those at risk of heart disease need even less) – the equivalent of about 1 tsp. Runners can get away with a higher intake of salt (since it's lost through sweat) but you'll still want to watch for it in canned goods, processed foods and sauces. Use fresh options whenever you can.

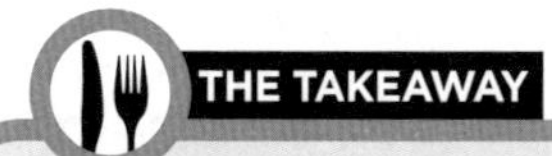

Remember your portions.
Some of the healthiest foods can still derail your diet if you eat too much of them in one sitting. Check serving sizes and make use of your kitchen scales to see what an actual portion looks like on your plate.

Don't get tricked by packaging claims.
Some claims have no legal definition, while others (eg, 'organic' or 'natural') may *sound* healthy, but that doesn't mean the food item is the best choice for you.

13.

VITAMINS AND SUPPLEMENTS

Vitamins and minerals play many important roles in your health: helping your body turn food into energy, keeping bones strong, boosting immunity, and repairing and rebuilding muscle.

And because exercise taxes many of the basic body functions and systems where vitamins and minerals play a key role, health authorities – including the American College of Sports Medicine and the Academy of Nutrition and Dietetics – have concluded that runners may need to make an extra effort to get those nutrients.[1]

It's always best to get vitamins and minerals from foods rather than supplements, as your body absorbs them better. Unless you're eating an unbalanced diet that consists of only one or two food items all the time, you don't run the risk of building up certain nutrients to toxic levels. And if you load up on fresh vitamin- and mineral-rich fruit and veg, you get other important nutrients such as phytochemicals and fibre you miss out on if you just pop pills.

> It's always best to get nutrients from food, not supplements

But when you simply can't consume enough foods to meet your nutrient needs – whether it's because you're cutting back your intake, have food allergies or just don't like certain foods – it's a good idea to take a supplement.

While no vitamin or mineral is magically going to help you lose weight, certain deficiencies can prevent you from meeting your weight-loss and racing goals. If you're not getting enough vitamin D or calcium, for instance, you could put yourself at risk of stress fractures, which can sideline you for months from running. If you're low in B12 or don't absorb it properly, you might feel chronically fatigued and unable to give your all to workouts and burn as many calories.

How do you know if you have a nutrient deficiency? You won't know until you run into a problem (say you start to get injured frequently or feel chronically run-down), see a doctor and get a blood test. So think of taking a multivitamin as having insurance; even if you don't need coverage for all the nutrients and minerals all the time, they'll be in good supply when you do need them.

Many sports foods are fortified with essential nutrients, so if you regularly eat foods such as energy bars or protein shakes, you're probably getting the nutrients you need.

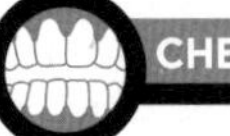

CHEW ON THIS

Because many vitamins can cause GI distress, you might want to take your vitamins before bed, when you have plenty of food in your stomach. If you've been prescribed a supplement by a doctor, find out whether a certain time of day is best to take it and if it should be consumed with food or on an empty stomach.

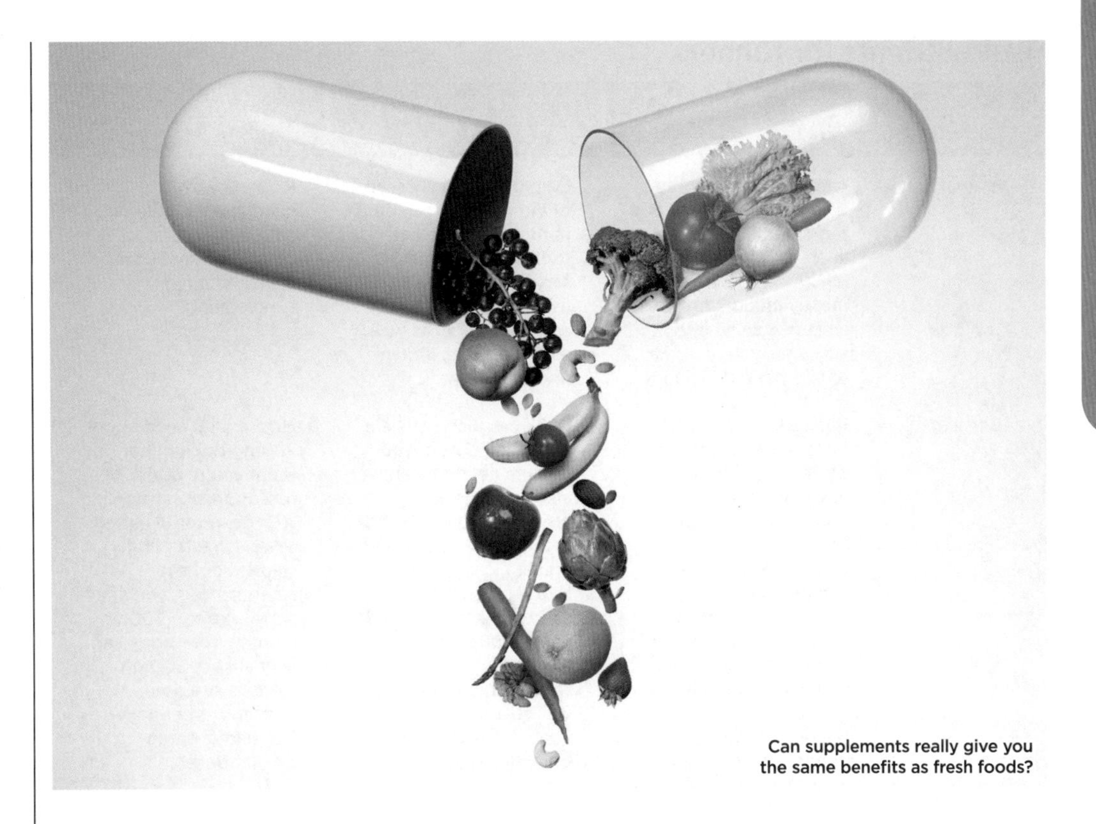

Can supplements really give you the same benefits as fresh foods?

The nutrients runners need most

If you've been cutting down on your calorie intake, increasing mileage, following a strict diet, doing a detox or eliminating food groups, you may be at risk of nutrient deficiencies, and a supplement might be right for you. See the table on the following pages for some of the nutrients runners need most.

Single supplements or multivitamin?

So is it better to take a multivitamin or a single supplement such as D3 or omega-3? In general, a multivitamin should meet your needs if you eat a varied diet and the supplement provides close to 100% of the reference intake (RI) of nutrients. However, certain nutrients – for example, vitamin D, calcium and iron – can be difficult to get in sufficient amounts in a multivitamin, so if you've been diagnosed with a deficiency, that may warrant taking a supplement. But if you haven't, just stick with a multivitamin. Single-nutrient supplements tend to supply much more than 100% of your needs and can build up to extreme amounts that you neither need nor can easily excrete. Talk to your doctor if you have questions about whether your multivitamin provides sufficient amounts of any given nutrient.

Don't go overboard

Many supplements contain excessive amounts of a certain nutrient – in some cases up to 433% of the recommended daily allowance. Unless your healthcare provider tells you otherwise, opt for a supplement that contains 100% or less of a nutrient and rely on your diet to supply the rest of your needs. In some cases, as with omega-3s, there is no specific recommended intake. Check out Consumerlab.com for reviews of the safest and most effective supplements.

Best nutrients for runners

	WHY RUNNERS NEED IT	BEST SOURCES FROM FOOD	DAILY DOSAGE
Vitamin D	The body needs vitamin D to absorb calcium and regulate phosphorus to keep your bones healthy. If you train mostly indoors or live in a place with limited sunshine, you're at risk of vitamin D deficiency.	Dairy is the main source of vitamin D. It can be hard to find in other foods but look for fortified products such as breads, orange juice and margarine, as well as mushrooms grown under UV light.	Runners with insufficient intake or who lack natural sunshine may benefit from a vitamin D supplement.
Calcium	Runners – especially female – who restrict calories tend to have low intakes of this bone-building and repairing nutrient. Calcium plays a role in many basic body functions, including muscle contraction and blood clotting. If your diet is low in calcium, you're probably draining it from your bones. If you don't get enough calcium and vitamin D, you increase the risk of low bone-mineral density and stress fractures.	Dairy products can help you meet most of your calcium needs. It can also be found in products made with milk (eg, certain crackers and breads), canned salmon, tofu set with calcium carbonate, and fortified orange juice. Leafy greens are a source of calcium, but it is not as well absorbed by the body as the calcium in other products.	Most adults need about 700mg calcium per day. But if you're at risk of osteoporosis, struggling with disordered eating, severely restricting calories or have amenorrhoea, you need more – up to 1,500mg per day. Your body can only absorb 500mg calcium at a time, so break your intake into two or three smaller doses.
B vitamins: thiamin, riboflavin, niacin, B6, pantothenic acid, biotin, folate and B12	All B vitamins are essential for energy metabolism. Thiamin, riboflavin, niacin, B6, pantothenic acid and biotin aid in energy production during exercise, while folate and B12 are required for red blood cell production, protein synthesis and tissue repair. Female runners, especially vegetarians or those with disordered eating patterns, are often low in riboflavin, folate and B12.	Enriched and whole grains are a potent source of many B vitamins. Other sources include meat, nuts, dairy and green vegetables.	Some data suggests exercise may increase the need for B vitamins by as much as twice the current recommended amount. Other experts suggest that as long as you're eating enough, you're fine. But if you're limiting calories to lose weight, you may want to consider adding a supplement. Look for one that provides 100% of your daily needs. If a supplement isn't for you, focus on consuming foods rich in B vitamins.

Iron	For runners, iron plays a vital role in forming oxygen-carrying proteins, haemoglobin, and myoglobin. Without enough iron, you'll fatigue easily and feel winded before you finish your run. Iron is one of the most prevalent deficiencies in runners – especially female. A number of factors can lead to this, including vegetarian diets, inflammation, heavy sweating, menstrual periods and foot-strike haemolysis.	It's easiest for the body to absorb haem iron—the kind that comes from animal products, such as beef, pork, poultry and liver. If you don't eat meat, non-haem iron sources such as black beans, kidney beans, fortified grains and breakfast cereals are good options. For best absorption, pair iron-rich foods with foods that are high in vitamin C, such as citrus fruits, leafy greens and red peppers.	For non-runners, it's recommended that women get 14.8mg iron per day; for men the figure is 8.7mg. Runners should aim for 1.3 to 1.7 times those levels, as they naturally lose iron during exercise. Vegetarians should also aim for that intake because vegetarian (non-haem) sources of iron are not as well absorbed as animal-based (haem) ones.
Zinc	Zinc plays a role in immune function, haemoglobin production, energy production, and building and repair of muscle tissue.	Find zinc in red meat, dark-meat poultry, raw oysters, whole grains, wheat germ, and enriched grains and cereals.	Men need 5.5-9.5mg zinc per day; women 4-7mg. It's not always readily absorbed, as other nutrients can affect its bioavailability. For example, non-haem iron supplements can inhibit zinc absorption. Haem iron (the kind in red meat) doesn't have the same effect. Try to keep your diet high in zinc through daily consumption of some of the foods listed in the column on the left.
Magnesium	Magnesium is a key mineral for strong bones; it helps to regulate calcium balance and vitamin D balance. Magnesium is also critical for nervous-system functions, blood-sugar control, protein synthesis and blood-pressure regulation. Marginal magnesium deficiency can actually impair performance, as well as amplify the negative effects of strenuous exercise.	Magnesium is found in leafy green veg such as spinach, as well as many whole grains, seeds and nuts. Seafood, beans and dairy products also contain some magnesium. Refined and processed foods are generally low in this nutrient.	Men should take 300mg per day, while women should aim for 270mg.

Probably not what your daily diet should look like

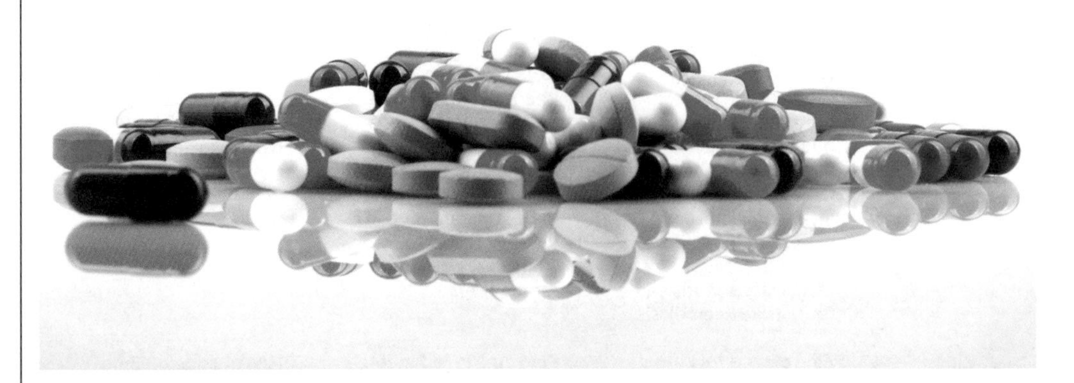

Are there *any* supplements that can aid weight loss?

Unfortunately, the answer to that is no. Some supplements – such as herbals – might be effective in promoting weight loss, but the side effects could be more than you bargained for. And these types of supplement are not closely regulated, which means the appropriate bodies don't provide the same level of oversight they give to food items. So be wary of any supplement that sounds too good to be true – it probably is. Your best bet is to make sure you're taking in adequate – but not excessive – amounts of B vitamins to keep your metabolism humming along.

If you feel you'd benefit from a supplement, choose one that's an extract of a real food, such as green tea. But as with all things, don't take excessive amounts.

A recent study published in the *Journal of Nutrition*[2] found that when study participants consumed a beverage rich (approximately 625mg) in the catechins found in green tea, they lost more weight and more abdominal fat than the control group. But do you need to run out and buy a green-tea-extract supplement? Probably not. One cup of green tea provides about 140mg and additional research has found that consuming about three cups a day is effective in promoting fat oxidation.

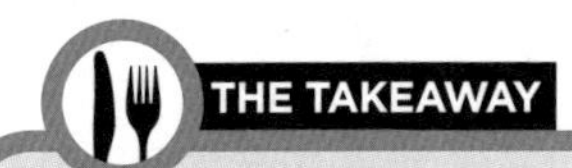

THE TAKEAWAY

Eat your fruits and vegetables.
Those foods are packed with the nutrients, vitamins and minerals you need. It's easier for your body to absorb vitamins and minerals from foods than from pills. Plus, with fruit and veg you also get fibre and hydration to keep your body running strong.

Take a multivitamin.
If you've been cutting calories, avoiding certain food groups or ratcheting up your exercise routine, it's a good idea to take a multivitamin to ensure you're getting the vitamins and minerals you need.

See a doctor.
If you're feeling chronically run-down, see a doctor and have your blood tested to determine whether you have any particular nutrient deficiencies that might be affecting your health and performance.

14.

ADAPTING MAINSTREAM DIETS

If you want to get fit and lose weight, you've got to make changes to what you eat and how you work out. So it's hard to resist the lure of diets that seem to promise instant, permanent results with little work or restraint.

The truth is that diets are a lot like training plans. No one diet is ideal for everyone; what you need is way of eating that's the best fit for *you* at any given time. Yes, most diets are similar in that they involve cutting calories and modifying the proportions of foods and food groups you might typically eat. But within these categories, each diet has certain parameters you must follow to reap the purported benefits.

You need a way of eating that's the best fit for *you*

Some diets have a laundry list of rules; others focus on simply eliminating a specific ingredient (or food group). Still others allow every food you can dream of – but in small portions – or require you to order the meals and snacks from a certain manufacturer. Or there are those that prescribe set calorie limits to help you avoid junk foods high in fat, salt and sugar. Each diet has its benefits and drawbacks for each individual, but the most important factor in any such plan is how well it helps you meet your goals, fits your needs and helps you maintain healthy eating habits for life.

Over the years, your own personal 'perfect diet' will evolve as you discover what works best for you. You'll gravitate towards the foods that make you feel healthy, lean, strong and energised for your workouts. Foods that leave you feeling tired, bloated or unsatisfied will ultimately lose their appeal.

Here's what you need to know about some of the more popular diets on the market and how to adapt them to fit your running goals.

Low-carb diets

The premise Technically, any low-carbohydrate diet is an eating plan consisting of less than 20% of a day's calories from carbohydrate, or approximately 20-60g per day. Each has a twist. Some diets call for a most drastic reduction – less than 40g carbs per day at first – reasoning that this forces the body to burn both stored fat and an energy source known as ketones. Others limit carbs to 40% of daily calories and call for the balance to be split equally between protein and fat.

The upside They're effective since you omit many of the empty-calorie junk foods (cakes, crisps, sweets) that are high in carbs and pack on the pounds. Proponents claim that weight loss will quickly and naturally follow restriction of sugars and carbohydrates. And indeed, you'll see results right away. When you slash carbs, you retain less water and the water in your system gets flushed out. Also, because many of these diets allow you unlimited fats

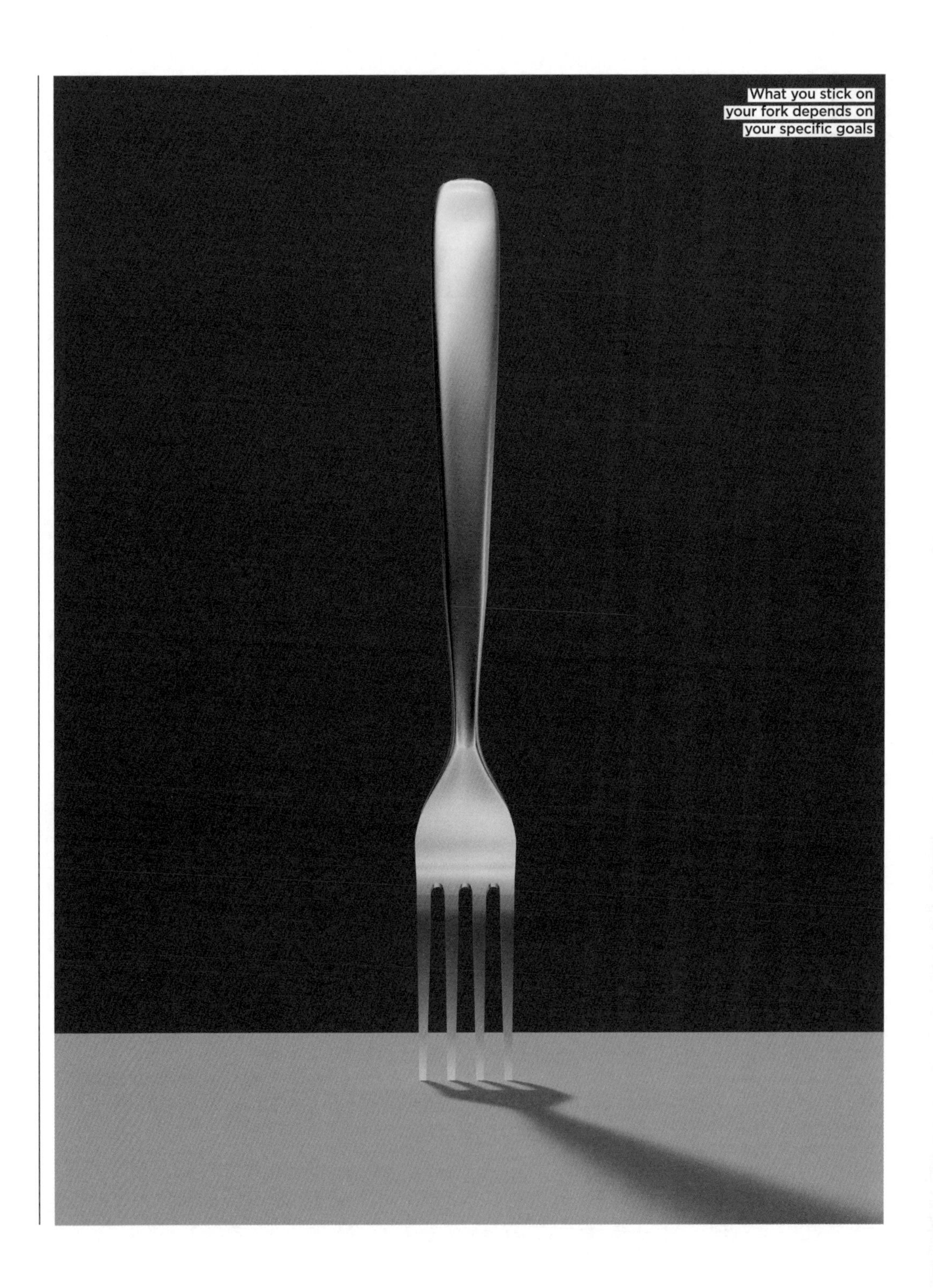

What you stick on your fork depends on your specific goals

and protein, you can indulge in carb-free foods you might have previously written off, such as eggs and bacon. And because fat and protein are digested more slowly, you'll feel fuller for longer and avoid feelings of deprivation that can lead to a binge down the road.

The downside Carbs are the nutrients your body can most efficiently convert into the energy you need to run strong, without causing GI distress. (Most runners should get at least 55% of their daily calories from carbs.) The body digests fats and protein more slowly. So if you're on a low-carb diet, you won't feel as energised on the run, and you may have to be more careful about what you eat before you run. In addition, many runners find these diets difficult to sustain. Finally, when you eliminate crucial food groups such as fruit and veg, you may be at risk of nutrient deficiencies. Can a multivitamin provide nutrients vitamin C and K? Yes. Can it provide the antioxidants and flavonoids, and other bioactive components essential to optimum health found in real foods? Probably not.

Is it safe? Short-term, these diets appear to be safe, but research has yet to determine their impact on the development of chronic diseases such as type 2 diabetes, osteoporosis and kidney disease. Because you eliminate many food groups when you go low-carb, you can develop certain nutrient deficiencies.

Will it work? Based on anecdotal evidence and peer-reviewed research, when practised in a sustainable way, low-carb diets can work. A study published in the *Annals of Internal Medicine* found that they were more effective for weight loss and reduced the risk of heart disease more than low-fat diets.[1]

How to adapt the diet to lose weight and run faster Low-carb diets can be effective if weight loss is your primary goal. But if you're running regularly or training for a race, you'll need to keep some carbs in your diet in order to achieve the results you're after. Rather than cutting out carbs as a group, you might use the principles of low-carb dieting to avoid simple junk carbs that might be dragging down your weight-loss efforts and, ultimately, hurting your long-term health.

You probably already know where these calories come from: processed, high-sugar, white-flour-rich choices such as breads, crackers and other quick snacks. (Read more about carbs in Chapter 1.) Work on replacing these refined carbs with carb-rich whole grains, low-fat dairy, starchy vegetables and fruit. And time your intake so those carbs will boost your running performance. Consume your most carb-rich foods when they're going to be quickly burned – in the hour before and the hour after a tough workout. The rest of the time, fill your plate with lean protein, vegetables and heart-healthy fats.

You might follow this rule: cut back carbs at all meals except the one before your running workout. Before a marathon, several days of carb-loading will probably pay off, but you don't necessarily need high carbs all the time during your regular training. (For more on carb-loading, turn to Chapter 17.)

High-protein diets

The premise Like other low-carb diets, these plans focus on replacing carbs with protein, reasoning that the body digests it more slowly – so you feel fuller for longer – and that it helps build and repair your working muscles. High-protein diets, which often fit under the umbrella term 'paleo', encourage foods that can be hunted, gathered or fished and are based on the theory that we're ideally suited to eat the foods that sustained our caveman ancestors. They generally advocate sticking with grass-fed meats, wild fish, poultry, eggs, nuts, fruit and vegetables – which are generally high in protein and fibre, and low in carbs – and avoiding grains and starchy vegetables. Healthy fats are also recommended. These diets tend to restrict certain foods, such as peanuts, lentils, beans, peas and processed sugar.

The upside No doubt about it, cutting out refined carbs and processed foods will help

Photography: Getty. **Sources:** 1. *Annals of Internal Medicine*

you lose weight and be healthier all around. After all, many processed foods are high in salt, preservatives and refined sugar, and offer little nutritional benefit. And with all that protein and fibre, you're not likely to go hungry. Studies have shown that people who eat more protein – about 30% of total calories – are less hungry, eat less and lose more weight then those who consume those same calories from carbohydrate or fat sources.[2] Other studies have shown that those who upped their protein intake were 50% less likely to regain the weight they lost, and lowered their percentage of body fat.[3]

The downside Because these diets are so high in fibre, while your digestive health may improve, it may be tough to get through a long run without a few pit stops or hitting the wall. Because the body runs most efficiently when it's using carbs, it has a harder time converting fat to fuel. So you may feel sluggish while you're adjusting to this new diet. And if you're running longer distances – say, up to a 10K or a half marathon – it may be challenging to find any energy gels or chews that meet the parameters of the diet. And because lean meats (the basis of paleo diets) cost more per pound than most grains, strictly following the diet may cause your grocery bill to swell.

Is it safe? Yes. But bear in mind that this diet is low in many essential vitamins and minerals you need to run strong. And you might find it difficult to maintain over the long term. If you're contending with any kidney conditions, talk to your doctor before trying a high-protein diet. If you're following such a diet, it's best to increase your intake of water; research has shown that a higher protein intake causes the kidneys to produce more concentrated urine, which can be a sign of dehydration. Check your urine: if it's the colour of light straw, you're hydrated; if it's darker, more like the colour of apple juice, drink more water.

Does it work? If you're replacing lots of junk food and refined grains with healthier options such as nuts, dried fruit and lean protein, you're likely to shed weight. Studies have shown that when obese men were given a variety of meals, those who consumed high-protein, high-fat and very-low-carb meals felt less hungry and more full (and lost more weight) compared with men fed moderate-carb, protein and fat meals.[4] Other studies have shown that those who cut their calories to lose weight while upping their protein intake to twice the US recommended daily value (0.73g protein per lb of body weight) lost more fat mass while retaining their hard-earned muscle.[5]

How to adapt the diet to lose weight and run faster There's nothing wrong with cutting out refined grains and junk carbs – it'll improve your weight and your overall health. But if you cut out *all* grains (including whole grains), you'll lose many essential vitamins – such as B vitamins – from your diet. And if you avoid dairy, you'll want to consider adding other sources of calcium and vitamin D.

To make a high-protein diet work for you, there's no need to go all-out; that could derail your training and your overall health. But there's something to be said for replacing fluffy, refined white bread with lean, satiating sources of protein. It'll keep you fuller longer and still give you that dose of B vitamins your body needs. For breakfast, have a protein shake or smoothie rather than a bagel. At lunch, skip the croutons and sweet dressing, and double up on the greens as well as low-fat cheese and meat. For a snack, grab some Greek yogurt and nuts instead of stacks of crackers and cheese. While cheese is low-carb, it's hard to stop at just one serving of crackers. At dinner, if you're hankering for seconds, grab another helping of chicken rather than pasta or breadsticks. At the end of the day, you'll have consumed more protein and less carbohydrate than if you weren't going 'low-carb'. Over time, you might consume fewer calories and a lot less junk food.

Detox diets

The premise It's easy to see why detox diets are so popular. After all, who wouldn't want to follow a diet that promises weight loss,

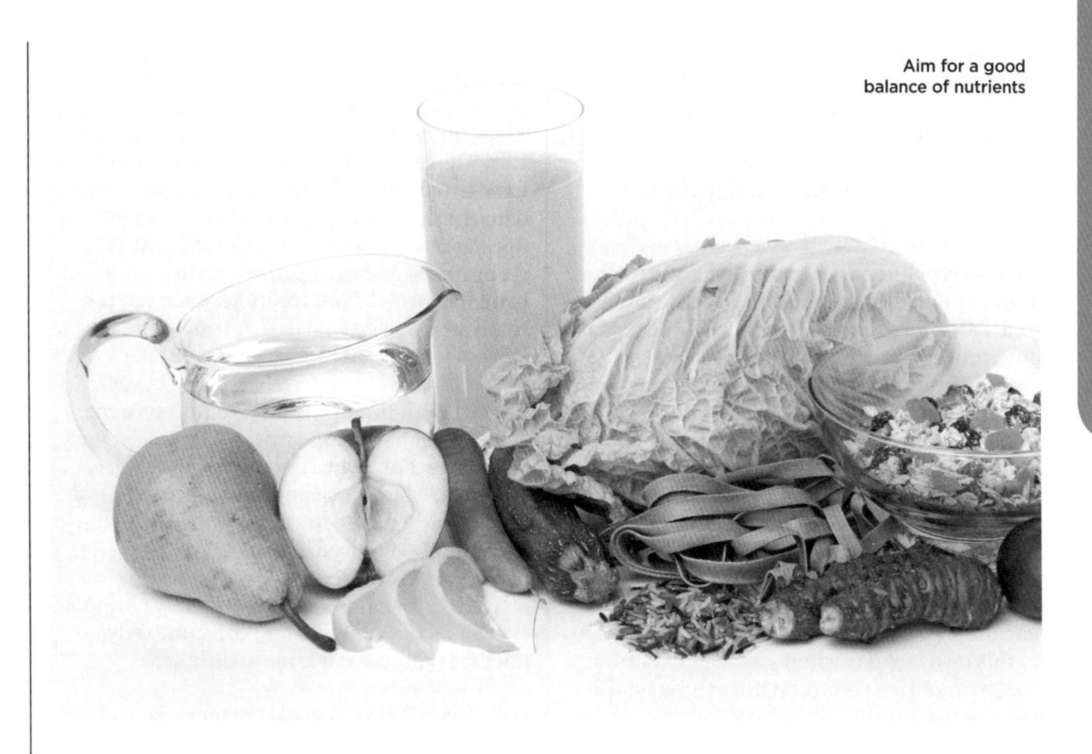

Aim for a good balance of nutrients

Photography: Getty. Sources: 2. American Journal of Clinical Nutrition. 3. International Journal of Obesity. 4. American Journal of Clinical Nutrition. 5. FASEB Journal

optimal health, clearer skin and shinier hair? These diets tend to be based on the premise that you just need to rid your body of toxins to feel and look your best. Some cleanses require followers to consume specific (branded) beverages for a specific period of time; others involve two-day fasts. There are also three-week schemes where dieters eliminate certain food groups, or drink 'cleansing' beverages daily. Generally these diets promise quick weight loss, healing, cleansing and a renewed sense of better health. While not all detox diets focus solely on weight loss, the eating is so restrictive that weight loss often follows.

The upside Quick results; because you're consuming so little, the weight immediately drops off. If you're struggling with weight or unhealthy eating, and need a hard and fast break from the life you've been living, a short-term detox in which you fast for a bit or eliminate certain foods can be a good way to get back on track.

The downside There's a good chance that an intense, severely restrictive or long-term detox diet will derail your training. You're likely to feel fatigued due to too few nutrients, and you may spend extra time darting for a portable toilet thanks to the 'cleansing products'. While you may lose weight in the short term, these diets don't nurture the kind of lifestyle change and nutrition improvement that are essential to keeping the weight off. Plus, you won't have the energy you need to work out, which is critical to sustainable weight loss. Probably the most frustrating part is that once you finish the detox and return to your old eating habits, the weight you lost will quickly return.

Is it safe? Some serious, negative long-term consequences can come from detox diets. Short-term, you might suffer some unpleasant side effects from so-called cleansing products. And if you suffer from a chronic disease such as type 2 diabetes, these diets could put you at risk of other complications if you forgo traditional, effective medical treatments while you 'cleanse'. But if you're following a short-term detox diet that calls for eating planned meals, or cutting some of the junk out of your diet, there's a good chance you can get the benefits without the harmful side effects.

How to adapt the diet to lose weight and run faster Struggling to get back on the wagon? Or need to jump-start a new pattern of eating? If so, a 'detox' of sorts might just work for you. But there's no need to run out and buy special shakes or secret ingredients; simply pick a date on which you will avoid all your trigger foods. This might be sugary products, fizzy soft drinks or salty snacks. Or you could pick a day on which you'll drink only water and eat only fruit and vegetables. Like any detox, this type should be short (since you're cutting out some important food groups), but it can be a good cleansing ritual and a day when you won't be 'cheating' or eating any junk. It's a good idea to do this on a rest day when you're not planning a big workout, as you won't be fuelling up the way you usually do.

Juicing

The premise Similar to detox diets, juicing diets call for incorporating fresh, raw or minimally processed juices into a regular diet. Proponents say juicing will make you feel more energised and healthy, fend off chronic diseases and even make you look better.

The upside If you're not getting enough fruit and veg in your diet, juicing can provide all the vitamins, minerals and phytonutrients you're missing out on. You can get the amount recommended in dietary guidelines and help boost cardiovascular health. While juicing might eliminate the fibre that our bodies also need, phytonutrients found in 100% fruit and vegetable juices can be beneficial for the general population and athletes. Juices are also a great source of energy and are highly portable. So if you're on the go all the time, it won't be difficult to take your juice along.

The downside If you're looking to lose weight and you enjoy fruit and veg, it's far better to keep consuming them in whole form, as that'll help you reach your weight-loss goals faster. Why? Research has shown that consuming fibre-filled raw produce, such as apples and bananas, in its whole form will satisfy your appetite far better than drinking it will. A study published in *Appetite* concluded that solid fruit makes you feel fuller than puréed fruit or juice, and that eating fruit at the start of a meal can reduce energy intake.[6] Researchers speculated that it may have to do with the amount of chewing required to eat an apple. What's more, raw, cold-pressed juice doesn't come cheap. If you're going to juice, be prepared to spend approaching £100 for a high-quality juicer, in addition to buying the ingredients required to juice regularly.

Is it safe? Yes. Unless you completely eliminate every other food group and consume only juices, a diet that contains juice is safe.

Will it work? If your goal is to increase your fruit, vegetable and nutrient intake, juicing is a good call. But juices aren't calorie-free and

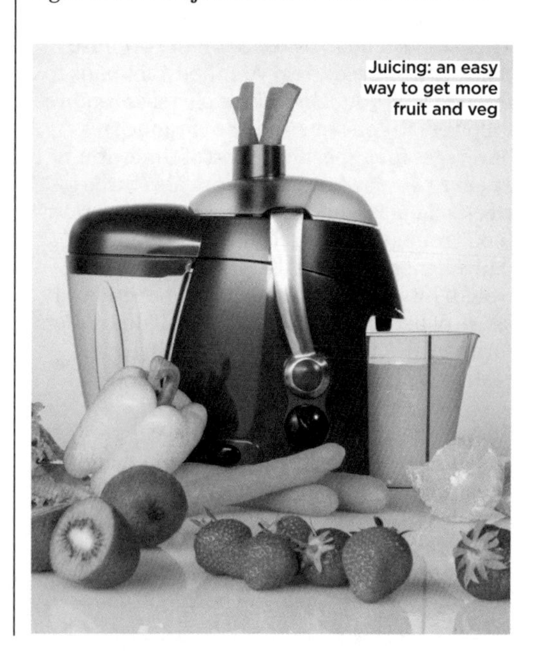
Juicing: an easy way to get more fruit and veg

they certainly don't include filling fibre. As we said earlier, consuming fruit and veg in their whole form will leave you feeling fuller longer.

How to adapt the diet to lose weight and run faster The best time to drink a juice is in the 30 minutes just after a tough workout, when your body is highly efficient at processing carbs and protein. Make a smoothie with fruit – using the whole fruit and peel – and include a scoop of protein powder to boost muscle repair and fill up faster. For other meals and snacks, consume fruit and veg in their whole form.

Intermittent fasting

The premise Fasting as a weight-loss tool has become popular in recent years. Supporters of such diets claim that it can help you lose weight, rev up your metabolism and improve blood-sugar control, all while allowing you to eat whatever you want during periods of non-fasting. Other related diets, which promote fasting or fat-burning periods each week, claim that these fasting periods reset your metabolism and help you lose weight.

The upside This diet does promote the consumption of healthy foods (lean meat, vegetable, etc), but it also allows periods of unrestricted eating of high-calorie foods. Creating windows for fasting requires careful thought and planning, which some experts suggest can lead to more mindful eating and therefore less habitual, mindless calorie consumption. You also have plenty of time while fasting to plan your next healthy meal.

The downside The diet is restrictive for certain periods of time, and during these periods, if you're sensitive to blood-sugar fluctuations, you might suffer from low energy levels and the symptoms that accompany low blood sugar. While you're free to consume whatever you want during certain designated periods, not every dieter has the willpower to avoid eating everything that's not tied down following a period of restriction.

Is it safe? While those sensitive to low blood-sugar levels will want to proceed with caution, some research has found that when men fasted every other day for two weeks, their insulin levels improved and they were more efficient at managing blood-sugar levels.[7] But, as with most trendy diets, there's still limited clinical research exploring this diet's effectiveness or safety. Most experts agree that intermittent fasting is probably safe for most individuals but shouldn't be followed long-term.

Will it work? If you find yourself grazing and mindlessly snacking at all hours of the day, you're probably consuming more calories than you realise and taking in lots of processed foods and other junk. Pausing your intake of food for several hours may lead you to eat more mindfully and make better choices when you return to a more conventional pattern. Athletes who've followed intermittent fasting report that it's difficult to adjust to but, once they get in the habit, they can adapt and function normally. Still others report that while they adapt and can function, all they can think about is food, and once they're 'allowed' to eat again, they have a hard time making healthy choices and returning to the wagon.

How to adapt the diet to lose weight and run faster If you're game to try intermittent fasting, you should know there's only limited scientific evidence supporting its claims. What makes this diet work is probably the fact that you're severely restricting calories. That said, if you think intermittent fasting is for you and this lifestyle syncs with what you're currently doing, you might give it a try. But try to time your meals so you're somewhat fuelled for your runs. It's fine to 'train low' for shorter, less intense workouts, but you'll want to time your meals so you have fuel on board before longer runs and harder workouts. And don't forget about recovery: time your 'fast' so you can fit in a meal or snack within 30 minutes of very hard exercise. And if you do try intermittent fasting, don't expect it to be a breeze at first. You'll need to give the diet time to take hold and work; aim for a trial of a few weeks before evaluating success or failure.

Photography: Getty. **Sources:** 6. Appetite. 7. Journal of Applied Physiology

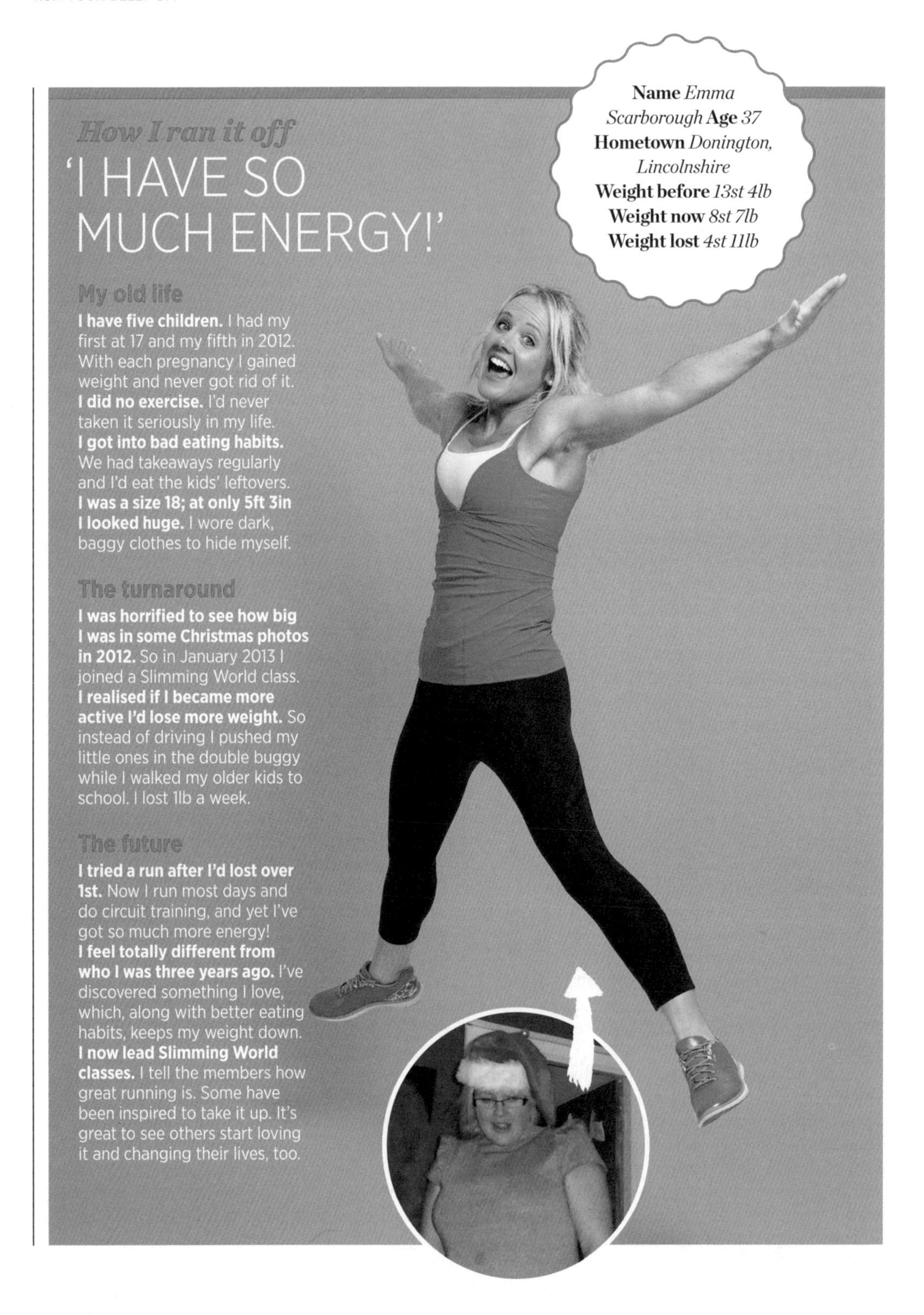

How I ran it off

'I HAVE SO MUCH ENERGY!'

Name *Emma Scarborough* **Age** *37*
Hometown *Donington, Lincolnshire*
Weight before *13st 4lb*
Weight now *8st 7lb*
Weight lost *4st 11lb*

My old life

I have five children. I had my first at 17 and my fifth in 2012. With each pregnancy I gained weight and never got rid of it.
I did no exercise. I'd never taken it seriously in my life.
I got into bad eating habits. We had takeaways regularly and I'd eat the kids' leftovers.
I was a size 18; at only 5ft 3in I looked huge. I wore dark, baggy clothes to hide myself.

The turnaround

I was horrified to see how big I was in some Christmas photos in 2012. So in January 2013 I joined a Slimming World class.
I realised if I became more active I'd lose more weight. So instead of driving I pushed my little ones in the double buggy while I walked my older kids to school. I lost 1lb a week.

The future

I tried a run after I'd lost over 1st. Now I run most days and do circuit training, and yet I've got so much more energy!
I feel totally different from who I was three years ago. I've discovered something I love, which, along with better eating habits, keeps my weight down.
I now lead Slimming World classes. I tell the members how great running is. Some have been inspired to take it up. It's great to see others start loving it and changing their lives, too.

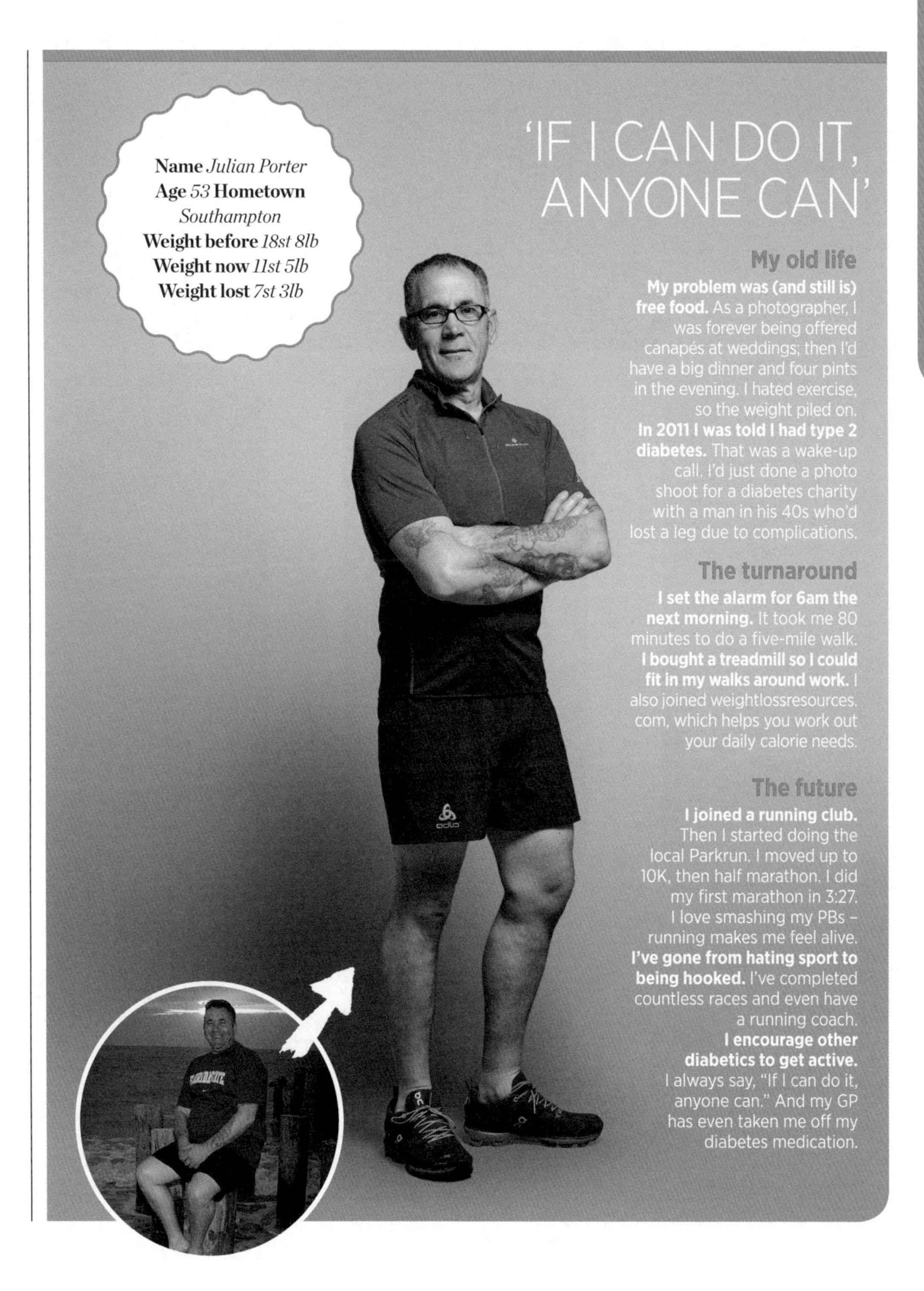

Name *Julian Porter*
Age *53* **Hometown** *Southampton*
Weight before *18st 8lb*
Weight now *11st 5lb*
Weight lost *7st 3lb*

'IF I CAN DO IT, ANYONE CAN'

My old life

My problem was (and still is) free food. As a photographer, I was forever being offered canapés at weddings; then I'd have a big dinner and four pints in the evening. I hated exercise, so the weight piled on. **In 2011 I was told I had type 2 diabetes.** That was a wake-up call. I'd just done a photo shoot for a diabetes charity with a man in his 40s who'd lost a leg due to complications.

The turnaround

I set the alarm for 6am the next morning. It took me 80 minutes to do a five-mile walk. **I bought a treadmill so I could fit in my walks around work.** I also joined weightlossresources.com, which helps you work out your daily calorie needs.

The future

I joined a running club. Then I started doing the local Parkrun. I moved up to 10K, then half marathon. I did my first marathon in 3:27. I love smashing my PBs – running makes me feel alive. **I've gone from hating sport to being hooked.** I've completed countless races and even have a running coach. **I encourage other diabetics to get active.** I always say, "If I can do it, anyone can." And my GP has even taken me off my diabetes medication.

Part II

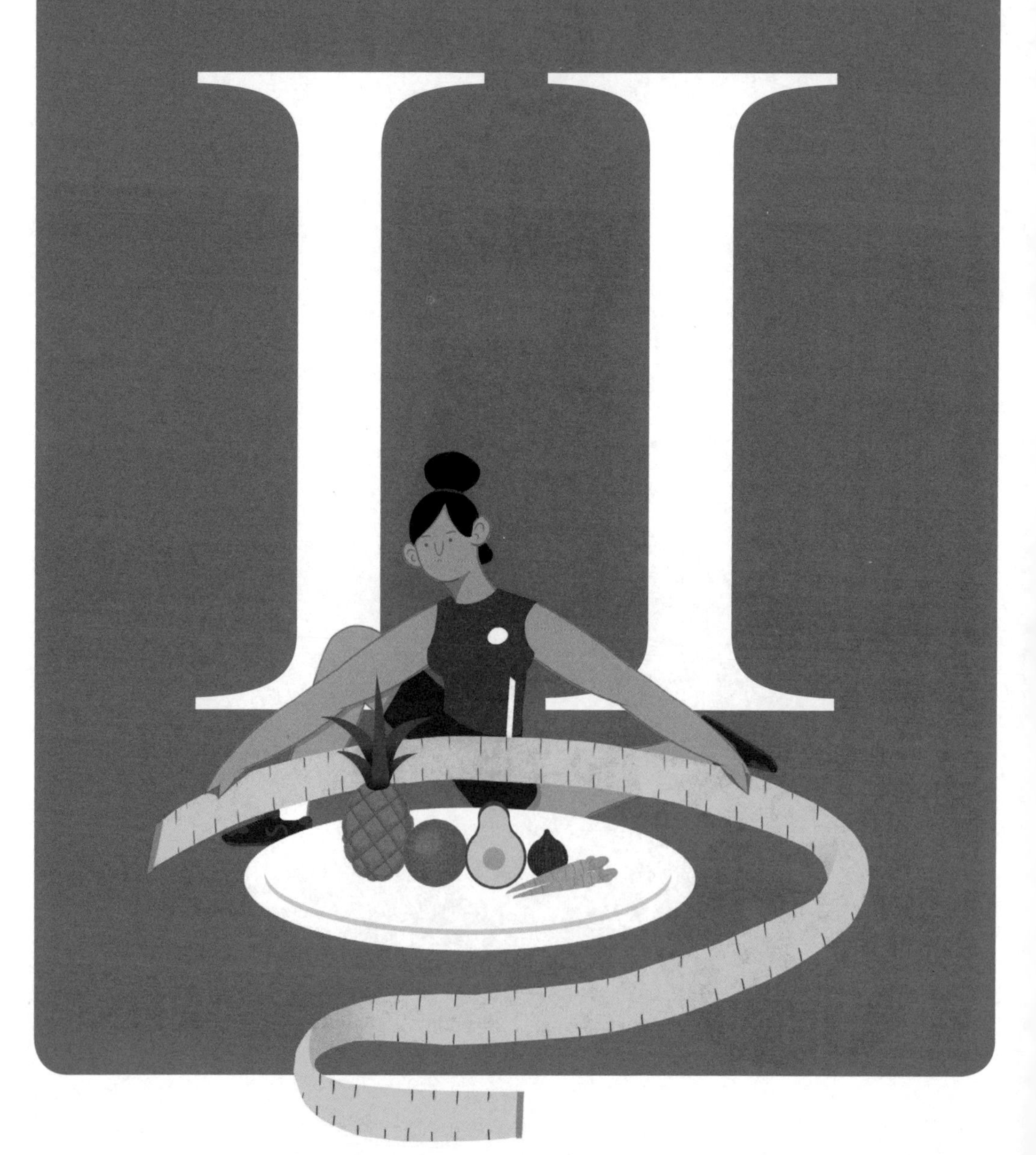

HOW MUCH TO EAT

This section gives you all the tools you need to determine how many calories you should consume each day to lose weight, stay energised and get faster. There are tips on sizing your portions to help you meet those targets, and we'll reveal the factors that affect your body's ability to burn calories – some of which have nothing to do with your running or eating habits...

15.

METABOLISM BASICS

Boost your metabolism is a popular headline on magazine covers and social-media channels. Stories that promise *'Eleven lazy ways to burn calories!'* and *'Nine foods that boost calorie burn!'*[1] suggest that if you simply eat more cayenne pepper, sprinkle every meal with cinnamon, guzzle more coffee and green tea, and set the heating in your home to 17°C, you can rev up the rate at which your body burns calories (even when you're not working out) and achieve the weight-loss breakthrough you're seeking.

Ah, if only it were that easy. Unfortunately, the reality is a lot more complex. Here's what you need to know about metabolism, the role it plays in your weight-loss efforts, and what you can – and can't – do to tweak it in order to achieve your feel-great weight.

The three ways your body burns calories

Between 50-70% of your metabolism is determined by what's known as your basal metabolic rate (BMR). That's the number of calories your body burns to keep your vital organs – lungs, heart, liver, kidneys and brain – doing their jobs. Another 10% of your metabolism comes from the number of calories you burn digesting food (this is called the thermic effect of food). It takes slightly more calories to digest protein than it does the equivalent amount of fat and carbohydrates.

The remaining 30% or so of your metabolism is determined by how much you burn through physical activity – whether that constitutes fidgeting at your desk or forcing yourself through a six-mile tempo run.

Factors that affect metabolism

Research has proved what you've probably witnessed in your own life: some people just seem to burn calories faster or more efficiently than others. Certain lucky types can pig out with abandon and never feel the impact; others gain 10lbs if they so much as smell a muffin. It's one reason why weight loss isn't just a simple matter of willpower, or even calories in versus calories out. "It's much more complicated than that," says Kim Larson, a spokeswoman for the Academy of Nutrition and Dietetics in Seattle, USA.

Certain factors affecting your metabolism are hard-wired – these include:

Gender

Men tend to have more muscle than women do, and since muscle burns more calories than fat, they tend to have a faster metabolism, too – anywhere from 3-10% higher than that of women, studies have shown.[2]

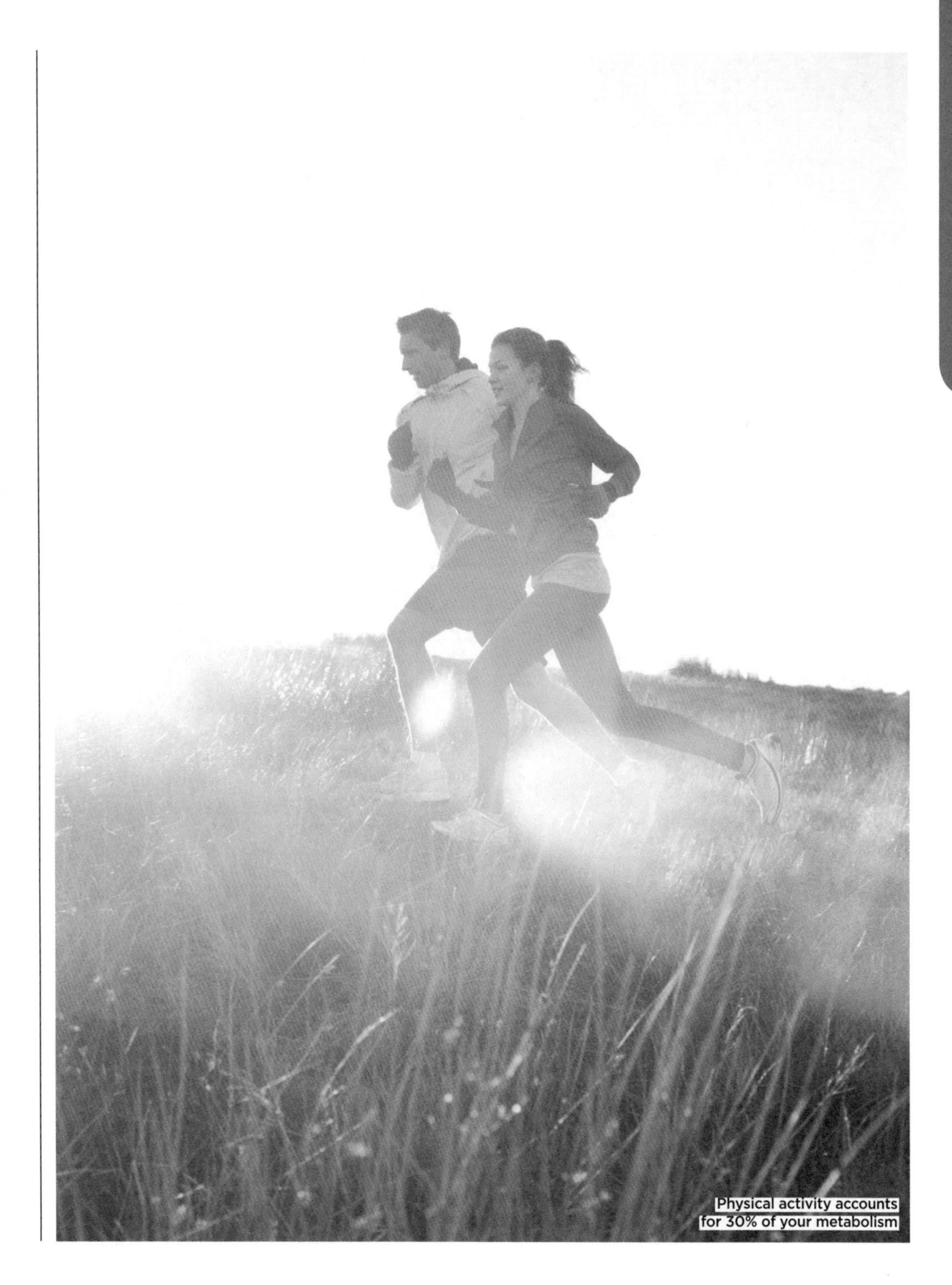

Physical activity accounts for 30% of your metabolism

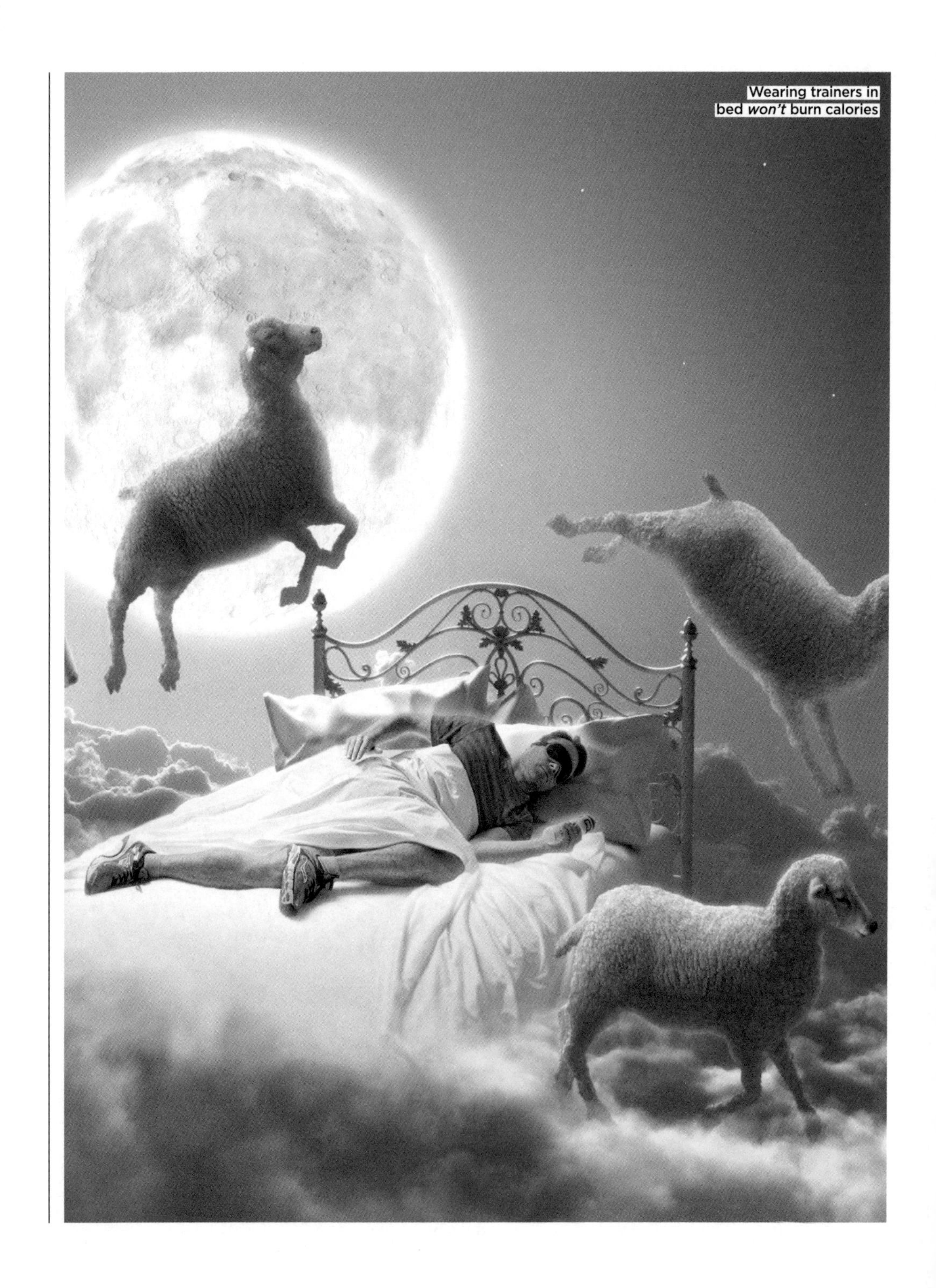

Wearing trainers in bed *won't* burn calories

Age

As you get older, your basal metabolic rate drops – between 3-5% per decade after the age of 18.[3] Part of that has to do with the fact that, as you age, your body composition changes. The proportion of calorie-burning muscle shrinks, while your proportion of fat rises. Plus, you tend to be less active as you age. When you're young, you're more likely to spend your free time physically active. As you get older, chances are you spend a large proportion of your life sitting in an office and much more of your free time in sedentary activities, such as watching TV.[4]

Menopause

While this is a relatively new area of research, scientists are learning more about how metabolism and fat gain are affected by the onset of menopause, which occurs the year after women stop menstruating (typically around age 50) and causes oestrogen levels to plummet. While menopause may not necessarily cause weight gain, researchers now know that it does change the way women store fat. The rate at which they store visceral fat – which surrounds the vital organs in the belly – starts to increase, according to a 2012 review of research by the International Menopause Society.[5] Another study showed that post-menopausal women burn less fat than younger women.[6] That's a problem, since increased belly fat increases risk of diabetes, heart disease, stroke and even some cancers.

That said, there's evidence that keeping up your running routine can help. In studies, women who gained the most weight – and the most belly fat – were the ones whose activity levels decreased the most. Those who kept a stable weight exercised for an average of an hour a day. What's more, those who were the leanest going into menopause had the lowest risk of experiencing weight gain.[7]

Room for improvement

You can't alter your age, much as you might like to, but there *are* certain ways you can rev up your calorie burn. They're no substitute for improving your diet, and they're not magic bullets, but taking these steps will help:

Sleep more

Studies have that those who sleep less than five to six hours per night have a higher risk of being overweight.[8] When you don't get enough sleep, the hormone ghrelin, which tells your body, 'I'm hungry!' spikes, while leptin, which tells it, 'I'm full!' drops.[9] A study published in the US journal *Proceedings of the National Academy of Sciences* (March 2013) showed that people who didn't get enough sleep tended to eat more. Researchers concluded that this was to get the energy they were lacking due to sleep

CHEW ON THIS

Ever wondered why crash diets don't work? Part of the problem is that they're tough to maintain; severe deprivation tends to lead to bingeing later on. But also, switching to an ultra-low-calorie diet of 500-800 calories per day actually slows down your metabolism by as much as 50% and lays the groundwork for weight gain, says Kim Larson of the US Academy of Nutrition and Dietetics. Starved of the calories it needs, the body shifts into survival mode, slowing the rate at which it burns calories. The result? You'll be depriving yourself but not seeing the scales budge, and you'll feel depleted even before you work out, unable to get the calorie-burning and muscle-building benefits. Even after you return to normal eating habits, your body will still be in survival mode, clinging to every calorie. And as you've probably lost muscle, you've further hampered your fat-burning capacity.

If you're stuck here, what can you do to get your body out of survival mode? Most people will respond to slowly increasing their calorie and carbohydrate intake and then keeping it under control. Aerobic exercise will boost metabolism, as will high-intensity interval training (HIIT), which not only burns more calories than a steady-state run but also continues to burn calories after the workout is over. This afterburn is known as EPOC, or excess post-exercise oxygen consumption. To read more about this, go to Chapter 24.

6. *Diabetes*. 7. *Obstetrics and Gynecology Clinics of North America*. 8. *American Journal of Epidemiology*. 9. *Annals of Internal Medicine*

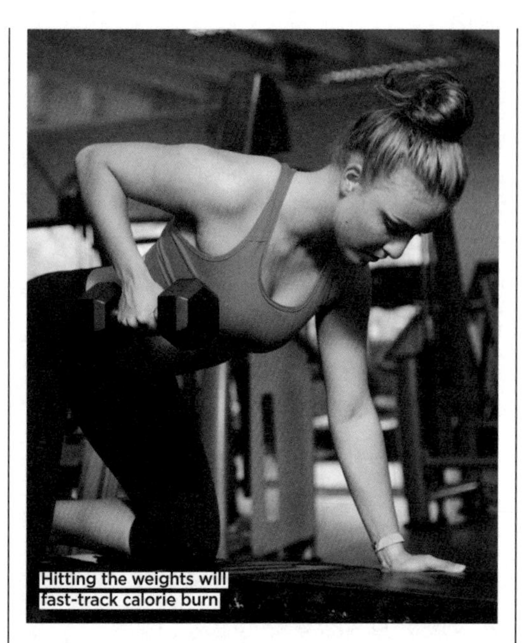
Hitting the weights will fast-track calorie burn

deprivation. So in the study, when food was plentiful they ate more than they needed.[10]

Weight train

You've probably heard that muscle burns more calories than fat. It's true. Some estimates say each lb of muscle burns anywhere from 4.5-7 calories per day, compared with two calories burned by 1lb fat. (See Chapter 25 for bodyweight exercises you can do at home.) "If you have a sluggish metabolism, the biggest way to make an impact is to increase your muscle mass," says Larson. "We have to be able to build more muscle because the more lean body mass you have, the higher your need for calories."

Drink caffeine, eat cayenne peppers, sprinkle cinnamon, etc...

Ingredients such as chilli, cinnamon, caffeine and green tea have been associated with boosting metabolism. And yes, research has shown that these foods do have a slight effect in the short term. But while the phrase 'fat-burning foods' may sell magazines and books, unfortunately none of these foods on their own is going to give you an express ticket to your feel-great weight unless you make some bigger changes at the same time. A review of caffeine studies published in *Obesity Reviews* in 2011 found that caffeine intake increased calorie burn, and that catechin-caffeine mixtures – such as that found in green tea – increased fat burn over a 24-hour period.[11] And various studies have shown that capsaicin – a compound found in chillies – boosts metabolism and increases feelings of fullness and satisfaction, so you eat less.[12] But because these ingredients have such a minimal effect on metabolism, says Larson, you'd be better off focusing on that 30% you can affect through physical activity.

Speed train

The faster you run, the more calories you burn per minute. While this might not have any impact on your resting metabolic rate, it can definitely increase your calorie burn, even after you're done working out. Obviously, you can't run fast every day – you'd get injured. But swapping your easy run for a tempo run or interval workout is a good way to burn extra calories. (See Chapter 24 for more on working out for weight loss.)

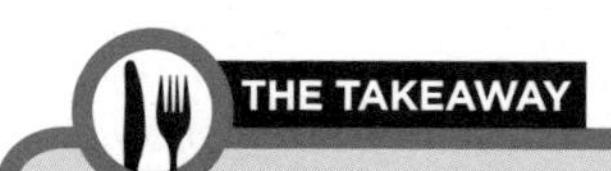

Get some sleep.
Get more than six hours' sleep a night; eight is ideal. And you'll need to rest up to rev up your energy instead of reaching for food.
Hit the gym and rev up your workouts a few times a week.
Building lean muscle mass and adding higher-intensity workouts can increase your calorie burn, even when you're done working out.
See a doctor if you're concerned.
If you're exercising, not losing weight and experiencing some symptoms of another medical condition, consult your GP.

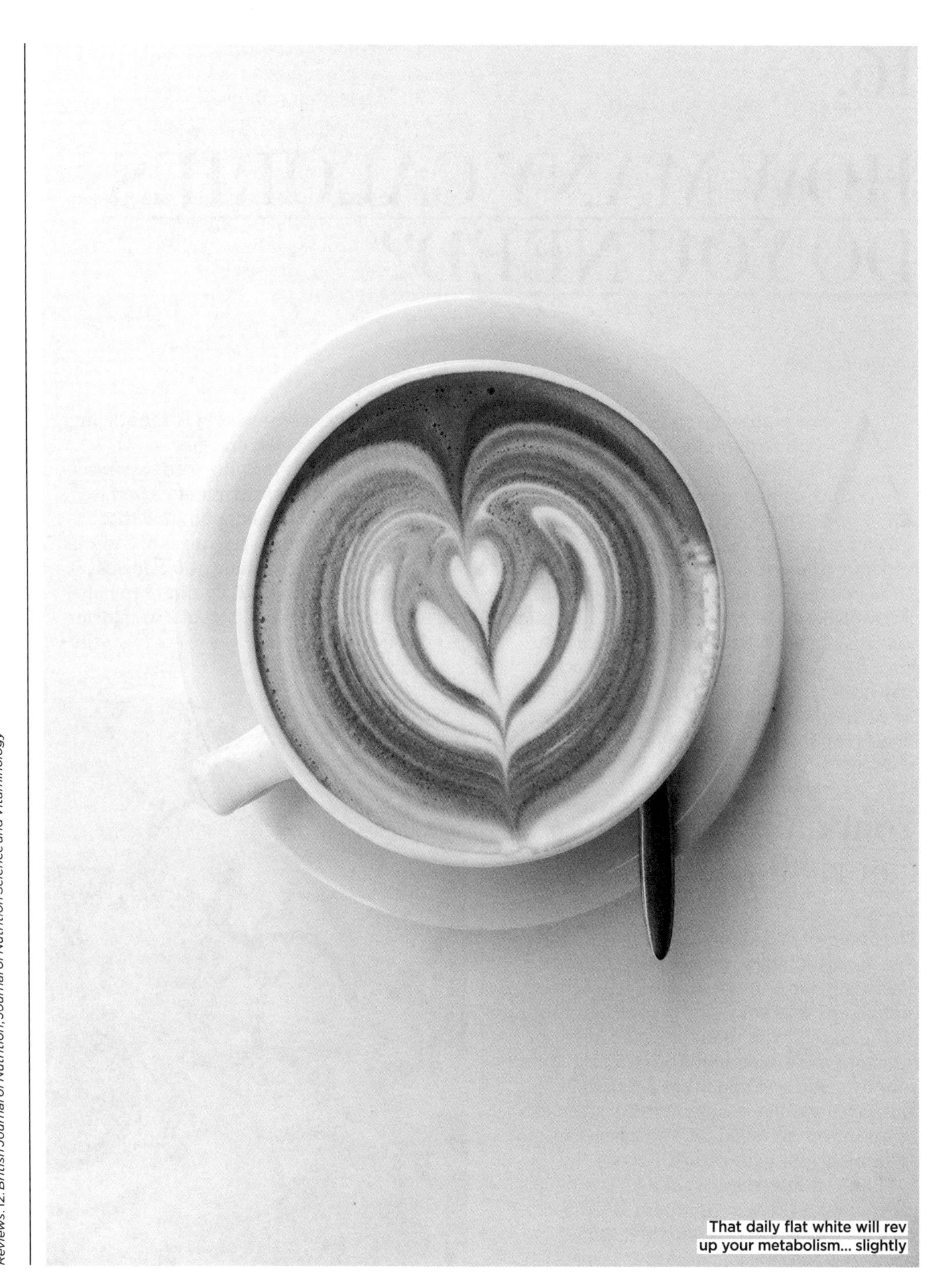

That daily flat white will rev up your metabolism... slightly

Reviews. 12. British Journal of Nutrition; Journal of Nutrition Science and Vitaminology

16.

HOW MANY CALORIES DO YOU NEED?

As with so many questions in nutrition, the answer to how many calories you should consume each day is rather complicated.

If you're trying to figure it out, your best bet is to have a body-mass assessment, with either a Bod Pod test or a DEXA scan. These tests are available at exercise physiology labs, many colleges and universities, and hospitals. But since they can be pricey and hard to access, many runners, trainers and nutritionists use formulas to estimate what their daily calorie targets should be to lose weight.

Your daily calorie formula

The first part of this process is figuring out your basal metabolic rate (BMR). This is essentially the number of calories you need each day to keep your vital organs functioning; it's the amount your body needs to keep your heart pumping, your blood circulating, and your liver, kidneys and lungs doing their jobs. Once you figure out your BMR, you can factor in your physical activity level (PAL) to determine your daily calorie needs.

When you determine what PAL is accurate for your daily life, multiply your BMR by your PAL. This will give you the number of calories you can consume every day to maintain your current weight while keeping up your current level of exercise.

To lose 1lb of body fat, you need to create a calorie deficit of approximately 3,500 calories. So if you're looking to shed that amount of weight over the course of a week, you would need to consume 500 calories per day less than your total. If you want to halve the rate of weight loss, subtract 250 calories per day from the total.

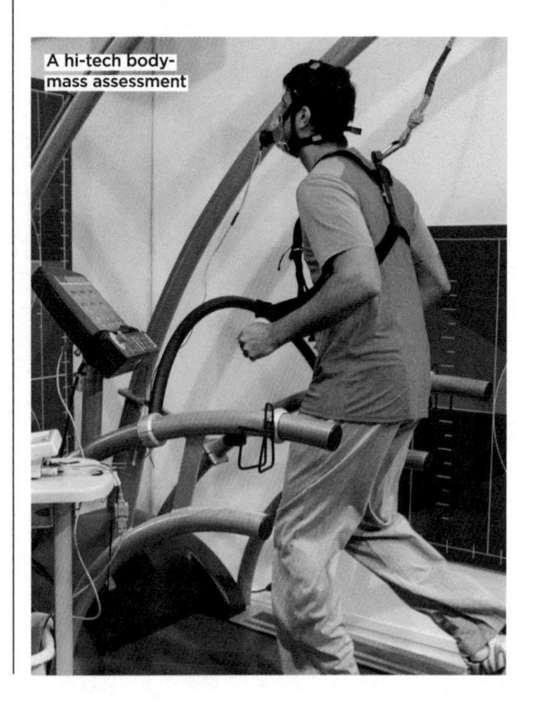

A hi-tech body-mass assessment

Determining your BMR

Many online BMR calculators use the Harris-Benedict equation to determine BMR. But over time, researchers have determined that this equation can overestimate daily calorie needs by as much as 5%, or 200 calories a day.[1] If you're counting calories, that's a lot!

We recommend that you use the Mifflin-St. Jeor equation.[2] Here's how:

YOUR BMR		SAMPLE BMR	
Height ____ Weight ____ Age ____		Woman: 5ft 4ins, 8st 8lbs (120lbs), 40 years old	
Height in ins x 2.54 =	cm	Height in ins x 2.54 =	162.56cm
Weight in lbs ÷ 2.2 =	kg	Weight in lbs ÷ 2.2 =	54.54kg
Height in cm x 6.25 =		Height in cm x 6.25 =	1,016
	minus		minus
5 x age in years =		5 x age in years =	200
	plus		plus
10 x weight in kg =		10 x weight in kg =	545.5
+ 5 for men or... - 161 for women	plus 5 or minus 161	+ 5 for men or... - 161 for women	minus 161
=	BMR	=	1,200.5 BMR

Photography: Getty Sources: 1. American Journal of Clinical Nutrition. 2. Journal of the American Dietetic Association

Factoring in your activity

Once you've determined your BMR, you have to multiply it by your physical activity level (PAL). Use this guide, from the US Institute of Medicine.[3]

Physical activity levels

PAL CATEGORY	MEAN PAL VALUE (RANGE)	EXAMPLE
Sedentary	1.25 (1.1–1.39)	You typically spend most of the day sitting.
Low level of physical activity	1.5 (1.4–1.59)	You typically spend most of the day sitting but walk around as you need to and perform activities of daily living.
Active	1.75 (1.6–1.89)	You exercise for approximately one hour a day or have a day job that's very active and requires the equivalent of walking six to eight miles per day.
Very active	2.2 (1.9–2.50)	You are a competitive athlete engaging in several hours of vigorous exercise each day.

Your weight maintenance/loss formula

FORMULA TO MAINTAIN WEIGHT		SAMPLE FORMULA	
BMR x PAL =	Calories	1,200.5 x PAL of 1.75 =	2,100.875

In order to maintain her current weight and activity level, this woman should consume 2,100 calories per day. If she wanted to lose 1lb per week, she could subtract 500 calories a day from the total and target 1,600 calories daily.

Portion help

It's way too easy to eat too much of the wrong things. Indeed, outsize portions are a common culprit in dragging down weight-loss efforts. The single-serving packages you buy or create with small zipper-lock bags have been proven to encourage portion control. But when that's impossible or impractical, try the following hints to help you downsize portions to meet your daily calorie targets.

Get your portion sizes right

Look it up

You can use a variety of calorie-tracking apps and websites to look up calorie counts of the foods you regularly eat or would like to incorporate into your diet. Using a calorie counter can help you meet your daily targets *and* make longer-term changes. Once you see that you're eating half your day's calorie portion at breakfast, you won't be able to look at that serving of eggs and bacon again.

Add it up

Don't rely on your memory. Writing down your food intake or recording it in an app or on a website can give help assure you you're staying on track. Seeing that you're near your daily calorie target will encourage you to eat a modest dinner and hold off on dessert. And every day you get a clean slate and a whole new batch of calories to work with!

Measure it

Keep measuring spoons and food scales at home or in your car so you can actually measure out the serving sizes detailed on the nutrition information label. You'll be surprised by how small some portions are.

Visualise it

If you don't always have such measuring devices handy or feel shy about carrying them around (don't worry, we understand), here are a few cues you can use to understand some common portions.

- **A phoneful of protein** A typical 85g serving of meat or fish should be about the size of the average smartphone.
- **A cricket ball of whole grains** A typical 180g serving of whole grains such as rice or quinoa is about the size of a cricket ball.
- **A tennis ball of fruit** 1 medium piece of fruit, such as an apple or orange, should be about the size of a tennis ball.
- **A golf ball of peanut butter** A typical 2tbsp serving of peanut butter or any other nut butter should be about the size of a golf ball.

Downsize your plates

Studies have shown that the smaller your plates and the more they contrast in colour with the food, the less you're likely to eat. So serve dinner on salad plates or those you'd typically use for starters. On the smaller plates, your serving size will seem abundant!

Take the guesswork out of portion sizing

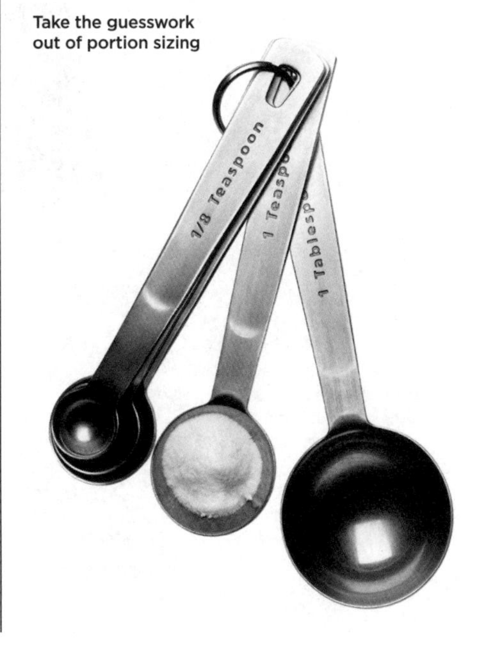

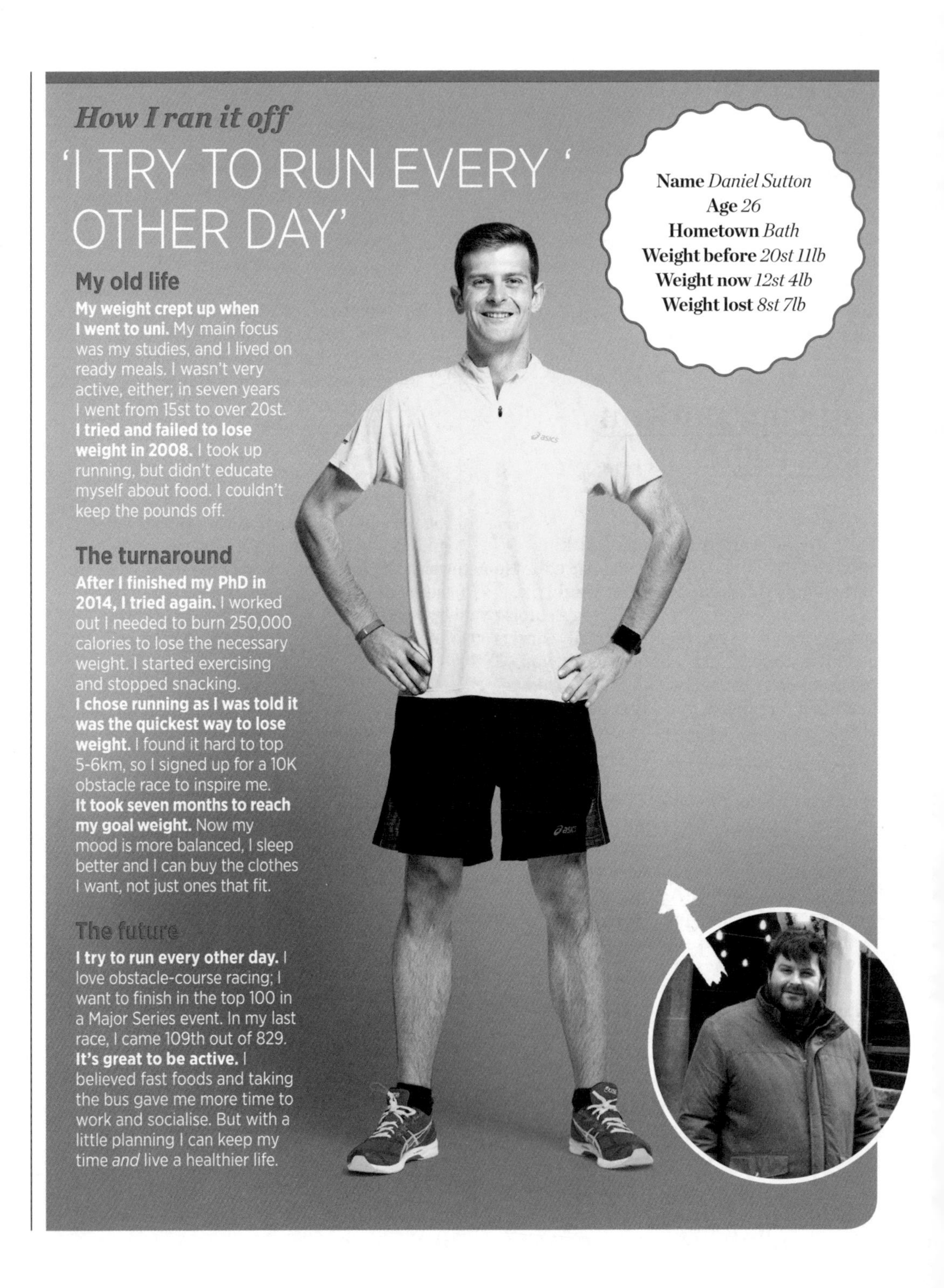

How I ran it off

'I TRY TO RUN EVERY OTHER DAY'

Name *Daniel Sutton*
Age *26*
Hometown *Bath*
Weight before *20st 11lb*
Weight now *12st 4lb*
Weight lost *8st 7lb*

My old life

My weight crept up when I went to uni. My main focus was my studies, and I lived on ready meals. I wasn't very active, either; in seven years I went from 15st to over 20st.

I tried and failed to lose weight in 2008. I took up running, but didn't educate myself about food. I couldn't keep the pounds off.

The turnaround

After I finished my PhD in 2014, I tried again. I worked out I needed to burn 250,000 calories to lose the necessary weight. I started exercising and stopped snacking.

I chose running as I was told it was the quickest way to lose weight. I found it hard to top 5-6km, so I signed up for a 10K obstacle race to inspire me.

It took seven months to reach my goal weight. Now my mood is more balanced, I sleep better and I can buy the clothes I want, not just ones that fit.

The future

I try to run every other day. I love obstacle-course racing; I want to finish in the top 100 in a Major Series event. In my last race, I came 109th out of 829.

It's great to be active. I believed fast foods and taking the bus gave me more time to work and socialise. But with a little planning I can keep my time *and* live a healthier life.

'RUNNING HAS CHANGED MY LIFE'

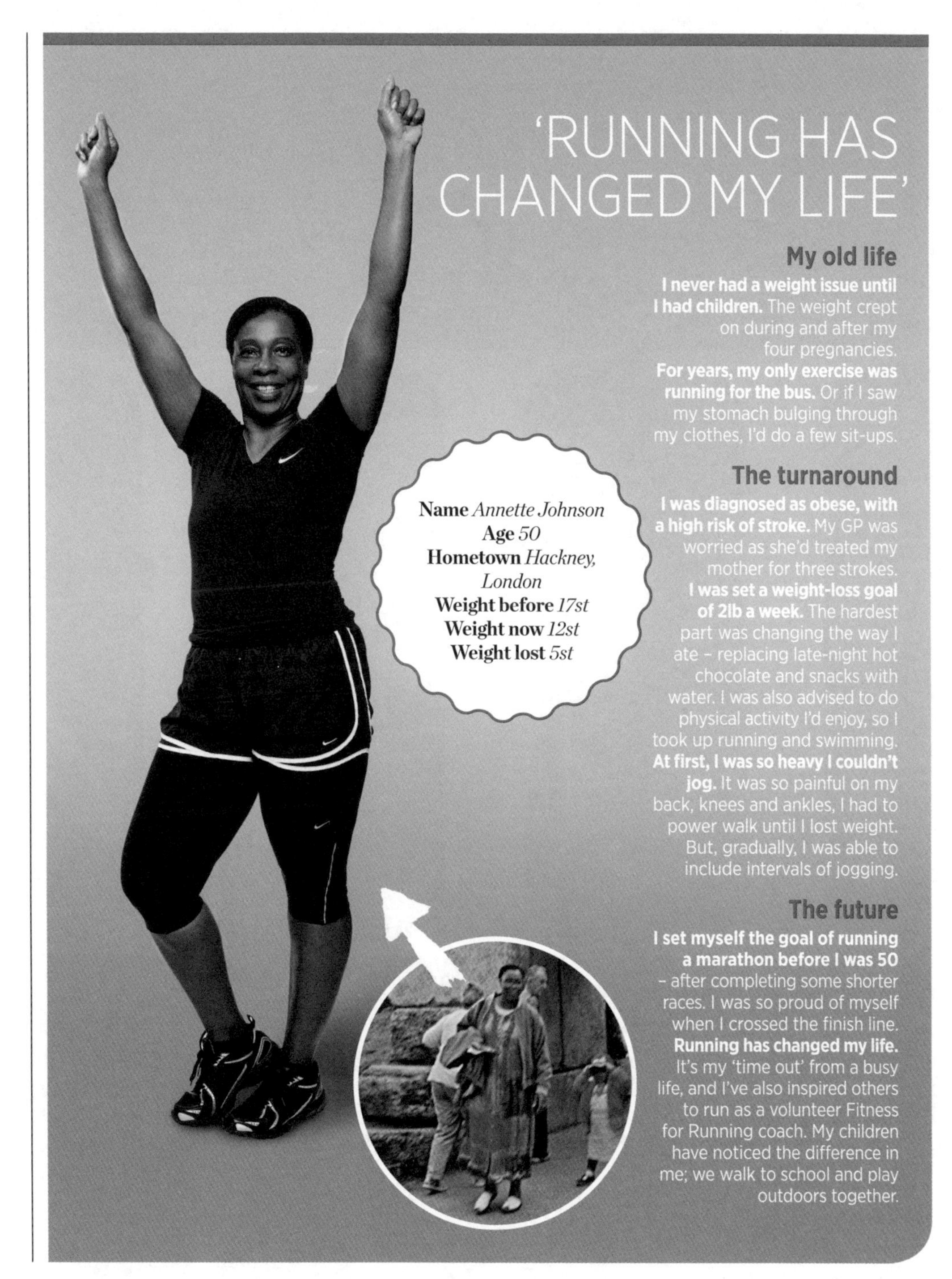

Name *Annette Johnson*
Age *50*
Hometown *Hackney, London*
Weight before *17st*
Weight now *12st*
Weight lost *5st*

My old life

I never had a weight issue until I had children. The weight crept on during and after my four pregnancies.

For years, my only exercise was running for the bus. Or if I saw my stomach bulging through my clothes, I'd do a few sit-ups.

The turnaround

I was diagnosed as obese, with a high risk of stroke. My GP was worried as she'd treated my mother for three strokes.

I was set a weight-loss goal of 2lb a week. The hardest part was changing the way I ate – replacing late-night hot chocolate and snacks with water. I was also advised to do physical activity I'd enjoy, so I took up running and swimming.

At first, I was so heavy I couldn't jog. It was so painful on my back, knees and ankles, I had to power walk until I lost weight. But, gradually, I was able to include intervals of jogging.

The future

I set myself the goal of running a marathon before I was 50 – after completing some shorter races. I was so proud of myself when I crossed the finish line.

Running has changed my life. It's my 'time out' from a busy life, and I've also inspired others to run as a volunteer Fitness for Running coach. My children have noticed the difference in me; we walk to school and play outdoors together.

Part

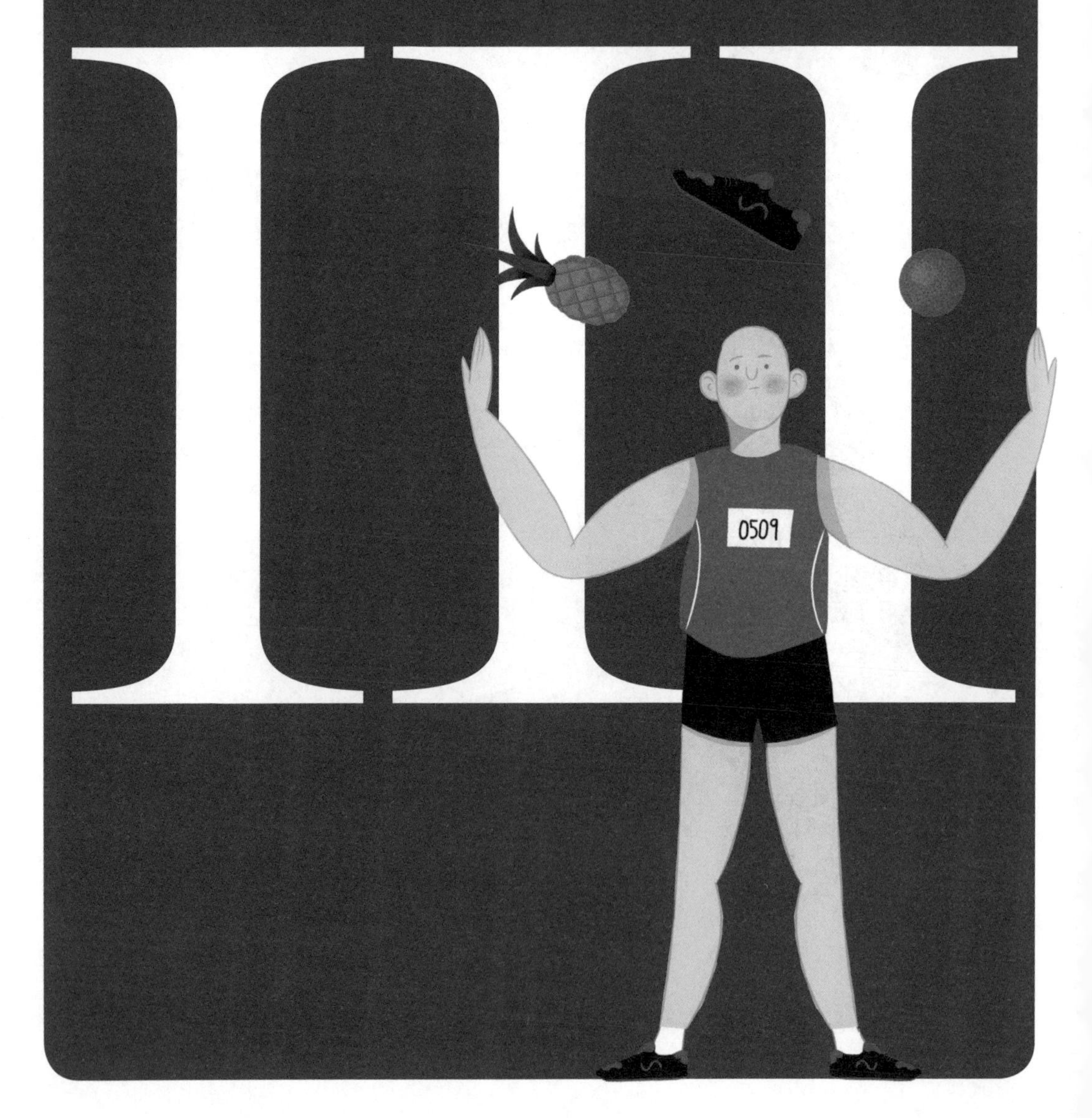

WHEN TO EAT

This section will teach you how to organise your nutrition to suit your running regime, the best times to eat, and how to manage your calorie intake before, during and after your workouts so you can run stronger and hit your goal weight. You'll also learn how to choose the foods that'll boost your energy without upsetting your stomach, so that you can fuel up without filling out.

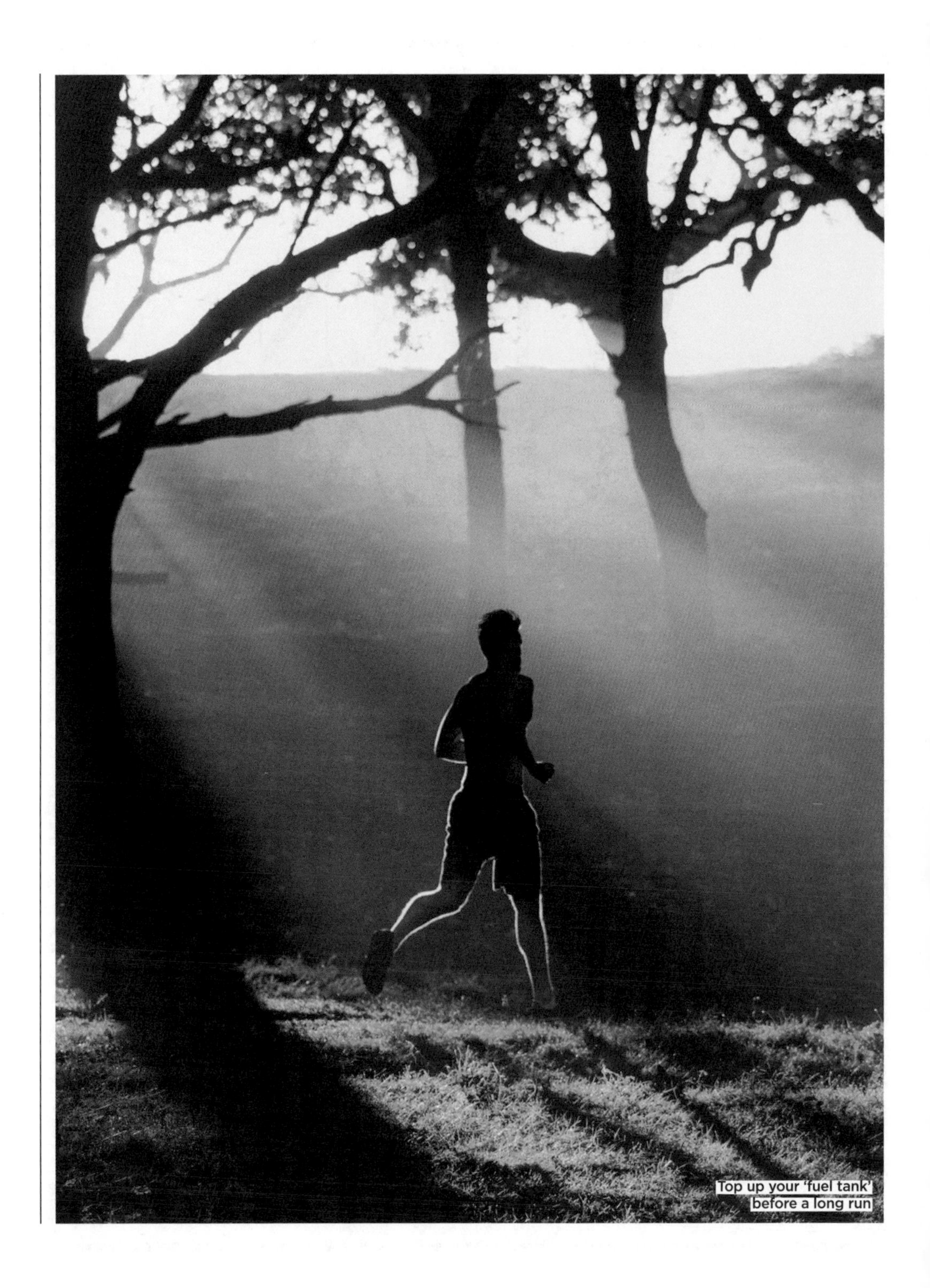

Top up your 'fuel tank' before a long run

17.

WHAT TO EAT BEFORE YOU RUN

It doesn't matter how good your genetics or your training are, what you eat and in what amount can make or break your workout. Your ideal pre-exercise eating plan depends entirely on what kind of workout you're doing. If you're heading out for an easy 30-minute run, you'll probably be fine without anything to eat; if you're planning to go faster (a tempo run or a speed session) or further (with a long run), it's best to eat first.

The perfect combo

Each runner's GI threshold is unique. Some runners are blessed with iron-clad stomachs; others can't even look at solids without feeling queasy. Over time, only you can experiment with different foods, flavours and brands to find what gives you an energy boost without upsetting your stomach.

In general, you want to keep your pre-run and pre-race meals higher in carbs – which your body quickly digests and turns into fast energy – and lower in fat, protein and fibre, which take longer to digest.

To avoid GI distress, keep your pre-run meal or snack to these per-serving limits:

- Less than 7g fibre
- Less than 10g fat
- Less than 10g protein

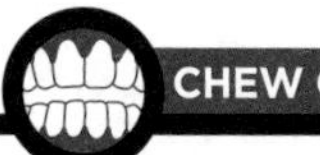

CHEW ON THIS

Fibre can help lower cholesterol and blood sugar, and lower your risk of heart disease and stroke. Plus, it can help keep your GI system in good working order. To get the benefits, men should consume 38g fibre per day, while women should aim for 25g. But steer clear of fibre right before you run; it takes longer to digest and could make for some unwanted pit stops. For pre-run meals and snacks, choose foods with less than 7g fibre per serving.

Get the timing right

When it comes to fuelling your workout, timing is everything. Before you head out for a run, you'll want something that'll give you a boost of energy without leaving you with an upset stomach on the road. In general, the bigger the meal, the more time you'll need to digest it. Each person is different, but most runners need at least 30 minutes between their meal and their run to avoid unwanted pit stops.

If your primary goal is weight loss, it's fine to head out the door for a short, easy run (less than 60 minutes) without having something to eat. If you tend to run out of energy on the road, you might consider a pre-run snack of 100 calories. After all, it's better to have 100 calories and finish that five-mile run, burning 400 calories along the way, than skip the pre-run meal in the hope of netting a higher calorie burn, but only manage two miles. If your main goal is weight loss, you might hesitate to consume a recovery snack or meal, worried about reloading the calories you worked so hard to burn. But as long as you don't overdo it, consuming carbs and protein immediately post-run can help you recover more quickly for the next workout so that you'll feel even stronger next time and you'll torch more calories. (For more on eating for recovery, see Chapter 20.)

What and how much you eat depend on the nature of your workout. Here's a guide:

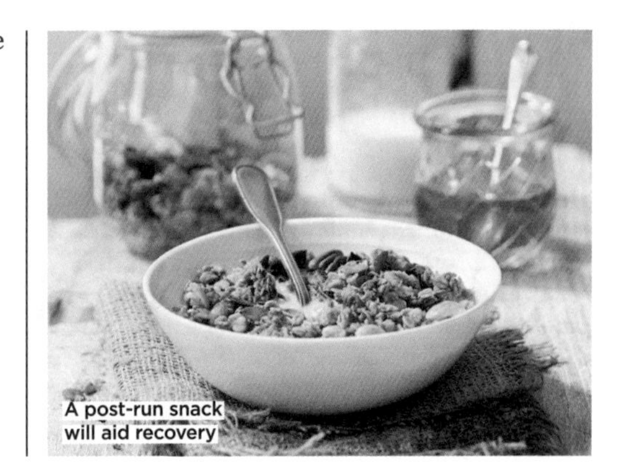
A post-run snack will aid recovery

Get your portions right

TYPE OF RUN	HOW MUCH TO EAT	WHEN TO EAT
30 minutes or less	Water is sufficient; no fuel necessary.	Drink 200-300ml, 10-20 minutes before you run.
30-60 minutes	If you're ravenous or low on energy, have a 100-200-calorie snack that's rich in carbs and low in fat and fibre. If you feel like 'training low', you can skip this snack to maximise your fat burn.	Eat and drink 30-60 minutes before you run.
60-75 minutes	Consume a 200-300-calorie snack that's high in carbs and low in fat and fibre.	Eat and drink 30-60 minutes before you run.
75 minutes or longer	Have a 200-450-calorie snack that's high in carbs. Aim for 0.5g carbs per pound of body weight for each hour before the run.	Eat and drink 60-120 minutes before you run.
Speed session (mile repeats, tempo runs)	Have a 100-200-calorie high-carb snack if it's been more than three hours since your last meal. Avoid 'training low' for these sessions; you'll miss the opportunity to build your fitness and maximise calorie burn.	Eat a full meal 2-3 hours before you run. If you need to have a snack, eat it 30-60 minutes before your workout.

Ideas for pre-run meals and snacks

Here are some nutrient-packed high-carb, low-fat, low-fibre meals and snacks that can provide the energy you need to run your best for a variety of different workouts. Use this as a guide, but listen to your body. Each individual is unique in terms of digestion time, so you may need to eat closer to your workout or a few hours earlier than what's prescribed here.

Eating before one-hour workouts

If you're exercising for up to an hour at an easy level of effort, it's perfectly OK to run on empty. But having a small snack or meal ahead of time may help you feel energised and strong throughout the workout. The snacks listed below are also ideal before shorter, quality workouts such as speed sessions and hill work.

Pre-run meals

FOOD	CALORIES	IDEAL TO EAT...	EXTRA NUTRIENTS FOR RUNNERS
40g low-fibre cereal with 250ml skimmed milk	195	30 minutes before workout	The milk provides protein; both the cereal and the milk have carbs to keep you energised.
3 fig rolls	192	30-60 minutes before workout	Easy to digest and packed with high-energy carbs, vitamins and minerals.
75g berries with 100g low-fat cottage cheese	160	60 minutes before workout	The berries offer carbs for energy, while the cottage cheese provides calcium, potassium and vitamin D – all of which come in handy when training.
1 digestive biscuit with 1 tsp honey	94	30 minutes before a workout or a shorter speed session	Packed with carbs to keep you energised for your workout.
175g low-fat fruit yogurt with 1 medium peach	275	60 minutes before workout	This snack has calcium, vitamin D and potassium to support bone and muscle health, plus antioxidants to boost immune function.

Eating before 60-90-minute workouts

Going longer? You'll need more fuel so you finish the workout strong and don't become tired out before you're done.

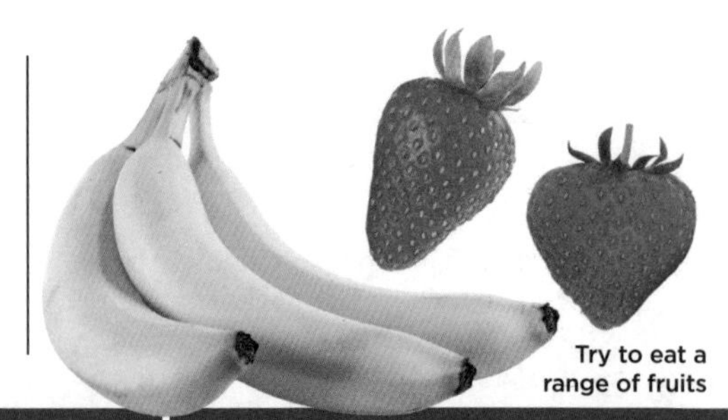

Try to eat a range of fruits

FOOD	CALORIES	IDEAL TO EAT...	EXTRA NUTRIENTS FOR RUNNERS
1 medium banana and 1 tbsp nut butter	200	1 hour before workout	The potassium and fluid in the fruit help you stay hydrated, while the nut butter offers heart-healthy fat and carbs.
1 bagel with 1 tbsp nut butter and 1 tbsp jam or honey	390	1 hour before workout	The bagel and toppings offer lasting energy so you can stay strong for longer.
120g pinhead oats with skimmed milk, topped with 170g sliced strawberries	256	1 hour before workout	Packed with carbs and B vitamins, this is an excellent choice for pre- or post-run recovery.
50g pretzels with 2 tbsp hummus	263	1 hour before workout	The pretzels provide easy-to-digest carbs for fast energy, plus sodium to keep you hydrated; the hummus offers iron for strength, plus protein.
2 whole-grain waffles (frozen) with 2 tbsp maple syrup	270	1 hour before workout	The syrup and waffles offer fast-digesting carbs to provide an energy boost; the syrup also has B vitamins to boost energy and bolster recovery.
Sandwich made with 2 slices whole-grain bread, 1 medium banana, 1 tbsp peanut butter	360	60-90 minutes before workout	All the ingredients provide carbs for energy. The peanut butter offers extra protein to fend off hunger, and the banana provides potassium to help stave off muscle cramps.
50g sweet and salty pretzel pieces dipped in 1 tbsp natural peanut butter	245	1 hour before workout	The pretzels provide carbs for energy and sodium to help keep you hydrated; the peanut butter offers protein to help muscles recover.

500ml sports drink	125	15-30 minutes before (or during) workout	Provides fluids and electrolytes to help keep you hydrated. Plus, if you're pressed for time or can't tolerate solid foods before a run, sports drinks can be a great option because they're digested quickly.
4 rich tea biscuits dipped in 1 tbsp peanut butter	250	30-60 minutes before workout	The biscuits are easy to digest and provide carbs for long-lasting energy. Peanut butter has vitamins and minerals such as potassium, and has been linked to a lower risk of coronary heart disease.
30g Cheerios with 1 cup skimmed milk and 1 medium banana	300	45-60 minutes before workout	The cereal and milk provide carbs for an energy boost. The banana provides potassium to support your muscles and the milk offers an extra boost of calcium for bone health.
75g deli turkey wrapped in a flour tortilla with 70g shredded veg	275	90 minutes before workout	Long-lasting energy with extra protein to aid muscle recovery.

What to drink before you run

Dehydration can drain your energy and ruin your workout, but so can a sloshy stomach or numerous wee breaks. So sip on calorie-free fluids throughout the day. That way you won't be tempted to quaff huge quantities of fluids immediately pre-run, which will leave you feeling queasy and prompt you to interrupt your run for pit stops.

In most cases, water is the best choice. But if it's hot out, you're a salty sweater or you're heading out for more than an hour's run, it'll probably benefit you to try a low-calorie sports drink, as this can provide electrolytes to aid your hydration and carbs to boost your energy. Look for a product that provides 25-50 calories per serving and vital electrolytes such as sodium and potassium.

Clearing the system

Many runners like to clear out their GI system (ie, go to the toilet) before they set out. It'll help you feel lighter and avoid pit stops. This is where the pre-run coffee, which also provides caffeine for an energy boost, can be useful. (For more on the benefits of caffeine, see Chapter 8.) But any hot beverage can help you move your bowels – including herbal tea or hot water with lemon. Allow at least 20 minutes for it to get through your system.

If this isn't as effective as you'd like, you might consider boosting the fibre content of your everyday diet. While you want to avoid packing in fibre just before a run, if you have enough in your general diet, your GI system will move more efficiently pre-run. Through meals and snacks, men should aim to consume 38g fibre per day, while women need at least 25g. For more on hydration, see Chapter 8.

Race-day fuelling for 5Ks and 10Ks

Runners put a lot time into preparing their legs and lungs for race day, but often underestimate the impact of what they eat on how well they race. If you show up at the starting line with an upset stomach or an empty fuel tank, or have to make a series of unplanned pit stops, it's going to be tough to unleash your potential – even if you're at your peak level of fitness.

For shorter races, such as 5Ks and 10Ks, there's no need to carb-load; that should be reserved for longer races – half marathons or marathons, for example – that typically take 90 minutes or more. (More on carb-loading later in this chapter.) At the same time, you don't want to start the race hungry or drained of energy. Here's how you can fuel up for a peak performance while making sure your stomach doesn't undo you on the race course.

Late-afternoon/ evening races

When your race is late in the day, you need to have a high-quality breakfast and lunch and sip fluids throughout the day so you're hydrated and well fuelled at race time.

Breakfast In the morning, consume a carb-rich meal with a small amount of protein. Good options include porridge with fruit, low-fat yogurt topped with fruit and granola, or dry breakfast cereal topped with dairy, almond, or soy milk. Or try a bagel topped with a scrambled egg, plus some fruit. Avoid cereals with more than 10g fibre per serving.

Lunch Avoid foods that are high in fat and protein, which take longer to digest (aim for less than 10g of each per serving). Great choices include pasta with tomato sauce, plus 250ml skimmed milk, or a turkey sandwich with a side of pretzels and a bottle of water.

Pre-race snack If you feel hungry en route to the race, have a snack that's rich in carbs but won't weigh you down. To avoid GI distress, keep it under 200 calories. You might grab a small banana, a few cream crackers or even some energy chews. If none of these appeals, reach for a sports bar; just make sure it has less than 10g each fat and protein, and less than 7g fibre. A sports drink can both boost your energy and carbs and help keep you hydrated.

Morning races

What you eat on the day before a morning race will affect how energetic you feel and how calm your stomach is. Aim for small, carb-rich meals throughout the day and avoid trying any new foods. Resist the temptation to gorge on carbs in the evening, as that could get in the way of a good night's sleep.

On race morning, have a light breakfast (200-300 calories) one to two hours before the event. The calories should mostly come from whole, unprocessed carbs, and the meal should be low in fibre and fat (under 7g each). It's also a good idea to avoid spicy stuff, which could upset your stomach. Try a bagel with a small apple plus 250ml sports drink; an English muffin topped with 2 tbsp jam and a piece of fruit, or a bowl of porridge topped with raisins and brown sugar.

Drink plenty of fluids, too: aim to consume 450-600ml, two to three hours before the race, and another 200-300ml 20 minutes before. It's OK to have coffee, tea or a sports drink if you regularly drink these before your runs and they don't upset your stomach.

Carb-loading for longer races

Many runners train hard for months preparing for a long-distance race, then undo all that hard work in the days before the race by eating the wrong things, or not eating enough

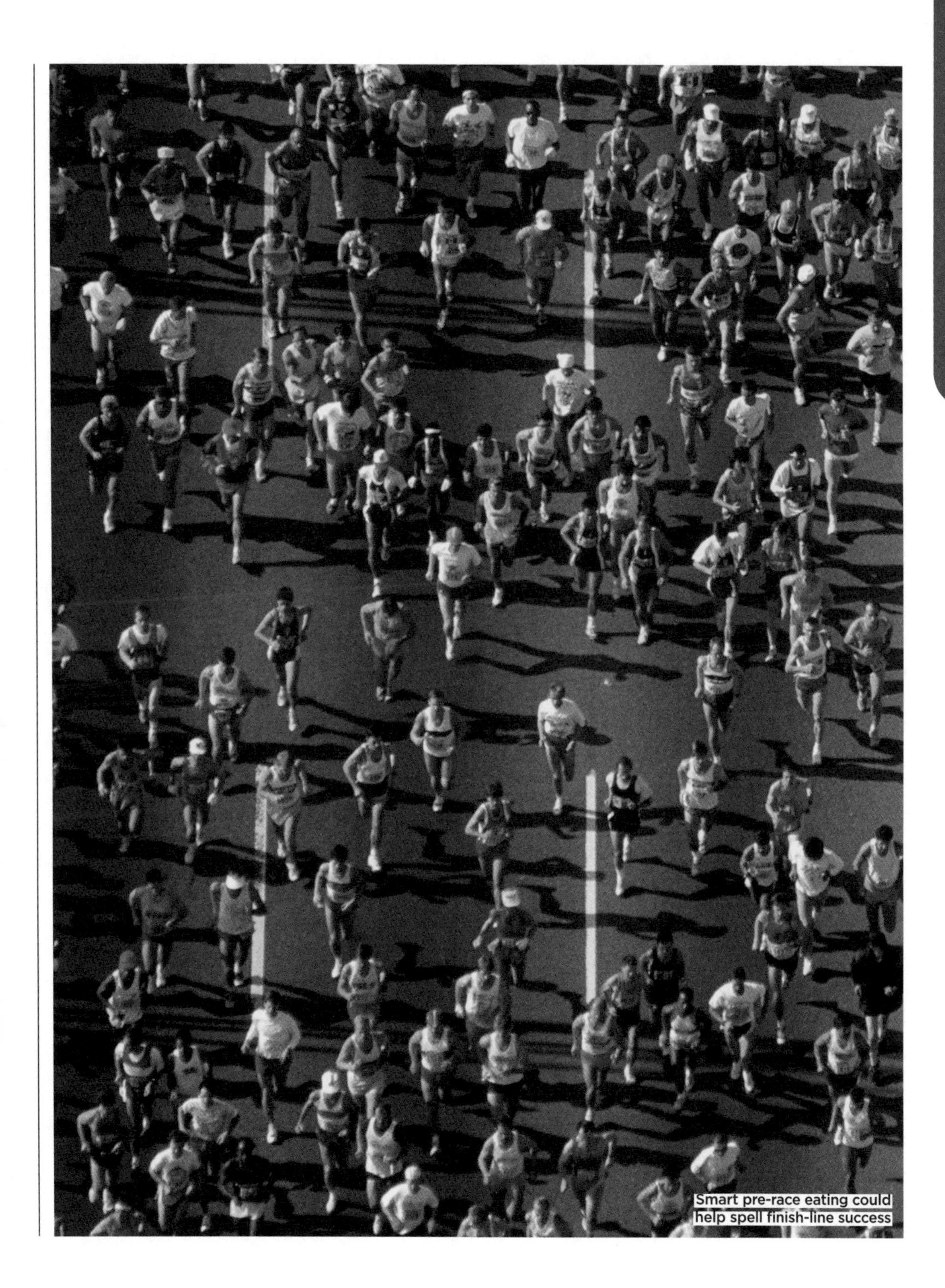

Smart pre-race eating could help spell finish-line success

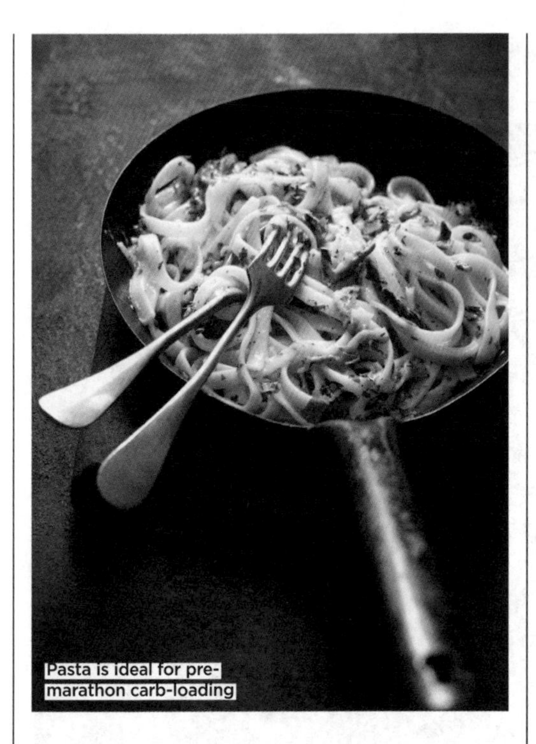
Pasta is ideal for pre-marathon carb-loading

of the right things. The term 'carb-loading' is bandied around a lot – typically any time a runner reaches for a bagel or is looking to rationalise a second heaped helping of pasta. But carb-loading isn't just about overloading on pasta and dessert the night before a race; it actually takes longer, requires more calories and is more complex than most people think.

Technically, carb-loading is the practice of loading the muscles with carbs in the three days leading up to a long race. The idea is to fill up your body's fuel stores so at the start your muscles are fully loaded but your GI system doesn't feel stuffed. It's like topping up with petrol before embarking on a long road trip.

As well as boosting your carb intake during these days before the race, you'll want to reduce how long you spend on your feet. As you taper in the days and weeks before your race, the carbs you consume will be stockpiled in the muscles. And the time off your feet lets your muscles fully recover and fill up on fuel so they're fresh and ready to go come race day.

Carb-loading for a full marathon is the best way to increase the chances of running your best race; for a half marathon, carb-loading is only marginally necessary, while for any run of less than 90 minutes, it's totally unnecessary, and could even hurt your chances of running well on race day.

You can be as casual or as precise as you like with carb-loading. Whatever approach you take, it's important to take good notes throughout the process so you have a record of what works and what doesn't for future races.

The casual carb-load

In the week before the marathon (and the three days before a half), the vast majority – up to 70% – of your calories should come from wholesome carbs, eg, bagel, pasta, rice or cereal. The balance of your calories should come from wholesome, low-fat, low-fibre foods, and lean proteins such as chicken, fish, beans and legumes. Avoid new or very spicy foods.

The calculated carb-load

If you want to take a more exacting approach to carb-loading, follow this proven formula for carb-loading success:

MARATHONS

7 days before the race: Consume 2.3g carbs per lb of body weight each day.
1-3 days before the race: Consume 3.6-5.5g carbs per lb of body weight each day.

HALF MARATHONS

1 to 3 days before the race: Consume 2.5-4g carbs per lb of body weight each day.

As long as you're trained to cover 13.1 miles, you should be able to make it through a half-marathon without carb-loading – as long as you have a few carb-rich meals in the days before the race and refuel at regular intervals while you're on the road. That said, carb-loading before a half marathon will certainly improve your chances of running fast. If you, say, forget to carb-load a few days out or simply can't stomach a high-carb diet in the days leading up to the race, you can taper in the three days before the event, then, the day before, aim to get most of your calories from wholesome carbs.

Here are some general rules to follow for both approaches.

Cut back on protein and fat To avoid starting the race overly stuffed and feeling sick, cut back on protein and fat while carb-loading. You may be eating as many calories as before, but a larger proportion will come from carbs, and less from protein and fat.

Be ready for side effects As fun as it might be to imagine loading up on all the carbs you can eat, especially if you've been following an otherwise low-carb plan, there are certain side effects – slight weight gain; stiffness due to muscles being fully stocked with glycogen – you might not find so pleasant.

Ditch the scale During a carb-load, you can expect to gain up to 4lbs. Water gets stored along with the glycogen when you eat high-carb foods. And many carb-rich foods are high in sodium, which will cause water retention. It can also make you feel bloated and heavy. The extra fluids you might be drinking to stay hydrated can also add weight. Resist the urge to get on the scales or to cut back your calories because you're running less.

Do a dress rehearsal. Loading up on carbs – especially if you're not accustomed to it – can feel downright uncomfortable. Many people report feeling stiff and sluggish during the carb-load. That's why it's best to practise this process at some point during your race preparation, in the days leading up to one of your longest runs. If you get used to it during training, it's one less worry during race week.

Embrace the process. If you're trying to reverse years of overeating, or going overboard on carbs, the idea of carb-loading to run fast can be tough advice to swallow. You may be worried about reigniting a craving you've worked hard to quell through dieting. But carb-loading *isn't* about letting loose and eating with abandon all the junk you've been trying to avoid; it's just a matter of replacing the protein and fat you'd usually have with healthy whole grains, starchy vegetables, fruit and low-fat dairy. And it's the final crucial step to unleashing your potential on race day.

Carb-loading has been found to postpone fatigue and extend the amount of time you can maintain your pace. If you skip it, you risk ruining your race and wasting all that hard work and time you put into preparing for it.

Once race day is behind you and you've had your celebratory meal, you can return to the healthy-eating practices that have helped you achieve your targets both on the race course and on the bathroom scales.

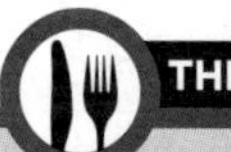

THE TAKEAWAY

Fuel up on low-fat, low-fibre fuel pre-run. Your pre-run meals and snacks should be high in carbs. Limit yourself pre-run to less than 10g fat, 7g fibre and 10g protein per serving.

Plan ahead and leave plenty of time. Hydrate well in the days and hours before a race. But remember, drinking loads immediately prior to a run is a bad idea and can lead to GI distress. Sip fluids throughout the day and give your body time to process them. A hot beverage 20-30 minutes before your run can help you move your bowels.

Do a practice run. While training, try a carb-loading 'dress rehearsal' so you get accustomed to the kinds of discomfort involved with eating a carb-rich diet. And try a variety of pre-run meals and snacks to figure out which give you the biggest energy boost without upsetting your stomach.

Fuel up with whole foods. These offer carbs for energy, plus nutrients and minerals, without the added sweeteners and fillers that could upset your stomach.

18.

THE WAR ON GI DISTRESS

Aside from being intensely uncomfortable, GI distress can be highly embarrassing and upsetting – especially if you run into trouble miles away from home. Just one bad experience with cramps, diarrhoea, a sloshy stomach, nausea or an emergency pit stop can make a runner too nervous to race, or even run with friends. But if you do tend to suffer stomach troubles on the run, you're not alone. Studies suggest that up to half of all runners are prone.[1]

One reason this happens is that when you run, the majority of blood flow is diverted away from the GI tract to get oxygen-rich blood to the working legs and muscles, and the skin. The tougher the run, the more blood is diverted. In addition, the jarring that running involves can further disrupt natural GI function. On top of that, dehydration – a particular risk when it's hot and humid – can add even more stress to your GI tract.

> Up to half of all runners are prone to GI distress

That's why it's best to stay hydrated throughout the day, leave plenty of time between your pre-run meal and your run, and make sure anything you do eat is low in fat and fibre, as these take longer to digest.

In a study published in *Sports Medicine*, researchers identified some of the most common culprits when it comes to GI distress, and provided these tips to avoid them.[2]

1/ Avoid high-fibre foods for several days before your event. In the lead-up to the race, choose foods with less than 7g fibre, 10g fat and 10g protein per serving.

2/ Avoid aspirin and NSAIDs such as ibuprofen... especially if you've had stomach issues while running. Both could help trigger GI distress.

3/ Avoid dehydration. Practise drinking while training to improve your comfort with fluids on board. But don't overdrink in races simply because there's so much handed out.

4/ Avoid overly sweetened drinks, gels, bars, etc. Increased sugar means increased risk of stomach distress – the gut can only process so many carbohydrates at once. If you opt for a sports drink, choose one with no more than 14-17g sugar per 250ml portion. If you consume an energy gel or sports beans, wash them down with water. If you try to chase an energy gel with a sports drink, you risk overloading your

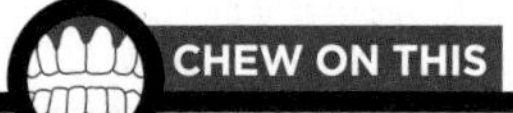

Wheat, dairy, fibre, artificial sweeteners and acidic foods can all irritate the gut. If you're having trouble with GI distress, try eliminating these ingredients and then keep detailed notes about how those changes affected the way you felt on the run.

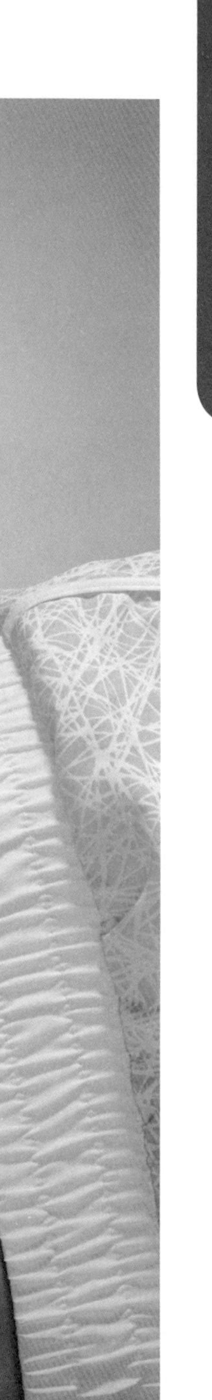
Part III | When to eat | GI distress

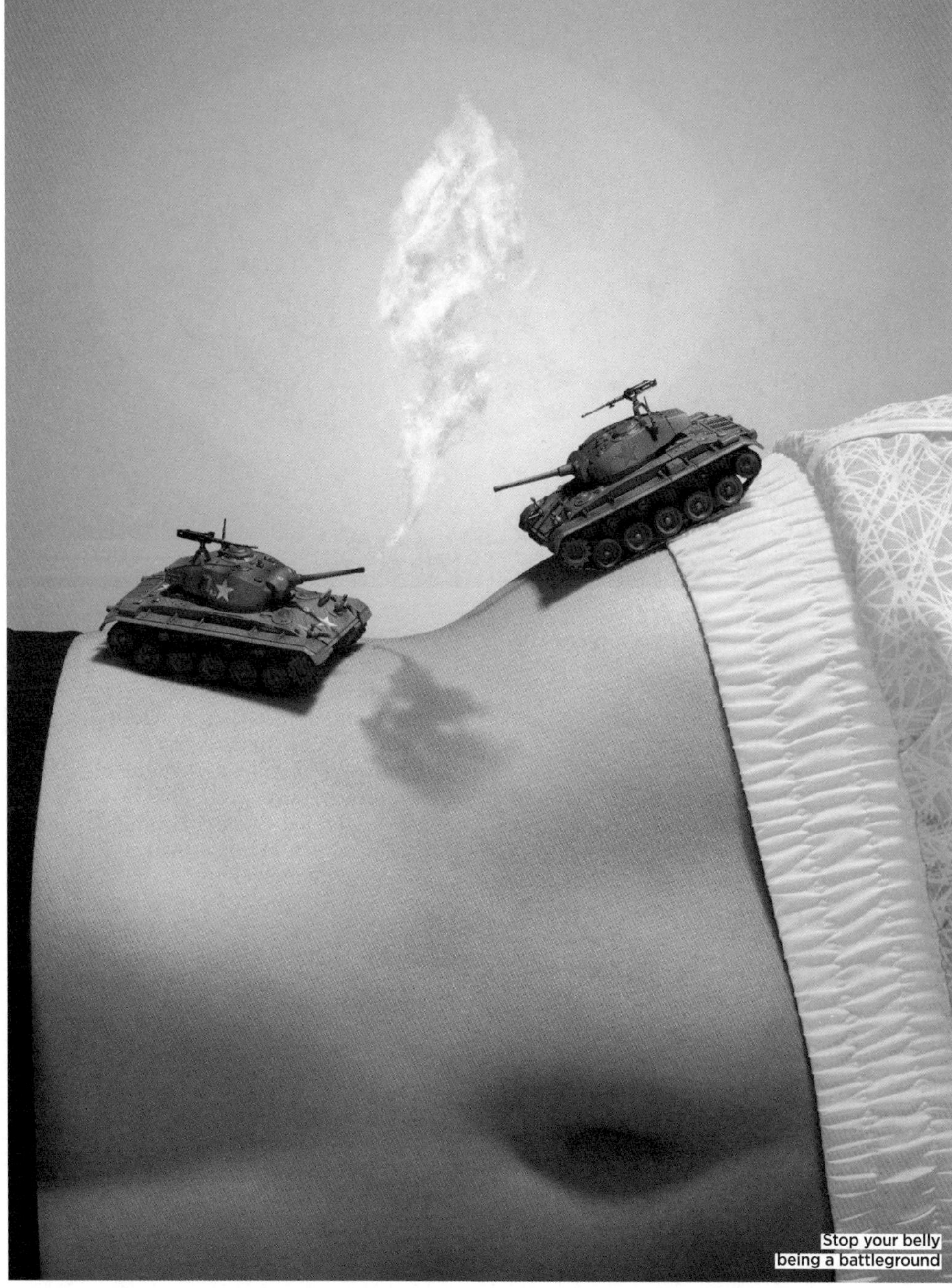
Stop your belly
being a battleground

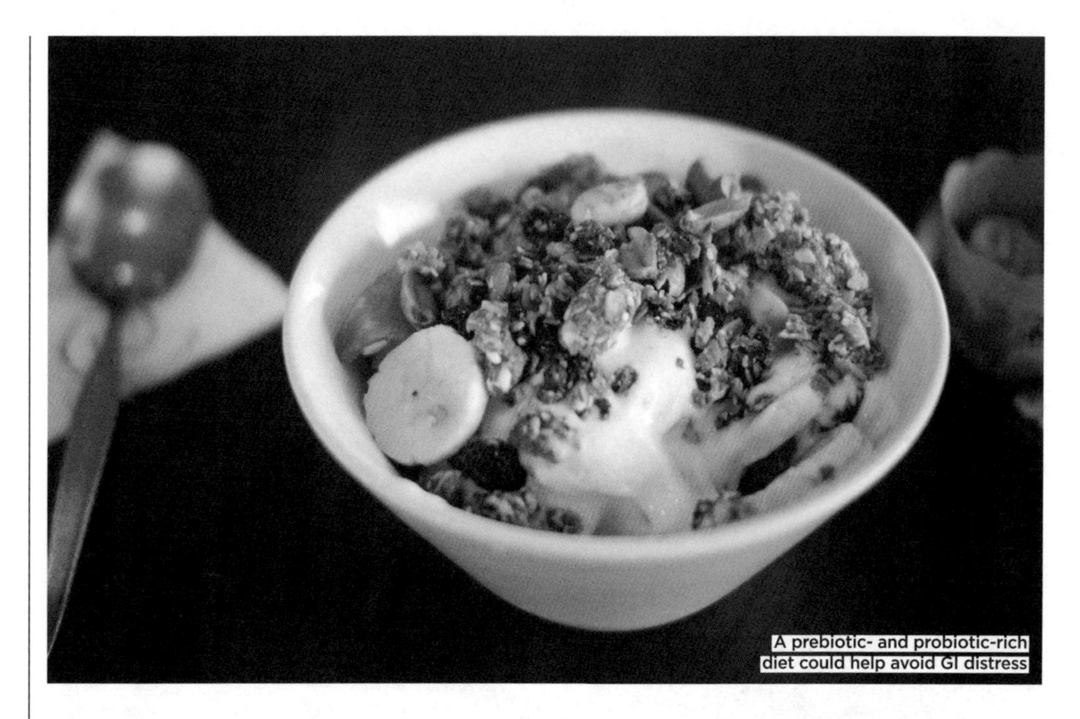
A prebiotic- and probiotic-rich diet could help avoid GI distress

gut, which could necessitate an emergency pit stop during the race.

5/ If you've had problems in the past, experiment with different foods during training. Try a variety of brands, flavours and foods to figure out what gives you a boost without upsetting your stomach.

Beyond food: prebiotics and probiotics

If you change your diet and still have problems, you might consider products with prebiotics and probiotics. These help strengthen your gut, boost your immunity and ultimately allow you to spend less time running for a bathroom. In addition to providing GI relief, whole foods that naturally contain prebiotics and probiotics tend to be nutrient dense, containing antioxidants, vitamins, minerals and phytochemicals that help you get stronger and more efficient.

Prebiotics stimulate the growth of beneficial bacteria in the gut to balance out the blend of helpful and harmful bacteria in the gastrointestinal tract. Common forms of prebiotics include fructooligosaccharides, galactooligosaccharides and inulin (also called chicory root or chicory root fibre). Go easy, though: research suggests that eating too much inulin can increase stomach distress.

You can take supplements or you can find prebiotics in natural foods, including onions, leeks, bananas, garlic, asparagus, soybeans, wholewheat foods and artichokes. Aim for a variety of these foods every day to help keep the GI tract healthy.

Probiotics enhance and replenish the good bacteria in your body that can be weakened by stress, illness, antibiotics or surgery. They're often used to treat diarrhoea, irritable bowel syndrome and inflammatory bowel disease. The two most common forms of probiotic are lactobacillus and bifidobacterium; you're likely to find them in yogurt and kefir, both of which contain calcium and protein.

When it's not about what you eat

In some cases, GI distress continues even when you correct your pre-run eating regime. While your diet leading up to and even during a run certainly affects the GI system, certain conditions and medications can irritate the bowels and cause problems on the road.

Crohn's disease This chronic inflammatory disease involves the small or large intestine and causes diarrhoea, narrowing of the intestine, malabsorption of nutrients, and the need for medical intervention. If you have symptoms of Crohn's, or a history of autoimmune diseases in your family that may be related to your GI distress, see your GP.

Irritable bowel syndrome (IBS) Runners with IBS typically complain of diarrhoea, constipation or abdominal pain, along with bloating, gas and highly irregular bowel movements. Some find it difficult to control the bowels and urine flow, especially during intense activity such as running. IBS causes no obvious tissue damage or inflammation; often the GI system is just sensitive to the presence, composition and volume of foods.

Runner's colitis This is an inflammation of the colon that can strike runners during or after longer and intense runs. The symptoms include severe cramping, diarrhoea, and runny and bloody stools. Symptoms can start in the hours after the run and last for days. Despite the prevalence of this condition, researchers still don't fully understand why it occurs.

Runner's trots If you suffer from diarrhoea on the run, it may be caused by diet, certain medications, weak pelvic-floor muscles or just the physical stress of running. It's a good idea to see a doctor to rule out any other potential causes.

Belching, flatulence, heartburn and diarrhoea All these are common among runners. Usually they're related to diet or the physiological changes that happen while exercising. Some runners report that their GI problems are due to pre-race nerves. If you're prey to any of these annoying symptoms, think about what you consumed in the 24 hours before the run. Too much fat, fibre or caffeine? Did you try a new spice? Some people find chocolate and citrus cause heartburn; for others, carbonated beverages can cause belching and flatulence. It may take some detective work to find the culprit.

Weak pelvic-floor muscles Especially common among mothers, this can make it difficult to control the bowels, especially on the run. If you've had children and suffer these symptoms, talk to your doctor. There may be exercises you can do to strengthen this area.

Medications Any medication could lead to nausea, diarrhoea and other GI symptoms, especially if they're new or in an altered dosage. If you think anything you're taking may be leading to GI distress, talk to your doctor about alternatives or whether it's possible to avoid these particular side effects while still getting any treatment you need.

THE TAKEAWAY

Shop around.
Try different foods and brands of mid-run fuel to find which ones give you a boost without upsetting your stomach. Stick with what works. Don't try anything new on race day.

Find the culprit.
If you've eliminated all possible dietary culprits and are still experiencing problems, talk to your doctor about whether any medical problems or medications may be leading to your GI distress.

Always be prepared.
Carry a few tissues or wet wipes in a ziplock bag on the run and pin it to your shorts or stuff it in a pocket. If you've got to go, do so ASAP to avoid further discomfort and irritation. Just in case, plan running routes that pass by public toilets.

19.

REFUELLING ON THE ROAD

When you're running to lose weight, refuelling while you're exercising can seem like defeating the purpose. Why would you restock the calories you're burning by consuming gels, blocks, beans and sports drinks?

But if you're running for more than an hour and you don't refuel while you're on the road, there's a good chance you'll be forced to cut your run short because you've run out of energy. Consuming carbs during a long workout has been proven to delay fatigue, improve endurance and fend off that negative inner voice that tells you you can't do it.

Hitting the wall when running a race can be devastating

And if you do run out of energy before you finish your run (often called 'hitting the wall' or 'bonking'), it can take days for your body – and your ego – to recover. Hitting the wall during a race you spent months or years preparing for can be devastating. We've heard from many runners who've experienced just that – a typical letter goes something like this:

'I was out for my long run. I was fine until about two-thirds of the way through, and then I just hit the wall. First I had to slow down, then I had to stop. What happened?'

Luckily, the wall is usually pretty easy to avoid by refuelling on the road at regular intervals. Here's everything you need to know...

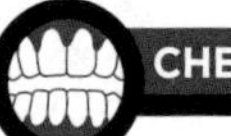

CHEW ON THIS

Be sure to wash down each gel, chew or block with water, which will help with digestion. Do *not* use a sports drink: your body can digest only so many carbs at once, and trying to wash down a gel with a sports drink is likely to send you running in search of a toilet.

The 75-minute rule

For any run of 75 minutes or more, you'll need to refuel on the go. You want to aim for 30-60g carbs per hour, beginning shortly after you set off, before you become hungry or starved for energy. Hitting the wall can be hard on the body. And if you wait until you run out of steam or your stomach is growling, it'll be too late to recover and bounce back. Refuelling at regular intervals – every 15-30 minutes – will keep your energy levels stable and help you avoid the blood-sugar crashes and spikes that could ruin your run.

It's important to nail down nutrition during training runs, because whatever works for you then is what should work for you on race day. Determining what gives you a boost without upsetting your stomach can take some trial and error; you may need to try out different brands, flavours and forms of fuel – gels, blocks, beans, chews, bars... and even real food. Each sports food has its own proprietary blend of ingredients, and each can affect you in radically different ways.

Experiment during training runs and note down what works and what doesn't. If you're preparing for a marathon or a half marathon, find out what will be provided on the race course. Try that out on training runs so you know if it sits well with you.

If you don't refuel, chances are you won't finish your run

If you don't refuel on the road, chances are you won't be able to finish your run. And if you're training for a long-distance event you're missing a key opportunity to develop the endurance you'll need on race day.

How electrolytes affect your weigh-in

Sports nutrition products contain both carbs and electrolytes to keep you well fuelled on a long run. The carbs give you energy; electrolytes such as sodium and potassium help your muscles work properly, but they also aid water retention. While under normal circumstances water retention is something to avoid, in this context it's a good thing, because the more fluid your body retains, the better hydrated you will be on the run. (Remember, dehydration can cause fatigue.)

But that fluid you're retaining *will* drive up the numbers on the scales (roughly 500ml fluid will add 1lb). So if you step on the scales after a 20-mile run – something we wouldn't recommend – your weight might have gone up. Try not to stress about it; within about 48 hours, these fluids will be flushed out of your system. But to avoid being disheartened when weighing in, you might want to skip the scales for a day or two after a long run. In short, there's no need to put your self-esteem through a beating when ultimately you're making all the right moves for weight loss!

Fuelling up with whole foods

For some people, specialist sports foods and drinks just won't do. Luckily, plenty of real-food alternatives can fuel you up just as well. Here are some rules to follow.

Keep it high in carbs and low in fat, fibre and protein. Beef jerky or a nut-heavy trail mix is not a good idea. While everyone's gut is different in terms of what it can tolerate, when it comes to fat, fibre and protein, opt for foods that contain less than 3-5g of each per serving. Start there and see how you feel. You might be able to tolerate more.

Consider its portability. Be sure the food is easy to carry on the run. While a bowl of spaghetti might be a great fuel source of fuel, lugging it with you isn't exactly practical.

Aim for 30-60g carbs per hour. Just as with sports foods, you should aim to consume 30-60g carbs during each hour of a long run. If your 'real' foods fall a little short, consider adding in some sports drink or maybe a sports chew or two. For a list of 'real' foods that meet the right criteria see the table opposite.

Match your fuel to your runs

The longer you're running the more carbs you should consume each hour. So if you're doing a 75-minute run, try consuming 30g carbs per hour. If you're heading out for 150 minutes, aim closer to 60g carbs per hour.

Each runner is unique in terms of how many carbs they need to stay energised. If you're new to long runs and refuelling on the go, start with 30g carbs per hour and see how you feel. You might finish your runs feeling strong, or find that 45g carbs per hour works better. If you follow a high-carb diet most of the time

Eating on the run

FOOD	CALORIES, CARBS AND FIBRE
3 fig rolls	195 calories, 37g carbs, 1.5g fibre
1 small box raisins (42.5g)	129 calories, 34g carbs, 2g fibre
160g mashed sweet potato (put in a zip-lock bag and tear a hole in the corner when ready to eat)	125 calories, 29g carbs, 4g fibre
45g dried sour cherries	133 calories, 32g carbs, 1g fibre
1 medium peeled and sliced apple	77 calories, 21g carbs, 2g fibre
25g low-fat bagel chips	128 calories, 19g carbs, 1g fibre
25g hard pretzels (go for extra-salty varieties if you're a salty sweater)	108 calories, 23g carbs, 1g fibre
1 large banana (try freezing it the night before and carrying it in a fuel belt or hydration pack. It will change colour, but if you consume it early in the run it shouldn't be too mushy. You can also mash a banana and carry it as you would the mashed sweet potato)	121 calories, 31g carbs, 3.5g fibre
Half a sandwich with 1 slice white bread, 1 tbsp natural peanut butter, 1 tbsp jam	220 calories, 30g carbs, 2g fibre
1 pouch apple sauce, original or mixed with other fruits (90g)	40–60 calories, 10–16g carbs, 2g fibre
25g boiled sweets	112 calories, 28g carbs, 0g fibre

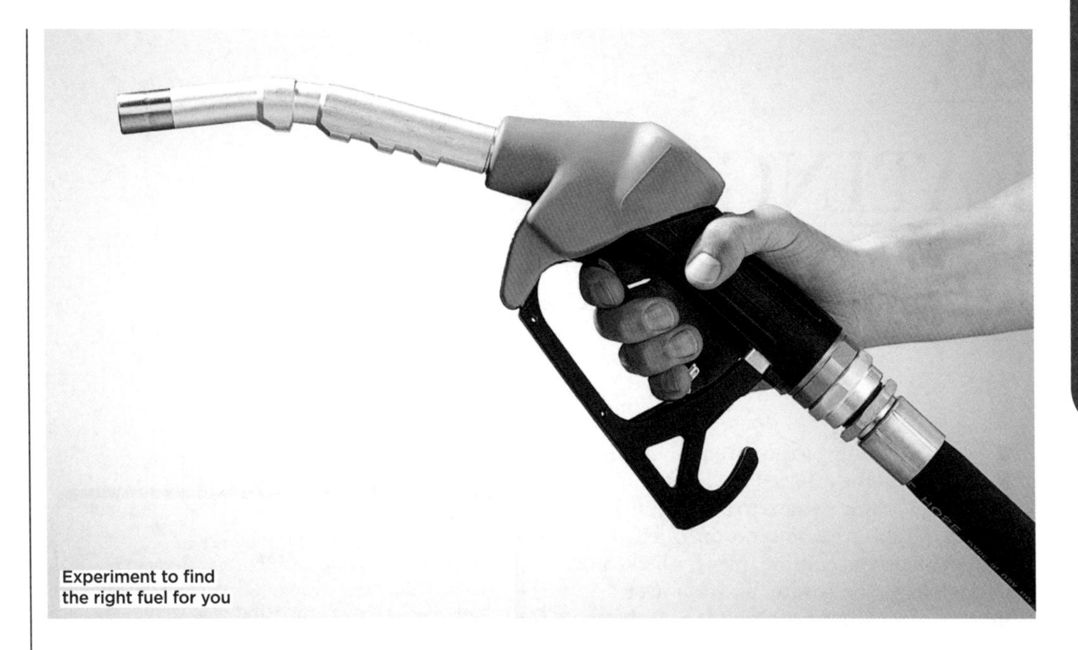
Experiment to find the right fuel for you

and fuel up well the evening before and the morning of a long run, you may be fine with 30g per hour. People who are targeting a PB and burn through fuel quickly might find they need more than 60g carbs an hour to run their best; some can tolerate up to 90g when running very long distances. But since the gut can only tolerate a certain level of carb intake, if you find you need more than 60g an hour, be sure to choose many different forms of fuel and ones that contain both glucose and fructose. They are digested differently and help prevent GI distress.

However many carbs you're using to refuel, don't forget to wash them down with water; the fuel needs to be diluted in order for your body to be able to absorb and deliver it to your working muscles.

Liquid replenishment

If you simply can't stomach anything solid while running, plenty of sports drinks provide all the carb, electrolytes and fluids you need to stay strong. Keep in mind that some drinks have more carbs than you need and may cause GI distress. Stick with ones that have no more than 14-17g carbs per 250ml serving. Look for drinks with multiple sources of carbs – such as glucose, fructose, sucrose or maltodextrin – which your body will absorb better than a single source by itself.

THE TAKEAWAY

Fuel up to go long.
On any run of 75 minutes or more, you'll want to refuel on the go. Have 30-60g carbs per hour. To keep your energy levels stable, consume them at regular intervals.

Test yourself.
On long runs, test different types of fuel to see what gives you a boost without upsetting your stomach.

Make a plan.
Once you find a long-run fuelling strategy that works for you, write it down and execute it on race day. This'll give you a better chance of reaching your finish-time goals.

20.

EATING FOR RECOVERY

If you're running to lose weight, the idea of consuming calories just after you've been working so hard to burn them isn't exactly intuitive. For most runners, the post-workout routine involves little more than stretching, some water and a shower.

But refuelling immediately after a workout can play a huge role in helping you bounce back quickly for your next session and stay healthy throughout your training, which means you keep your weight-loss efforts on track.

Timing matters

It's important to refuel within 30 minutes of finishing a workout. During this window, your muscles are primed to take in nutrients and glycogen so they can begin to rebuild from the stress they just endured.

When designed correctly, a recovery meal or snack prevents further muscle breakdown, helps optimise muscle and liver glycogen stores, and ultimately helps the body adapt to training. If you skip this meal, your body will remain in a state of breakdown, and you're likely to suffer more intense muscle soreness in the hours and days after your workout.

Chances are you won't feel hungry after exercising. Most runners don't. In fact, a study published in the *American Journal of Clinical Nutrition*[1] found that running causes a decrease in ghrelin (which increases appetite) and an increase in peptide YY (which is known to dampen appetite). So it's important to find foods and drinks that you can stomach and that will give your body the recovery it needs. Follow these guidelines to aid the process:

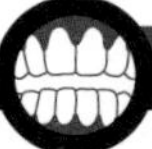

CHEW ON THIS

Don't take refuelling for recovery to extremes. Lots of people fall into the trap of overindulging post-workout, eating back all the calories they burned and then some. (For more, see Chapter 30 on mindless eating.)

Get it quick. Plan your post-workout meal before your run, so you can grab it as soon as you get back and take advantage of the 30-minute refuelling window.

Steer clear of junk food. Any carbs will help restock your glycogen stores, but you'll recover better if you refuel with healthy, wholesome choices. Whole foods such as sweet potatoes, milk, porridge and whole grains have the vitamins and nutrients your body needs to stay healthy and injury-free. Junk foods have lots of additives you just don't need. A banana and a chocolate bar might have the same number of calories and similar carb counts, but with potassium, fibre and other nutrients, a banana will help you bounce back better.

Make it routine. While refuelling isn't as critical after a short, easy run as it is following

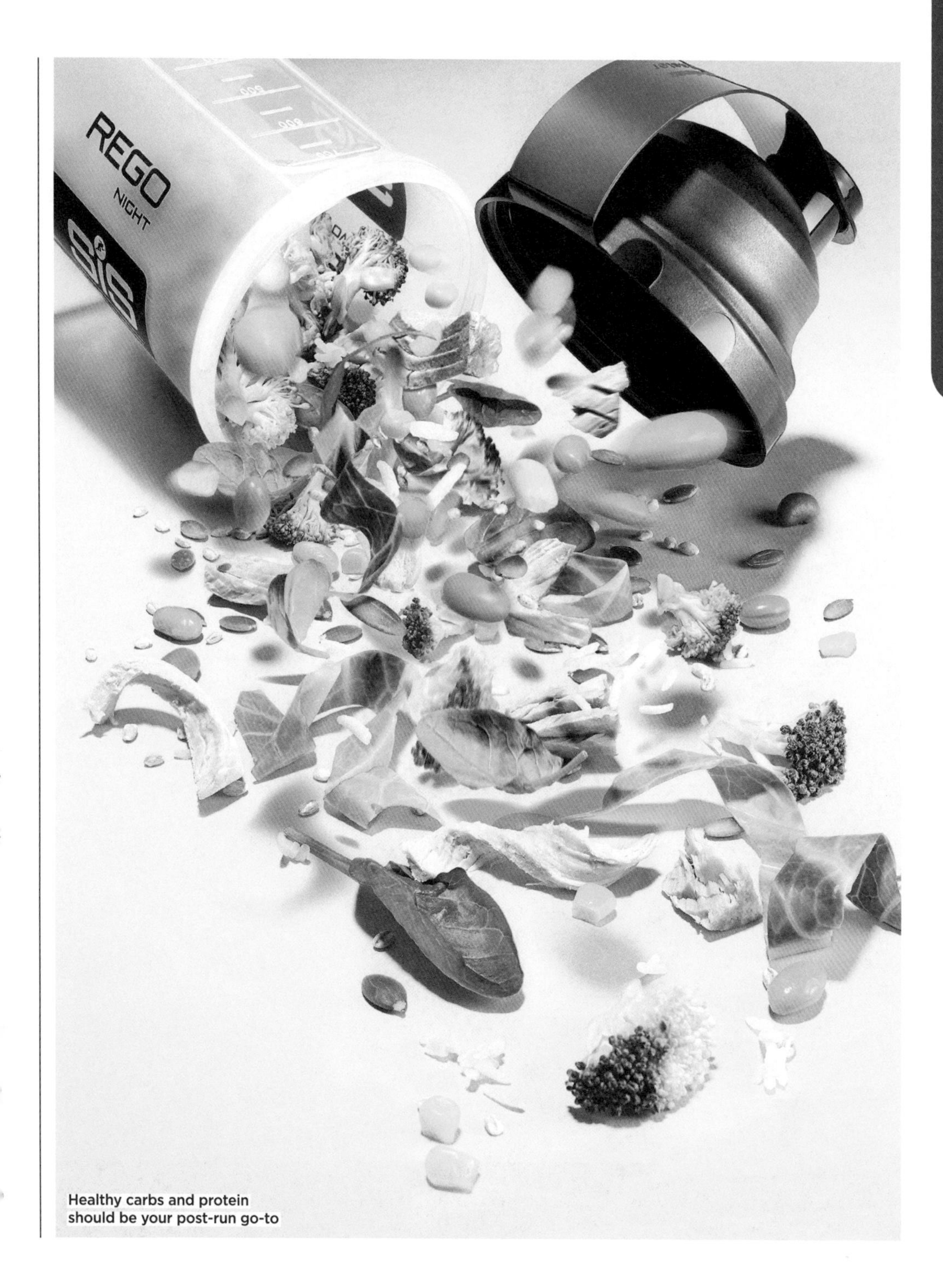

Healthy carbs and protein should be your post-run go-to

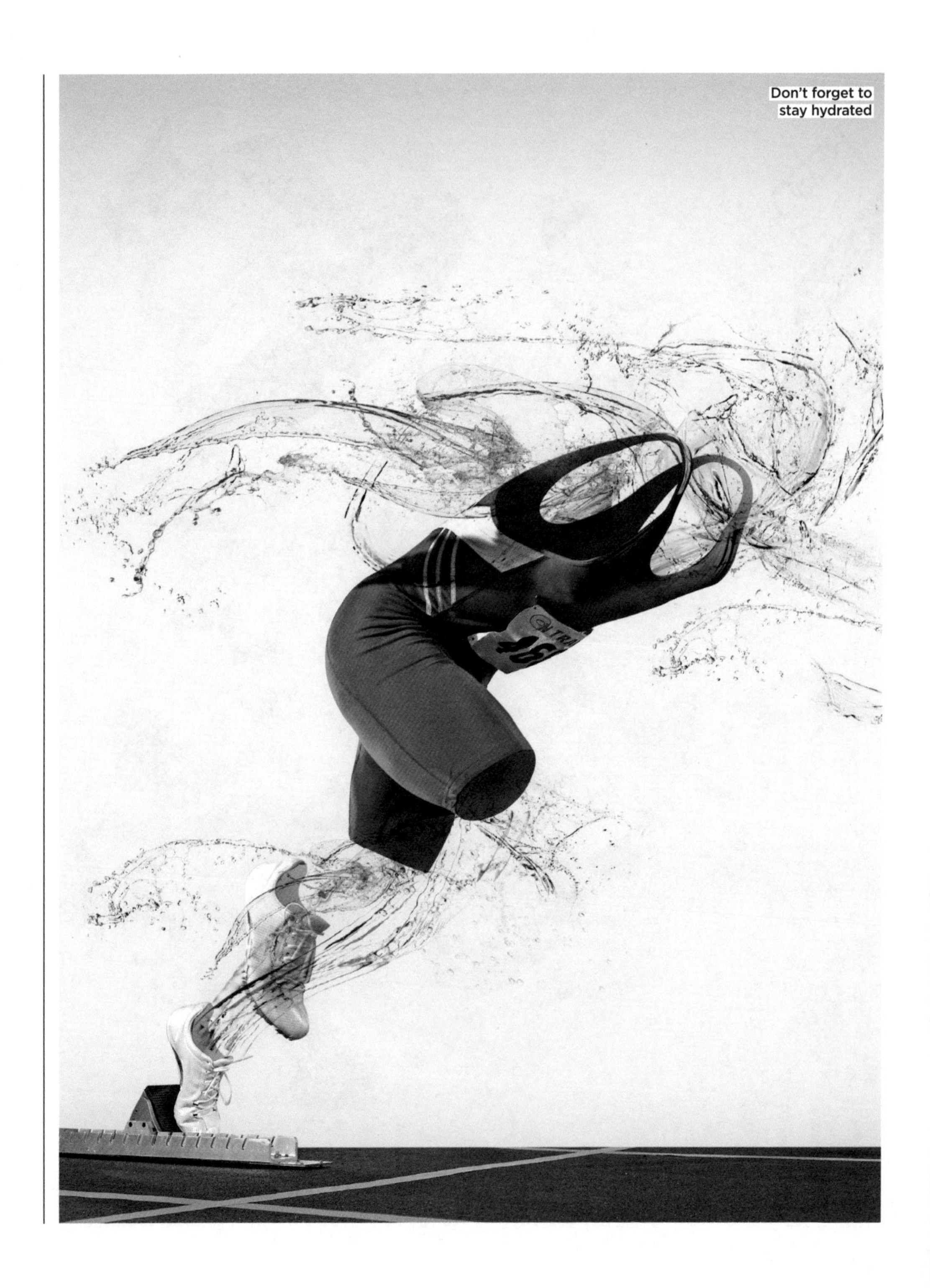

Don't forget to stay hydrated

a speed workout or a long run, it's a good idea to establish a habit of refuelling right after every workout so it's second nature when it really counts – after those more intense runs.

Carbs and protein: the perfect post-run combo

Research has shown that carbs and protein are the best nutrients for helping the body recover after a workout. The carbs in your recovery meal restock your spent glycogen stores. Aim for approximately 0.5g carbohydrate per lb of body weight. So if you weigh 150lb (10st 10lb), have a recovery meal with 75g carbs.

Adding a small amount of protein – 15-25g – to a recovery meal will speed your recovery. It'll aid muscle repair and help you adapt to your training, so your next workout will feel a little bit easier.

Rehydrate Drinking after your workout is just as critical to recovery as refuelling. Fluids are critical to so many of your body's basic functions, including transporting nutrients to your cells and flushing waste products out of your muscles. If you're dehydrated, your body has to work even harder to recover. It's a good idea to reach for a drink with electrolytes to help rehydrate your body as effectively as possible. To ensure you're properly rehydrated, drink until your thirst diminishes and your urine runs a light straw colour.

Ideas for post-run recovery snacks

When you're eating for recovery, try to consume at least 15-25g total protein along with 0.5g for every lb of body weight. Try mixing and matching some of the following foods to find your perfect recovery meal or snack.

Carbs
The following foods have 25-30g carbs:

- 1 small bagel or 2 slices bread
- 3-4 rice cakes
- 150g rice or corn
- 500ml sports drink
- 1 energy bar (check label for total carb and protein content)

Protein
Each of these foods has 20-25g protein:

- 4 whole eggs or 6 egg whites
- 3 tbsp reduced-fat peanut butter
- 700ml milk – choose skimmed or semi-skimmed
- 225g low-fat cottage cheese
- 250g fat-free Greek yogurt
- 75g chicken, fish, pork or beef
- 75g low-fat cheese (not cream cheese)
- 700ml soya milk
- protein drinks and powders (typically 15-45g/serving)

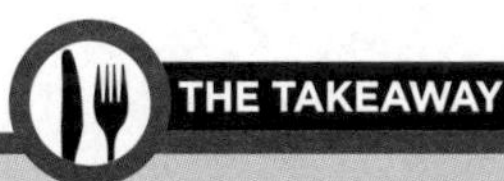

Plan ahead.
If you're going out for a long run or a speed session, plan your post-workout meal and have it ready to grab as soon as you finish. Make sure it contains 15-25g protein. Consume it with a food that has 0.5g carbohydrate for every lb of body weight. (So if you weigh 150lb, aim for 75g carbs.)

Act fast.
Consume your recovery snack within 30 minutes of finishing your workout. That's when the body is primed to use the fuel to restock spent glycogen stores and repair muscle tissue.

Don't forget to drink.
Wash your recovery meal down with water. Fluids help all your vital organs function, and we lose a lot of moisture when we sweat during tough workouts.

Recovery suggestions Turn over for our great recipes to revive you ▶

Recovery-boosting recipes: go with the grain

Looking beyond ordinary white rice can give you a taste *and* a nutrient boost. These dishes, designed by nutritionist Matthew Kadey, combine whole-grain varieties of rice with creative, tasty toppings for perfect post-run recovery meals.

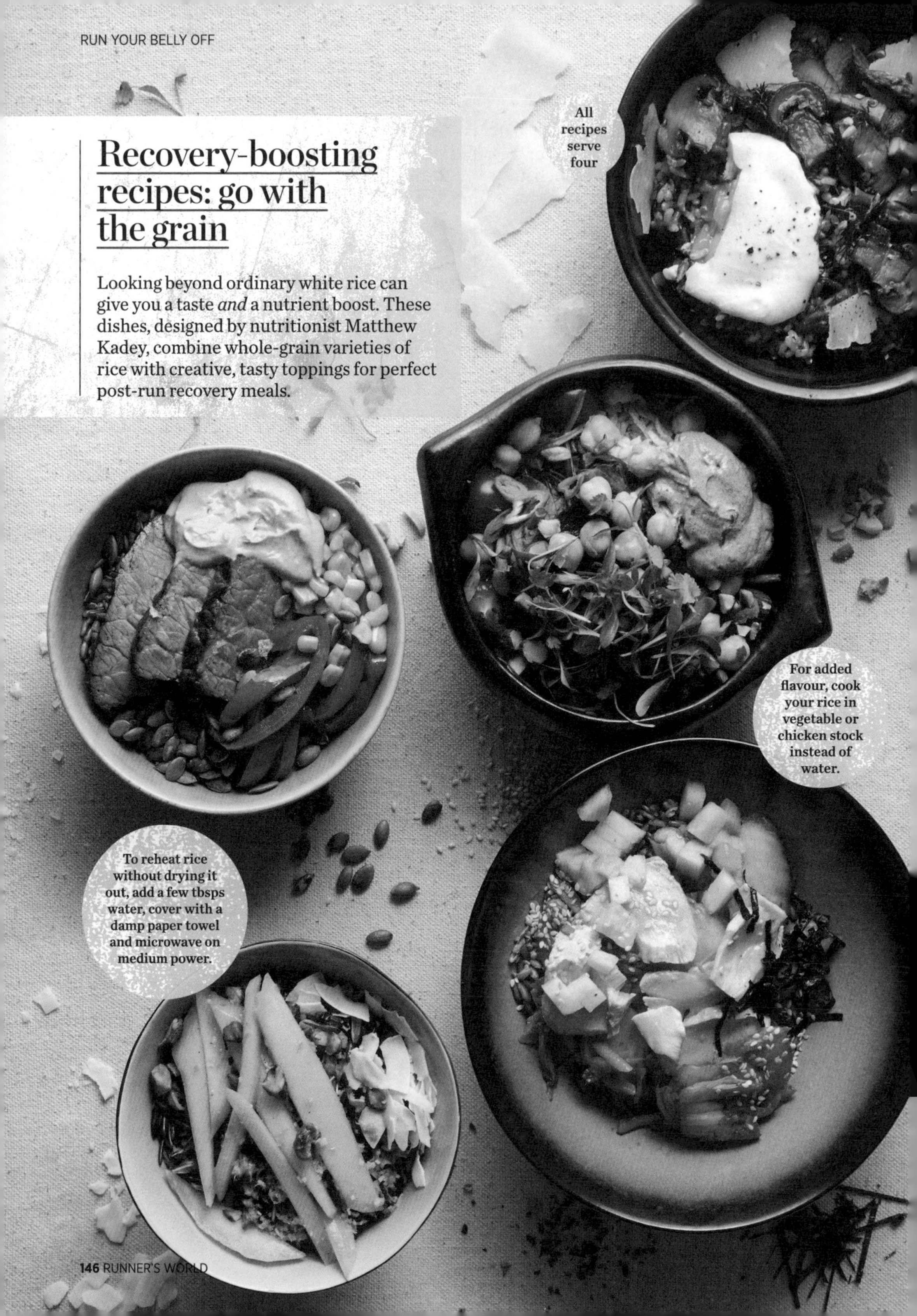

All recipes serve four

For added flavour, cook your rice in vegetable or chicken stock instead of water.

To reheat rice without drying it out, add a few tbsps water, cover with a damp paper towel and microwave on medium power.

Wild rice with asparagus

Technically a grass, wild rice has a nutty, smoky flavour and an impressive range of nutrients, including phosphorous, zinc, magnesium and B vitamins.

Cook your rice
- 170g wild rice

Add your toppings
- 1 bunch asparagus, chopped and sautéed
- 225g chestnut mushrooms, sliced and sautéed
- 4 poached eggs (1 per serving)

Drizzle your dressing
Whisk together:
- 3 tbsp extra virgin olive oil
- juice of 1 lemon
- 2 tbsp chopped dill
- 1 clove garlic, minced
- ½ tsp salt
- ¼ tsp red pepper flakes
- ¼ tsp black pepper

And garnish with...
- Grated Parmesan

Indian chickpea basmati bowl

Basmati rice is a staple in Indian cooking, and the whole-grain variety packs a powerful bundle of fibre, vitamins, minerals and antioxidants that can help the body recover from exercise and fight off illness.

Cook your rice
- 195g basmati rice

Add your toppings
- 425g canned chickpeas, drained and rinsed
- 900g baby spinach
- 300g cherry tomatoes, halved
- 2 spring onions, thinly sliced

Drizzle your dressing
Stir together:
- 250g plain yogurt
- 1½ tsp garam masala
- 1 tsp lime zest
- ¼ tsp cayenne or chilli powder

And garnish with...
- Chopped toasted almonds
- Chopped coriander

Kimchi salmon on red rice

Red rice gets its rosy hue from a pigment in its husk, and has a subtle sweetness. Since only the husks are removed, red rice retains its natural vitamin and mineral levels. Kimchi is a Korean staple made from fermented cabbage that's rich in probiotics.

Cook your rice
- 225g red rice

Add your toppings
- 230g kimchi
- 1 carrot, grated
- 200g pineapple
- 450g grilled salmon

Drizzle your dressing
Whisk together:
- 2 tbsp reduced-salt soy sauce
- 2 tbsp rice vinegar
- 2 tsp sesame oil

And garnish with...
- Chopped nori (seaweed) sheets
- Toasted sesame seeds

Chipotle steak with wehani rice

Wehani is a russet-coloured rice that fills the kitchen with the aroma of buttery popcorn as it steams. It can take up to an hour to cook, so make a big batch and freeze the leftovers.

Cook your rice
- 200g wehani rice (amazon.co.uk)

Add your toppings
- 450g sirloin steak, cooked as desired and thinly sliced
- 2 red peppers, sliced and sautéed
- 325g corn kernels, cooked

Drizzle your sauce
Blend together:
- 230g soured cream
- Juice of ½ lime
- ½ avocado
- 1 tsp minced chipotle chilli in adobo sauce (mexgrocer.co.uk)
- 1 clove garlic, minced
- ½ tsp ground cumin
- ¼ tsp salt
- ¼ tsp black pepper

And garnish with...
- Toasted pumpkin seeds or coriander

Black rice and mango

Black rice adds visual appeal and a great chewy bite. It also packs a hefty amount of anthocyanin antioxidants – the same molecules found in blueberries that mop up cell-damaging free radicals.

Cook your rice
- 170g black rice

Add your toppings
- 1 mango, peeled and sliced
- 35g chopped, unsalted pistachios

Drizzle your sauce
In a saucepan, heat together:
- 350ml coconut milk
- 2 tbsp honey
- 2 tsp orange zest
- 1 tsp grated fresh ginger
- 1 tsp vanilla extract
- ½ tsp ground allspice

And garnish with...
Coconut flakes

Recovery-boosting recipes: bounce-back-faster pasta

These easy-to-prepare and very tasty pasta-based combos, also devised by Matthew Kadey, provide a valuable post-run mix of carbs and protein, plus other key nutrients.

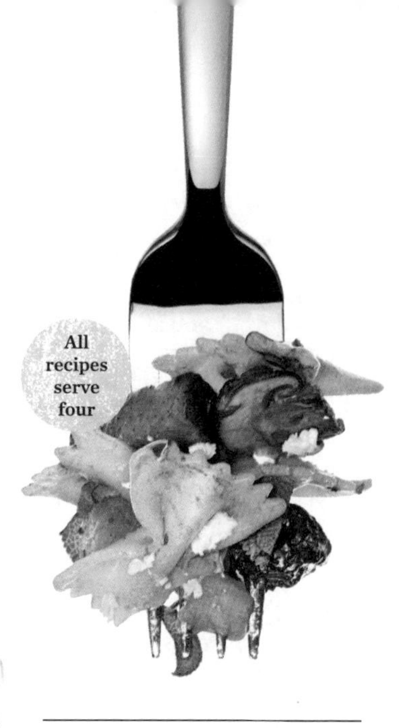

All recipes serve four

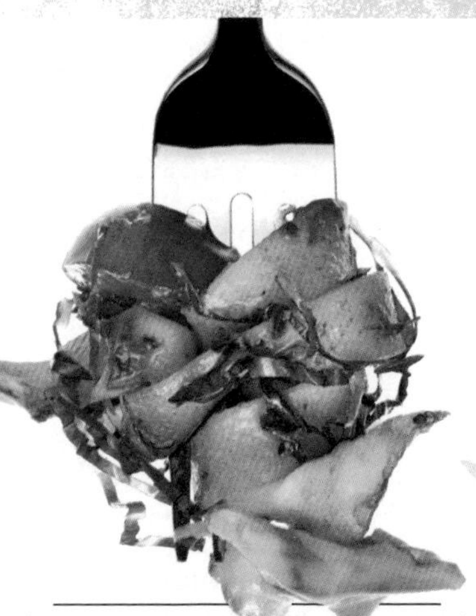

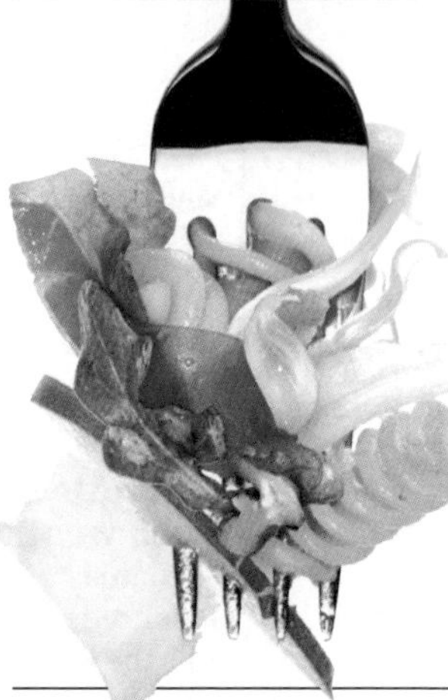

Green eggs and tomato

Top your pasta with a fried egg for gooey richness and plenty of vitamin B12, which is needed to keep your nervous system functioning. The olive oil in pesto supplies oleocanthal, an anti-inflammatory compound.

Cook your pasta
- 500g linguine, spaghetti or tagliatelle

Then mix in...
- 80g shredded radicchio
- 450g cherry tomatoes, halved

Toss with the sauce
- 3 tbsp fresh pesto

And garnish with...
- 4 fried eggs (1 per serving)

Pear prosciutto

Pears and fennel are a fibre-packed, hunger-taming duo. Walnuts add a healthy dose of essential omega fats.

Cook your pasta
- 500g fusilli or penne

Then mix in...
- 85g prosciutto, chopped
- 2 pears, sliced
- 180g thinly sliced fennel
- 2 big handfuls rocket
- 50g walnuts, chopped

Toss with the dressing
- 2 tbsp extra virgin olive oil
- 1 tbsp cider vinegar
- 2 cloves garlic, minced
- ¼ tsp black pepper

And garnish with...
- shaved Parmesan

Cranberry squash

Turkey sausage is leaner than pork, while butternut squash provides carotenoids that may improve brain function.

Cook your pasta
- 500g farfalle or orecchiette

Then mix in...
- 800g cubed roasted butternut squash
- 225g cooked turkey sausage
- 400g sliced mushrooms, sautéed
- 60g dried cranberries
- small handful chopped fresh sage

Toss with the dressing
- 2 tbsp walnut oil
- 1 tbsp balsamic vinegar
- 2 cloves garlic, minced
- ¼ tsp black pepper
- ¼ tsp chilli flakes

And garnish with...
- crumbled goat's cheese

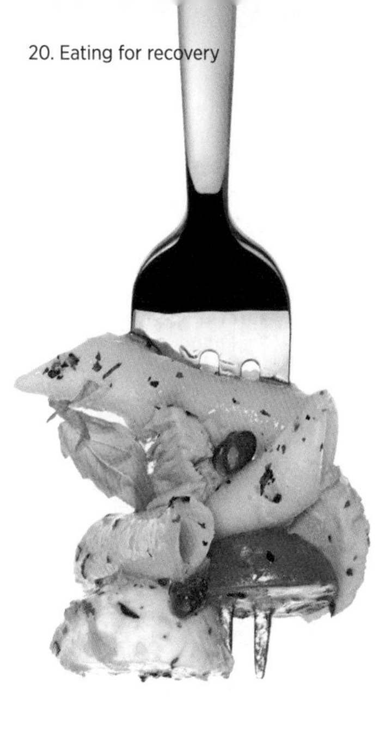

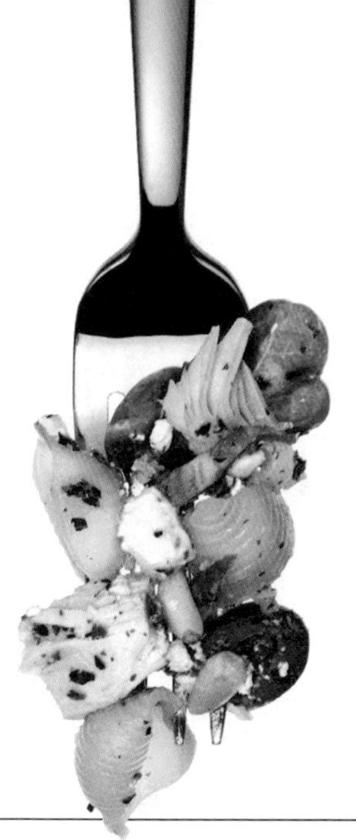

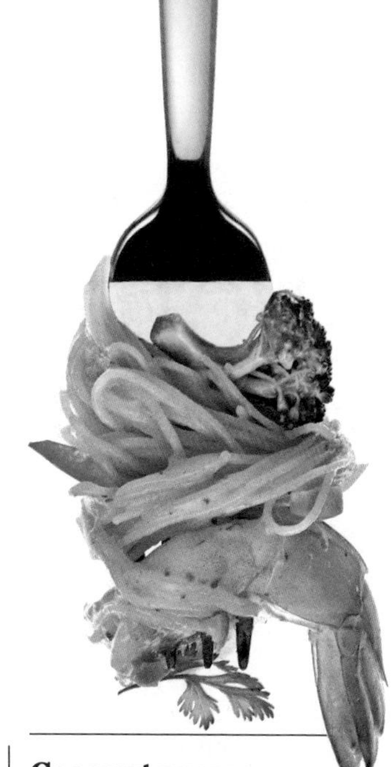

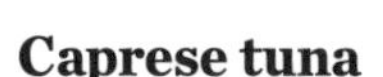

Caprese tuna

Sustainably fished albacore tuna (available at waitrose.com) provides protein and selenium, an antioxidant that may ease post-exercise oxidative cell damage.

Cook your pasta
- 500g penne or fusilli

Then mix in...
- 285g albacore tuna, drained
- 450g cherry tomatoes, halved
- 170g buffalo mozzarella balls, halved
- 1 tsp lemon zest
- 1 tbsp capers, drained

Toss with the dressing
- 2 tbsp extra virgin olive oil
- 1 tbsp lemon juice
- 2 cloves garlic, minced
- 2 tsp Italian seasoning
- ¼ tsp salt
- ¼ tsp black pepper

And garnish with...
- fresh basil

Mediterranean chicken

Chicken packs protein, B vitamins and zinc to boost the immune system. The nitrates in spinach help deliver oxygen to your muscles.

Cook your pasta
- 500g shells, fusilli or penne

Then mix in...
- 300g chopped cooked chicken
- 400g baby spinach
- 125g sliced marinated artichoke hearts
- 55g sliced sun-dried tomatoes
- 40g diced feta cheese
- 35g chopped kalamata olives

Toss with the dressing
- 2 tbsp extra virgin olive oil
- 1 tbsp red-wine vinegar
- 2 cloves garlic, minced
- 2 tsp Italian seasoning
- ¼ tsp black pepper

And garnish with...
- toasted pine nuts

Coconut prawn

Prawns are a source of heart-healthy omega-3 fats and vitamin D, a nutrient shown to reduce inflammation following a workout. Broccoli is packed with key anti-cancer phytochemicals.

Cook your pasta
- 500g rice vermicelli noodles

Then mix in
- 450g prawns, peeled, deveined and cooked
- 700g steamed broccoli florets
- 1 red pepper, sliced

Toss with the dressing
- 235ml reduced-fat coconut milk, warmed
- 1 tbsp yellow curry paste
- juice of ½ lime

And garnish with...
- chopped peanuts and coriander

21.

AVOIDING WEIGHT GAIN IF YOU CAN'T RUN

It happens to all of us at some point, usually when we least expect it. Our exercise and weight-loss efforts are humming along, when suddenly something – injury, a work project or a family illness – sidelines our exercise routine.

When your running gets derailed, it can be easy to pack on the pounds. Some people keep up the eating routines that fuel their running even though they're not lacing up. For others, the absence of the stress release that running provides makes it even easier to give in to the call of junk food.

But weight gain when you can't run doesn't have to be a foregone conclusion. Here's how to prevent the number on the scale from going up while your mileage goes down.

Identify the culprit Where are your extra calories coming from? Have your portions grown too large? Have you got into the habit of taking second helpings, or mindlessly snacking in the afternoon or in front of the TV? Are you continuing to indulge in your post-long-run ice cream even though you're not running long? Be honest with yourself. It may be humbling, but to get back on track you need to face the truth about what you're consuming.

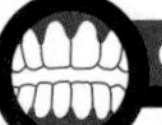

CHEW ON THIS

When our standard calorie burn gets stifled, we often fail to adjust our calorie intake accordingly. It's just a matter of maths: decrease your workouts and you'll need to put the brakes on your calorie intake if you want to keep your weight the same.

Stop emotional eating Consider when you might be snacking simply to procrastinate or relieve boredom, stress, restlessness or any other uncomfortable emotion. Make a list of calorie-free strategies you could use to relieve those feelings and pin it up where you can see it. Clean out a drawer, do the dishes or laundry, or just get out of the house. Studies have shown that waiting as little as two minutes after the 'I want to eat' urge is enough to make the craving dissipate. (For more on this, go to Chapter 27 on emotional eating.)

Set yourself up for success If you've got a weakness for chocolate and know it's the first thing you go to when you're stressed, don't buy it. Don't even walk down the supermarket aisle where it's kept. Keeping temptations out of sight and out of reach drastically reduces the chance that you'll eat them when you're stressed. Something as seemingly minor as eating from smaller plates has been shown to help downsize portions (for more on this, go to page 119).

Just keep moving If you can still work out – even if it's at a lower intensity – do it at the same time of day you'd usually run, so you get the comfort from your routine. And you do get some calorie burn. If you can't work out, try to incorporate more activity whenever you

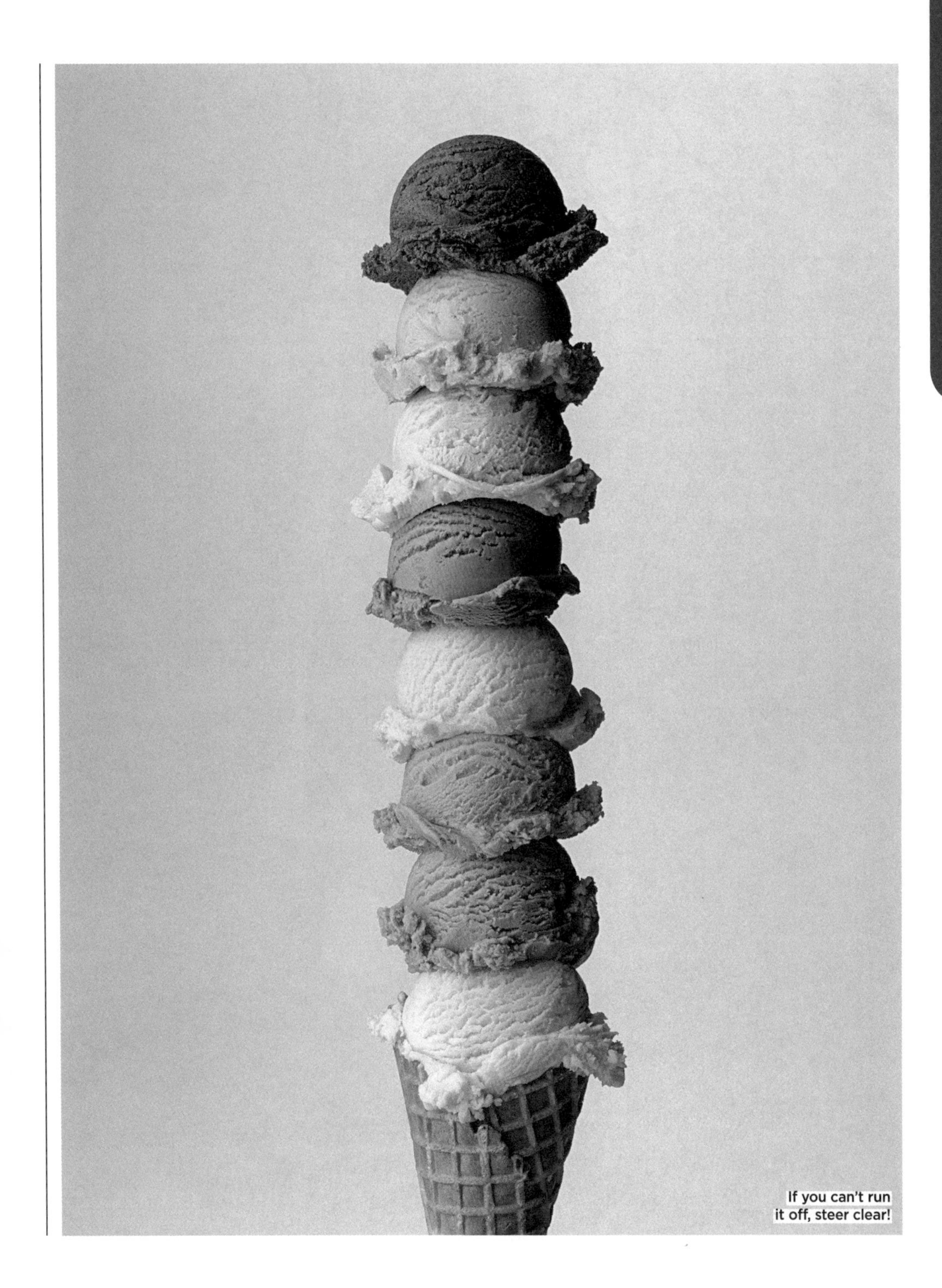

If you can't run it off, steer clear!

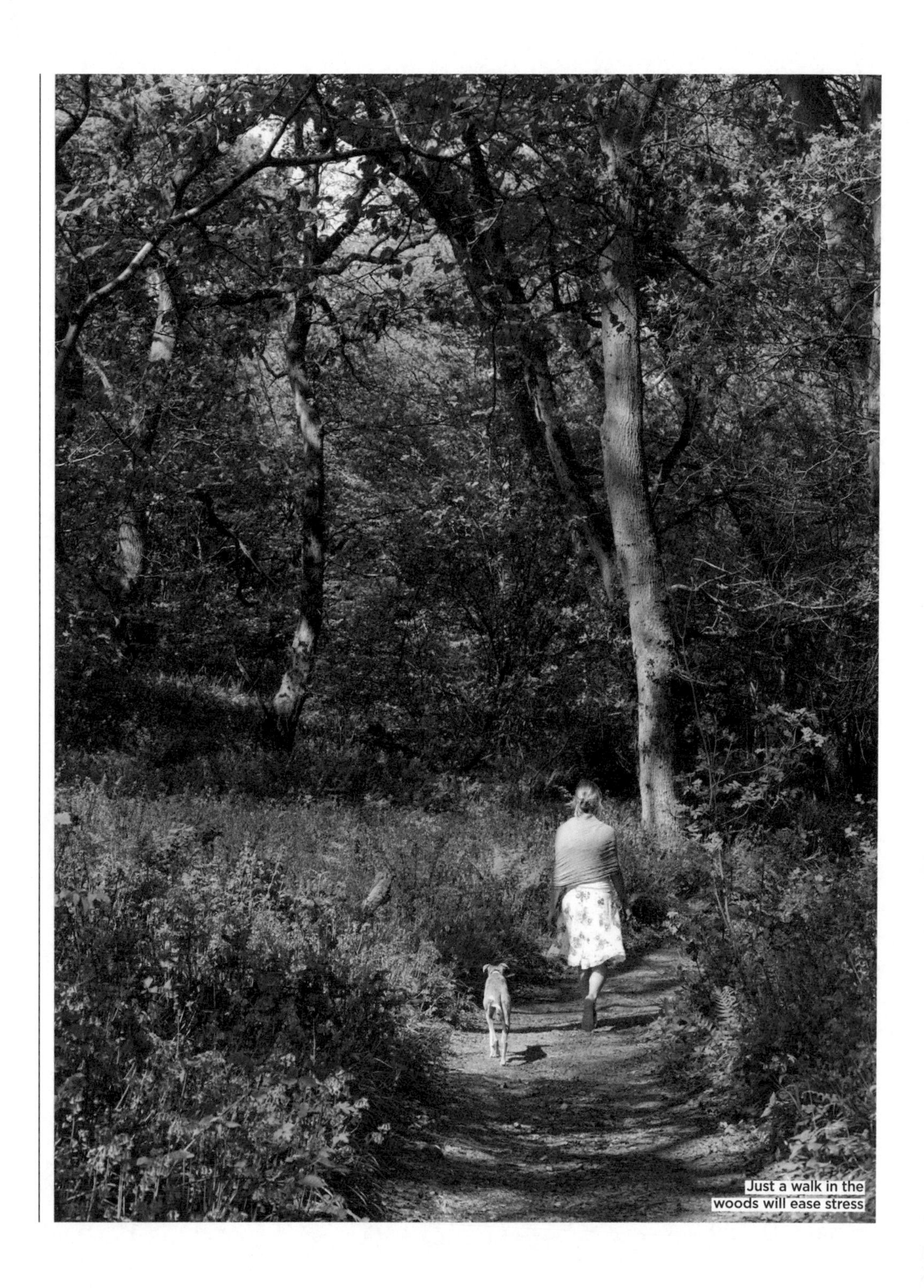

Just a walk in the woods will ease stress

can. get up from your desk and walk to the water dispenser, go the long way to the toilets, take the dog for a walk, take the stairs instead of the lift, or park far away from the shops to sneak in extra activity. These extra minutes of moving add up, and every calorie burned helps.

Get help Explain the situation to family, friends and anyone in your support system. Tell them you're trying not to lose your mind or gain weight while sidelined and it'll be easier for you to do both if there are no snacks or sugary foods in the house. You might get some resistance at first from those you live with, so try to explain it in terms they can relate to: you can't do something you enjoy that gives you a sense of accomplishment and fun on a daily basis – and that'd put anyone in a bad mood. If you're not happy because you're not running and are overindulging, they probably won't be happy either.

Seek the benefits elsewhere Remember that aside from a calorie burn, running also provides a daily biochemical reset. Studies have proven that just 30 minutes of physical exercise inoculates you against stress later in the day. If you're used to running with friends, it also provides social time, laughter and a connection you might not otherwise get. And just a few easy miles are enough to give you a sense of accomplishment that can boost your mood and confidence for the day. So if you're facing a time when you can't run, make a list of the benefits running provides, and work out how you could reap similar benefits. Maybe meet with friends on Saturday mornings when you'd usually join a group run. Or set aside that time to write or do some other reflective practice that'll allow you to relieve stress or meditate. Even a low-impact activity such as walking or swimming could help.

> Meet with friends when you'd normally go running

Plan ahead It's hard to make a healthy choice when you walk in the door from work, still shouldering the stresses of the day. If you're feeling ravenous because you skipped a meal or missed your usual 3pm snack, making a healthy choice is going to be even harder. By planning ahead you'll increase the chances of eating right. Try mapping out the week's dinners on Sunday evening. Do some of the prep (or enlist help) ahead of time so dinner is ready within minutes of walking in the door. This way you won't be tempted to give in to crisps, crackers and cheese.

Fill up on low-cal fruits and vegetables When compared with other foods, most vegetables and many fruits are low in calories while high in essential nutrients, fibre and water. Aside from the health benefits, fibre and water keep you fuller longer. Fill your plate with fruit and veg and round out each meal with lean meat and whole grains. If you're thirsty, avoid drinking your calories and instead hydrate with a calorie-free beverage such as water with a slice of lemon or a relaxing cup of tea.

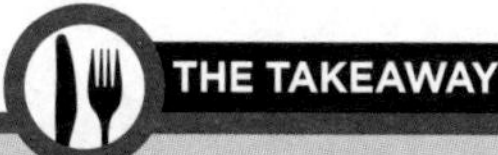

Expect some discomfort.
When you're accustomed to your daily dose of running for fresh air, personal time and biochemical reset, expect to feel off and stressed when you can't run. List some activities that will give you the same sort of mental and emotional release running provides. Use the time you'd usually go running for a fulfilling personal or social activity, or something that gets you outside.

Watch your intake.
When you're not running regularly, you have to be extra vigilant about your calorie intake. Fill up on fruit and veg. Avoid junk food in the house, and work hard to find alternative strategies for stress release so you're not tempted to indulge in the wrong foods.

Address your weaknesses.
Use the time off from running to strengthen the areas of fitness where you might be weak. It's a good time to start a strength-training programme or start a routine of cross-training or massage.

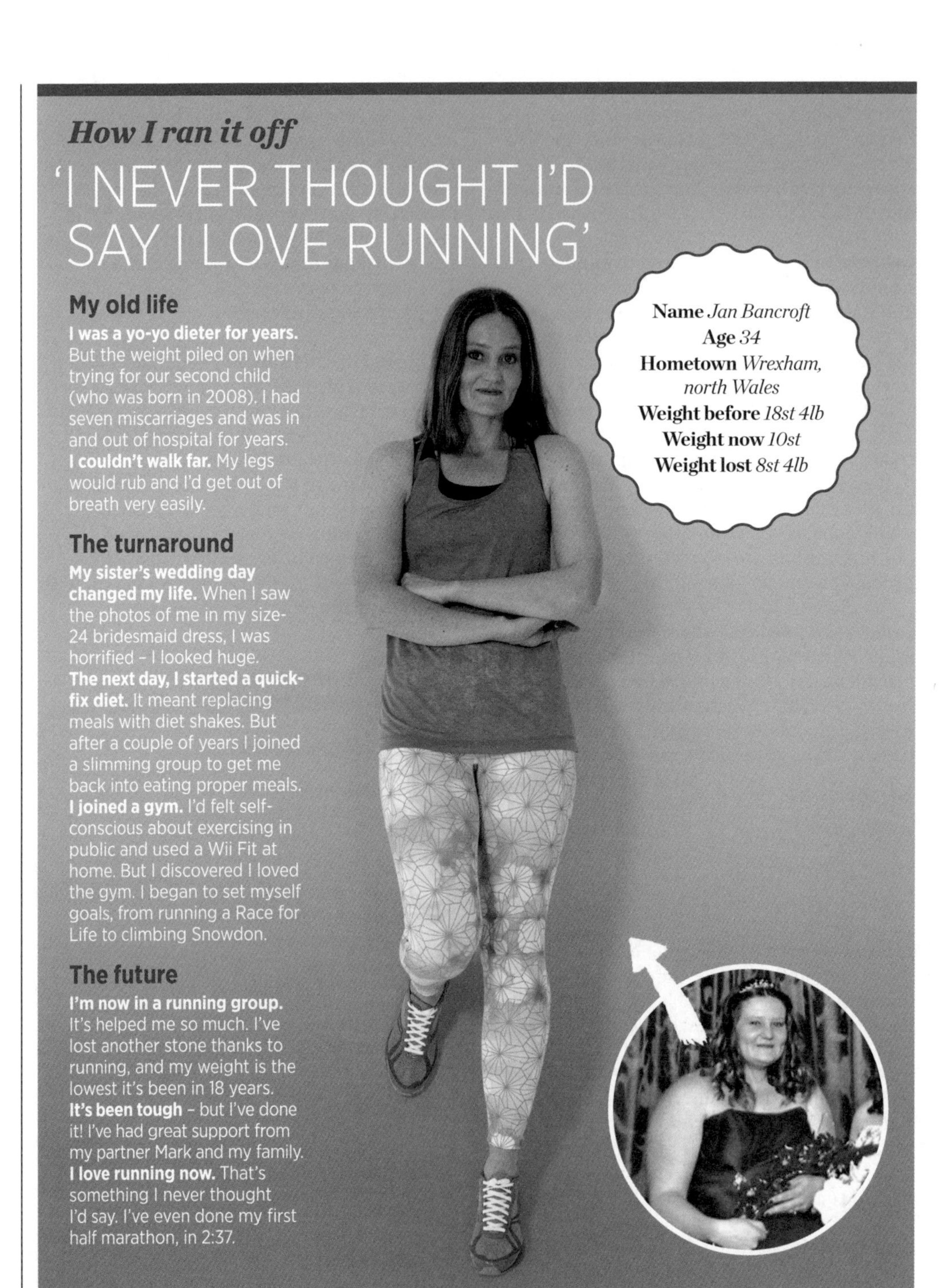

How I ran it off

'I NEVER THOUGHT I'D SAY I LOVE RUNNING'

Name *Jan Bancroft*
Age *34*
Hometown *Wrexham, north Wales*
Weight before *18st 4lb*
Weight now *10st*
Weight lost *8st 4lb*

My old life

I was a yo-yo dieter for years. But the weight piled on when trying for our second child (who was born in 2008). I had seven miscarriages and was in and out of hospital for years. **I couldn't walk far.** My legs would rub and I'd get out of breath very easily.

The turnaround

My sister's wedding day changed my life. When I saw the photos of me in my size-24 bridesmaid dress, I was horrified – I looked huge. **The next day, I started a quick-fix diet.** It meant replacing meals with diet shakes. But after a couple of years I joined a slimming group to get me back into eating proper meals. **I joined a gym.** I'd felt self-conscious about exercising in public and used a Wii Fit at home. But I discovered I loved the gym. I began to set myself goals, from running a Race for Life to climbing Snowdon.

The future

I'm now in a running group. It's helped me so much. I've lost another stone thanks to running, and my weight is the lowest it's been in 18 years. **It's been tough** – but I've done it! I've had great support from my partner Mark and my family. **I love running now.** That's something I never thought I'd say. I've even done my first half marathon, in 2:37.

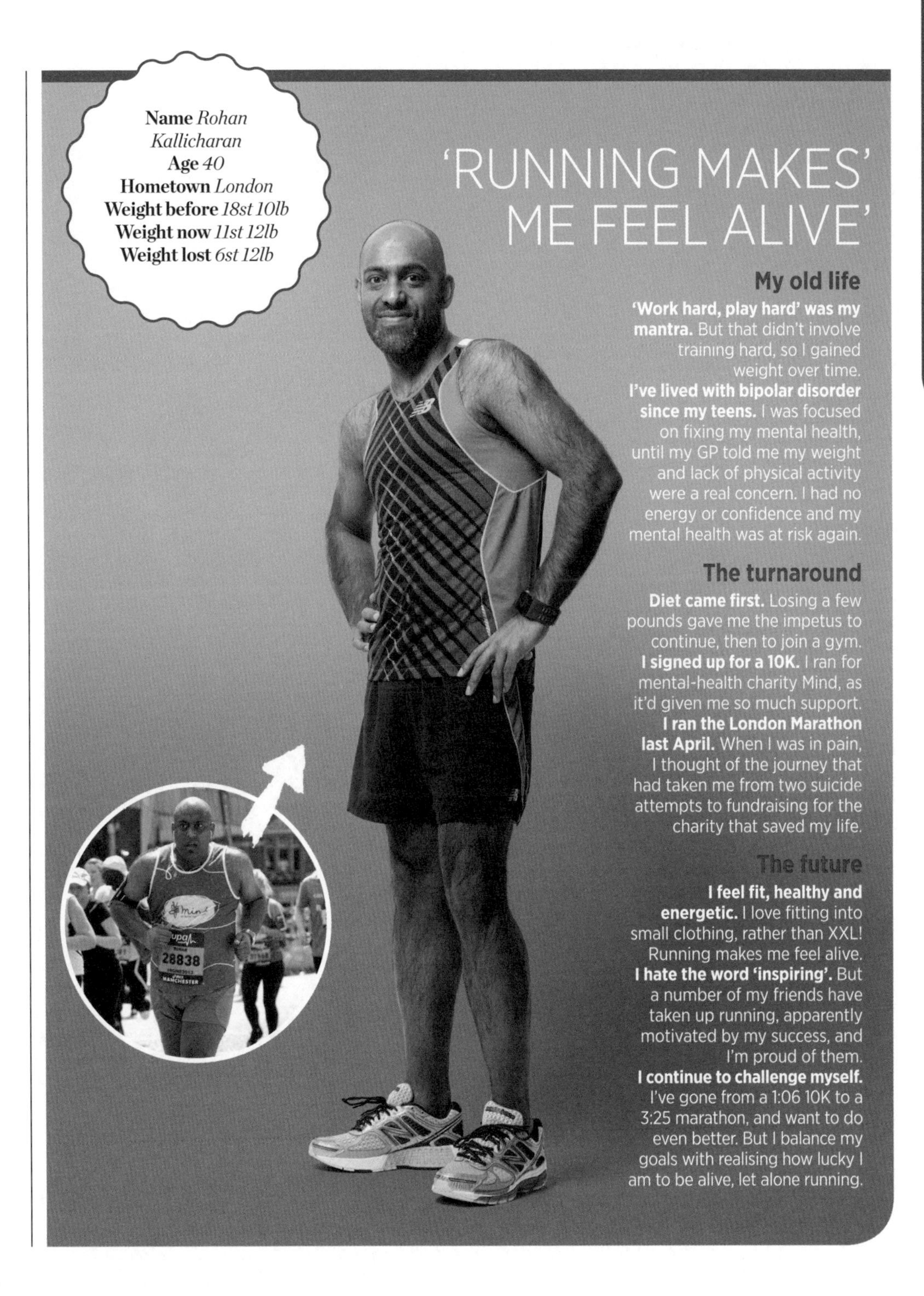

Name *Rohan Kallicharan*
Age *40*
Hometown *London*
Weight before *18st 10lb*
Weight now *11st 12lb*
Weight lost *6st 12lb*

'RUNNING MAKES ME FEEL ALIVE'

My old life

'Work hard, play hard' was my mantra. But that didn't involve training hard, so I gained weight over time.

I've lived with bipolar disorder since my teens. I was focused on fixing my mental health, until my GP told me my weight and lack of physical activity were a real concern. I had no energy or confidence and my mental health was at risk again.

The turnaround

Diet came first. Losing a few pounds gave me the impetus to continue, then to join a gym.

I signed up for a 10K. I ran for mental-health charity Mind, as it'd given me so much support.

I ran the London Marathon last April. When I was in pain, I thought of the journey that had taken me from two suicide attempts to fundraising for the charity that saved my life.

The future

I feel fit, healthy and energetic. I love fitting into small clothing, rather than XXL! Running makes me feel alive.

I hate the word 'inspiring'. But a number of my friends have taken up running, apparently motivated by my success, and I'm proud of them.

I continue to challenge myself. I've gone from a 1:06 10K to a 3:25 marathon, and want to do even better. But I balance my goals with realising how lucky I am to be alive, let alone running.

Part

IV

RUNNING TO LOSE WEIGHT

In this section, you'll learn how to redesign your running routine to rev up your calorie burn when you're on the road and even after you're done. You'll also find a gut-busting strength-training routine you can do anytime, anywhere – no gym or equipment required. And it'll allow you to get fit without the risk of injury. The bonus? You'll have a routine that'll help you enjoy running more, and deliver better results on the scales and at the finish line.

22.

GETTING STARTED

If you're new to running, getting started can be daunting and you will have questions. Lots of them. One of the best ways to get answers is by talking to other, more experienced runners. They'll be excited to see you taking up the sport, and there's a very good chance you'll walk away with both the information you need and a sense of the camaraderie you can expect if you stick with it.

However, assuming you don't live in a high-altitude training camp in the Rift Valley, there may be times when there's no experienced runner on hand to chat through your queries. Don't worry: you'll find time-tested answers from a panel of experts on training right here.

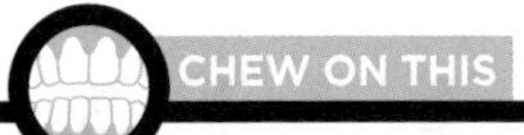

It's rare to find a runner who doesn't want to talk about running. Everyone has a friend or colleague who never misses a chance to discuss their latest race, or the bells and whistles on their fancy new GPS watch. If you're just taking your first strides in running you may not find this chat all that riveting. But you should put on your best 'interested' expression and pay attention, because for a new runner, the knowledge and experience of the run geek is a very valuable resource.

'I'm not a runner yet... what's so great about running, anyway?'

Actually, you already are a runner. You probably ran around the playground as a kid. Humans are built to do it. In fact, our bodies, with their long legs and lack of fur, are *designed* for running. And the good news is that it doesn't require a lot of pricey equipment to get into it, and it beats other activities when it comes to not just losing weight, but also fending off disease. Want some specifics? Since 1991, the National Runners' and Walkers' Study at Lawrence Berkeley National Laboratory in California has followed more than 154,000 runners and walkers. It's found that running as little as three to seven miles per week reduces your risk of stroke, heart disease, diabetes and high cholesterol. As a rule, the more you run, the more your risks decrease. The study found that running also offers the following benefits...

Promotes joint and bone health

Contrary to popular belief, running might actually prevent osteoarthritis and the need for joint replacements, with the body responding to the impact of our footfalls by thickening cartilage and building bone-mineral density. Those who averaged more than 1.2 miles per day of running were found to be at 18% less risk of osteoarthritis and 35% less risk of needing a hip replacement than non-runners.

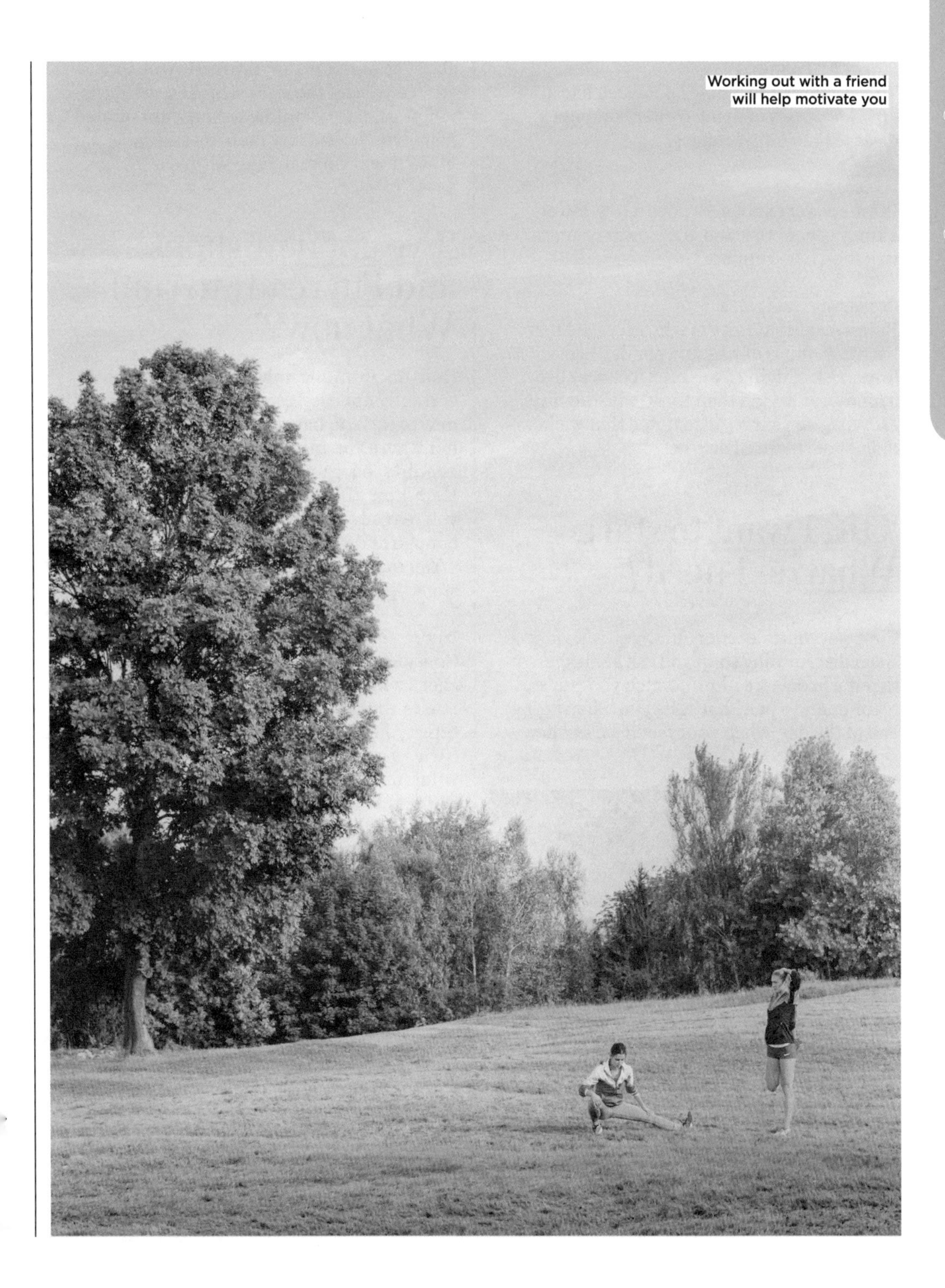

Working out with a friend will help motivate you

Fights Alzheimer's

Those who ran 15.3 miles per week had a 40% lower risk of dying from Alzheimer's disease than non-runners.

Lowers cancer risk

Runners were shown to have a 76% lower kidney cancer risk and 40% lower brain cancer risk than non-runners.

Boosts survival rates

Breast-cancer survivors who averaged more than 2.25 miles of running per day had a 95% lower risk of dying from breast cancer over a nine-year period than those who did little exercise. The survey also noted that walkers did not decrease their risk.

'OK, I want to start. What do I need?'

First, get some decent running shoes. Go to a specialist running shop and ask a salesperson to put you on a treadmill, watch you run and recommend a pair that suits you. Shop at the end of the day, when your feet have swollen about as much as they normally will, to ensure you get the right size. And resist the temptation to go online to find a discounted pair – you need to try them on and shoes can break down when they're sitting in the box.

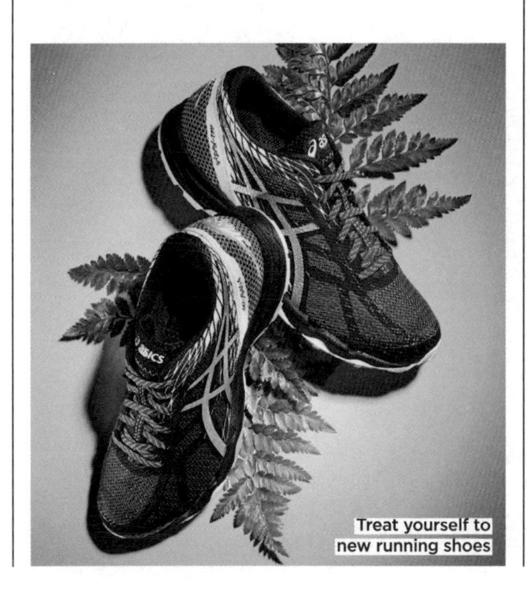

Treat yourself to new running shoes

'I've got new shoes and I'm ready to run! What now?'

Hold on. Running might by simple, but it's certainly not easy, especially when you're new to it. "You have to start where you are, not where you think you should be," says running coach and exercise physiologist Janet Hamilton. "If you go further or faster than you're ready for, your body can't adapt quickly enough and you'll get injured."

You may need to take some preliminary steps before you start a running programme if:

You're very overweight

Consider losing a little, via diet and walking, and check with your doctor before you start to run. Each step you take when running presses three times your body weight down on your joints (twice as much as walking), leaving you more vulnerable to injury. One study found novice runners with a body mass index (BMI) of 30-plus were 17% more likely to get injured than leaner new runners. See our Stage 1 Plan on page 164 for a detailed guide to getting started.

You're completely inactive

Spend 3-4 weeks doing any gentle aerobic exercise several times a week, working up to where you can walk briskly for 30 continuous minutes. Again, see our Stage 1 Plan.

Even if neither of these applies to you, if you're new to running, start slowly. Begin by alternating between running and walking. It keeps your muscles from tiring too quickly and delivers less impact on your joints and tendons, while still giving you the heart-health benefits of a longer workout. Plus, those walk breaks split the run into segments, making

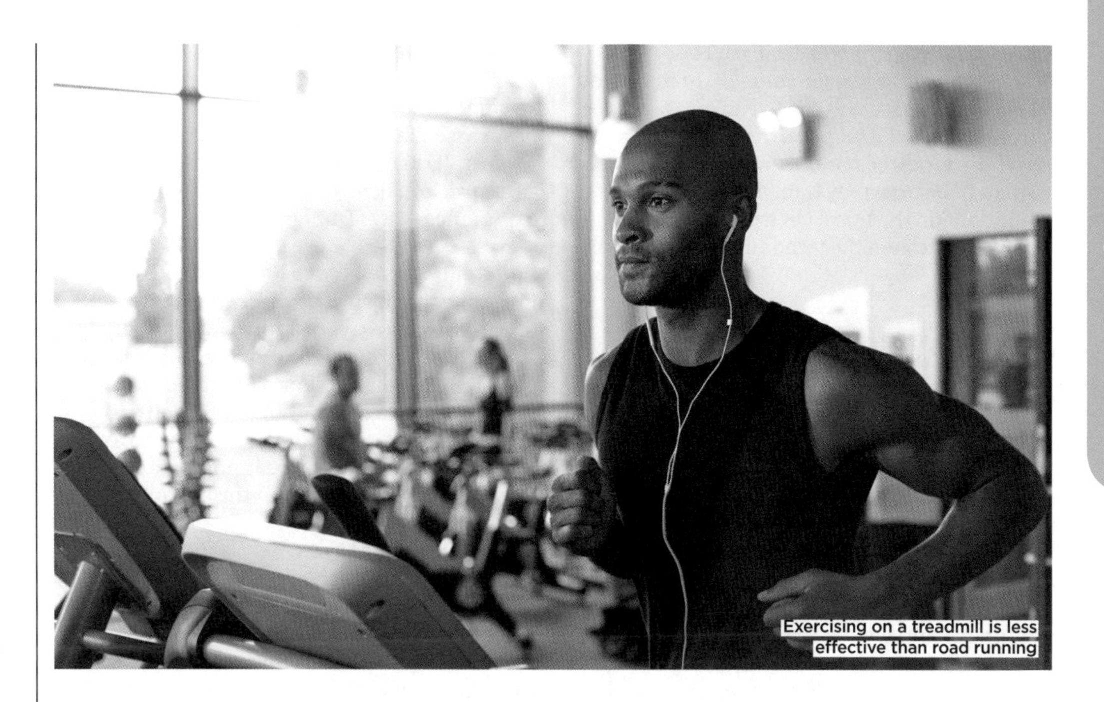
Exercising on a treadmill is less effective than road running

it mentally easier to go the distance. See our Stage 2 plan on page 166 for more.

'Ouch. Is running meant to hurt this much?'

A little muscle soreness is normal, and often it won't even kick in for a day or two after you run. But if you have pain that sticks around for more than 48 hours, or restricts your movement, that's a red flag. Take some time off and consider seeing a physio. You might need to re-evaluate your regime. New runners tend to get injured when they ramp up their mileage too quickly, or run too fast or too often.

'My skin is rubbed raw!'

Runners call that 'chafing,' and it's certainly not one of the sport's selling points. Put a little petroleum jelly (or an anti-chafe balm, such as Bodyglide) on sensitive areas before you run. If you've lost weight and have extra skin causing chafing, compression garments – tights, base layer – can keep everything in place. And whatever you do, don't wear cotton, which traps moisture and worsens chafing. Look for shorts, tops and socks made of technical fabrics that will wick sweat away from your skin, keeping it dry.

'I've started running on a treadmill. Is it the same as road running?'

Not quite. Treadmill running can feel harder than running outside as it takes balance and coordination (and some willpower) just to stay on the thing. In reality, it doesn't give you as much of a workout as running on varied terrain, fighting against the wind. Also, because it sets the pace for you, the treadmill isn't very good at teaching you how to pace yourself. In one study, 21 participants were asked to run on a track for three minutes at a set pace, then to run on a treadmill for three minutes, adjusting the speed to match the pace they thought they'd been running at on the track. On average, runners ran 32% slower on the treadmill.

'I enjoy running once I get going, but I have trouble motivating myself to start'

Lots of runners have that problem before they work out how to plan their runs. First, it helps to know what time of day you most enjoy running, then, schedule your runs as you would a meeting at work or a date with a friend. And try to create a pattern. If you can get yourself into the habit of running at a certain time, eventually the absence of it starts to feel weird.

"Once exercise becomes a habit, it just feels easier," says Charles Duhigg, author of *The Power of Habit*, (£8.99, Random House). "When you don't feel like it, it doesn't take as much willpower." Use the following tips to help you kick into the running habit, and stay at it over the long run.

Make a plan

According to Duhigg, every habit we acquire is made up of a group of cues (time, place, mood, music, other people...); a reward (chocolate, massage, smoothie...); and a routine (the workout). So write out a plan with cues and rewards that will incentivise you, then post it where you can see it.

Keep it regular

Create a pre-exercise routine to cue your body and mind, then repeat it. Run at the same time of day and put on the same pre-run music. "The cues have to be consistent," explains Duhigg. "You're creating neural pathways that make the activity into a habit."

Reward yourself immediately

Treat yourself to something you enjoy straight after you've finished your run, so your brain associates exercise with an immediate reward. "You can't intellectualise your way to a reward. You have to teach the brain through experience," says Duhigg.

And treat yourself in the long run, too

Put some money in a jar after each run to go towards a trip (maybe to run a race) or buy some new running kit once you reach a certain milestone. Research shows that while the distant promise of lost weight and better health may not motivate us to stick with an exercise programme, more immediate material rewards do – particularly in the beginning.

Build your support system

Equip your routine with activities that will make you feel good about it, suggests Duhigg. Meet up with friends so the run doubles as socialising time and you can run and chat along the way. And consider joining a beginner's running group. It helps you realise you're not alone in this thing and provides a place to swap advice on the challenges you're facing. Plus, there's nothing more motivating than knowing someone's waiting for you at the crack of dawn to go for a run.

Track your runs

Keep a diary, or log your activity via a tracking site such as strava.com or myfitnesspal.com. Research shows that people who track what they eat and when they exercise tend to eat less and exercise more.

Don't just run

Listen to a favourite podcast, or use your run time to think through a problem you're having in your job or relationship. "Running can be a great time to daydream or come up with solutions," says running coach Rik Akey.

Go public: tell the world you're a runner

Set a mileage goal or sign up for a race and share your plans on social media. Then you'll have a network of people to help keep you accountable.

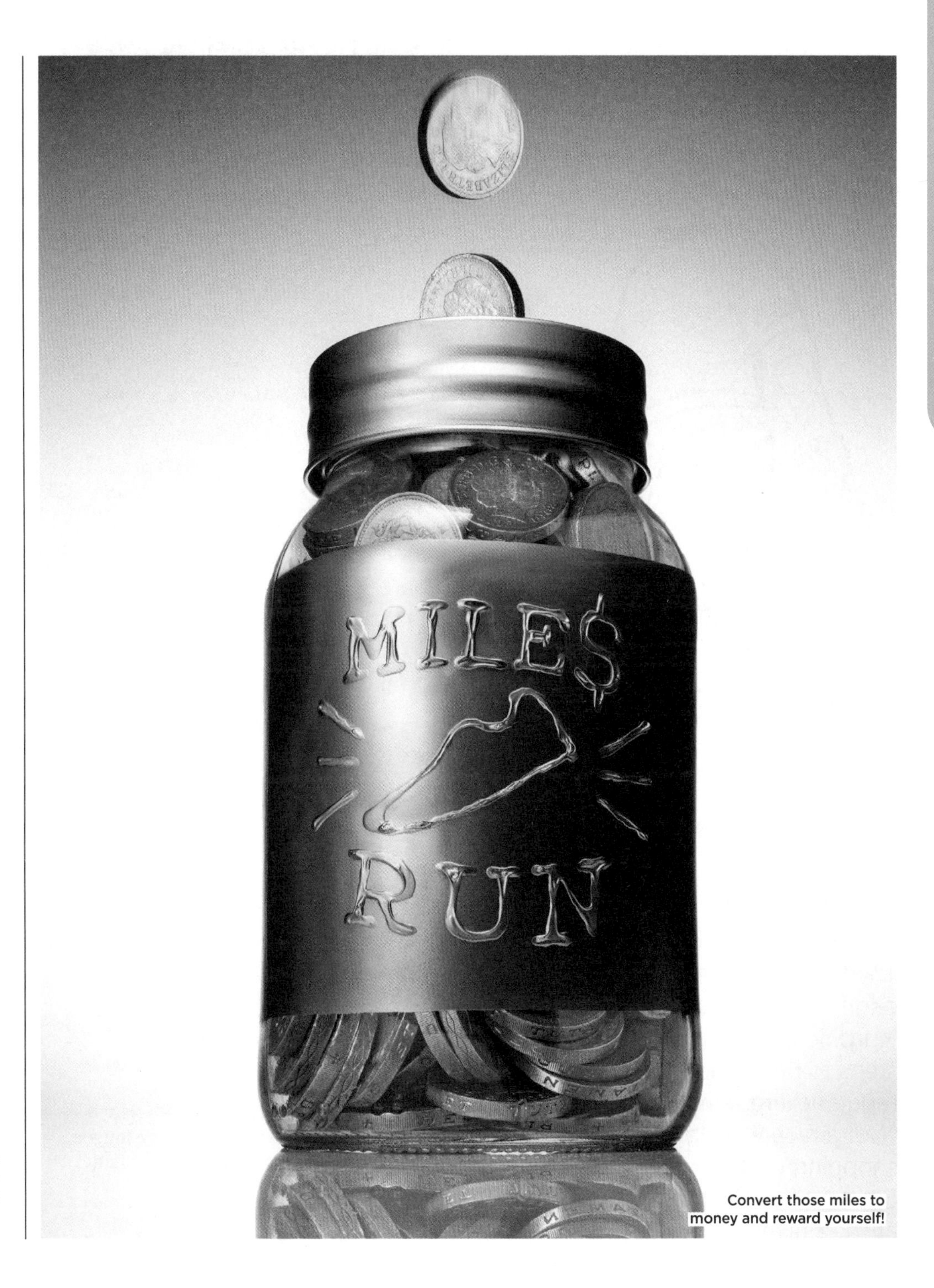

Convert those miles to money and reward yourself!

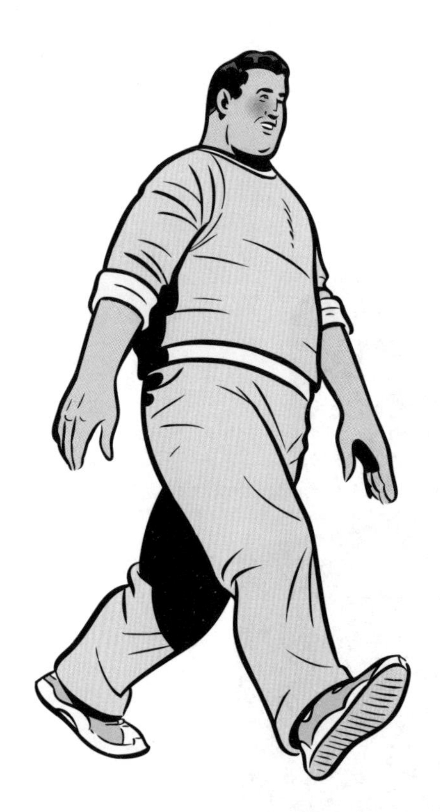

Plan*	MON	TUE
Week 1	15 mins	25 mins
Week 2	15 mins	28 mins
Week 3	20 mins	30 mins
Week 4	20 mins	35 mins
Week 5	20 mins	40 mins
Week 6	20 mins	40 mins
Week 7	20 mins	45 mins

Stage 1
Just get moving

The five plans over the next 10 pages, by running coach Sam Murphy, will take you from your first steps to being race-fit. But get in the regular exercise habit by walking: "Not a race walk, but not a window-shopping walk either," says Steven Blair, professor of exercise science at the University of South Carolina.

Length of plan Seven weeks. (If your BMI is 35 or higher, you're over 60 or just want gradual progression, use this plan for eight to 12 weeks.)
First workout Walking for 15 mins
Goal workout Walking for 60 mins
Are you ready? This plan is for anyone who has yet to exercise at all. It involves only walking, to give your bones, muscles, tendons and general fitness the base they need to progress to running without injury.
Room to manoeuvre No time for a longer session? Split the week's longest in half between morning and afternoon.

WED	THU	FRI	SAT	SUN	Total
Rest or 15 mins	25 mins	Rest	35 mins	Rest	100-115min
Rest or 15 mins	28 mins	Rest	38 mins	Rest	109-124 mins
Rest or 15 mins	30 mins	Rest	40 mins	Rest	120-135 mins
Rest or 15 mins	35 mins	Rest	45 mins	Rest	135-150 mins
Rest or 20 mins	40 mins	Rest	50 mins	Rest	150-170 mins
Rest or 20 mins	40 mins	Rest	55 mins	Rest	155-175 mins
Rest or 20 mins	40 mins	Rest	60 mins	Rest	165-185 mins

*All workouts in this plan are walking only

No more excuses!

THE EXCUSE I just don't have time!
BEAT IT Find a time of day when exercise is non-negotiable, advises coach Susan Paul. For many, that's the morning. "If you do it first thing, you don't have time to think up an excuse," says Paul.

THE EXCUSE People will laugh.
BEAT IT Everyone feels self-conscious at first, and it's easy to believe you're being negatively evaluated by others. Just bear in mind people are much more concerned about themselves.

KEY TO SUCCESS

Get checked. If you're over 40, have a family history of heart disease or a BMI of 35or more, see your GP before you begin running.

Get good gear. Go to a specialist running shop and get fitted for trainers; a bad pair will ruin your running. Also, invest in socks with sweat-wicking fabric to avoid blisters.

Sneak in activity. Take 15 minutes of your lunch break to go walking outside, or even use your office corridors. And set an alert every hour to remind you to get up: taking a five-minute walk break once an hour burns 132 calories over an eight-hour day.

Plan	MON	TUE
Week 1	Walk 30 mins	30 mins cross-training (cycling/elliptical trainer)
Week 2	Walk 30 mins	30 mins cross-training
Week 3	Walk 5 mins; run 1 min/walk 4 mins for 15 mins; walk 5 mins	Walk 5 mins; run 1 min/walk 4 mins for 25 mins; walk 5 mins
Week 4	Walk 5 mins; run 1 min/walk 3 mins for 20 mins; walk 5 mins	Walk 5 mins; run 1 min/walk 3 mins for 25 mins; walk 5 mins
Week 5	Walk 5 mins; run 2 mins/walk 3 mins for 20 mins; walk 5 mins	Walk 5 mins; run 2 mins/walk 3 mins for 25 mins; walk 5 mins
Week 6	Walk 5 mins; run 2 mins/ walk 2 mins for 20 mins; walk 5 mins	Walk 5 mins; run 2 mins/walk 2 minutes for 25 mins; walk 5 mins
Week 7	Walk 5 mins; run 2 mins/ walk 1 min for 15 mins; walk 5 mins	Walk 5 mins; run 2 mins/walk 1 min for 25 mins; walk 5 mins

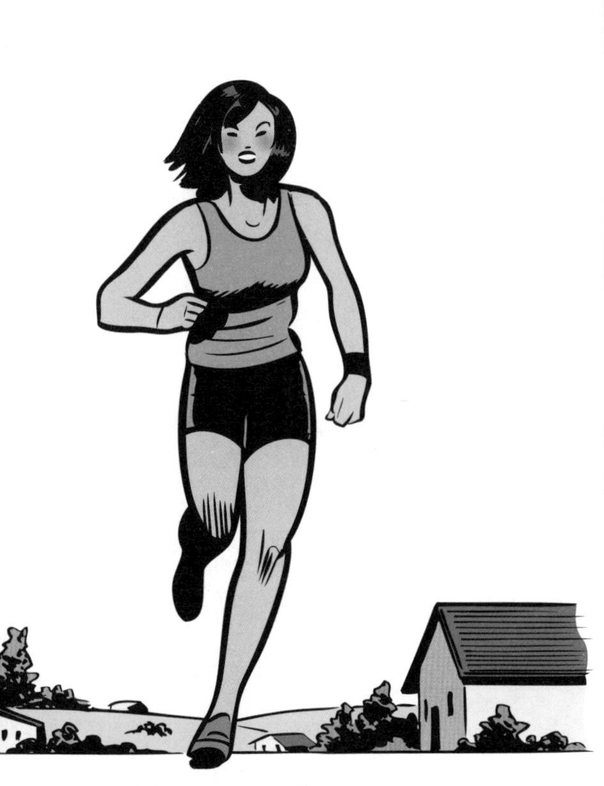

Stage 2
Start running

You're ready to run. And here's the good news: because you'll be moving faster, you'll cover longer distances without adding workout time to your schedule. At the end of this seven-week plan, you'll be able to complete 175 minutes of exercise per week, running for about twice as long as you walk.

Length of plan Seven weeks
First workout Walking for 30 minutes
Goal workout 1 hour with run/walk ratio of 2:1
Are you ready? This plan is for the already active, including Stage 1 finishers. In the first two weeks, you'll exercise for roughly 30 minutes, five days per week. You start running in week three.
Room to manoeuvre Want more of a challenge? On any given day, work out for the same amount of time, but gradually build to a run/walk ratio of four minutes to two minutes, then six minutes to three minutes. Want to take it easier? Repeat any week for as long as you like.

WED	THU	FRI	SAT	SUN	Total
Rest	Walk 30 mins	20 mins cross-training	Walk 40 mins	Rest	150 mins
Rest	Walk 30 mins	20 mins cross-training	Walk 50 mins	Rest	160 mins
Rest or walk 20 mins	Walk 5 mins; run 1 min/walk 4 mins for 25 mins; walk 5 mins	Rest	Walk 5 min; run 1 min/walk 4 mins for 40 mins; walk 5 mins	Rest	145-165 mins
Rest or walk 20 mins	Walk 5 mins; run 1 min/walk 3 mins for 25 mins; walk 5 mins	Rest	Walk 5 mins; run 1 min/walk 3 mins for 40 mins; walk 5 mins	Rest	150-170 mins
Rest or walk 20 mins	Walk 5 mins; run 2 mins/ walk 3 mins for 25 mins; walk 5 mins	Rest	Walk 5 mins; run 2 mins/ walk 3 mins for 40 mins; walk 5 mins	Rest	150-170 mins
Rest or walk 20 mins	Walk 5 mins; run 2 mins/ walk 2 mins for 25 mins; walk 5 mins	Rest	Walk 5 mins; run 2 mins/ walk 2 mins for 40 mins; walk 5 mins	Rest	150-170 mins
Rest or walk 20 mins	Walk 5 mins; run 2 mins/ walk 1 min for 25 mins; walk 5 mins	Rest	Walk 5 mins; run 2 mins/ walk 2 mins for 50 mins; walk 5 mins	Rest	155-175 mins

'I lost 7st and became a marathoner!'

Andrea Ball, 31

Secret of my success What really helped me was making my goals public. It's a giant boost to have people 'like' your status when you've completed a tough workout.

I wish I'd known... To go slow. I was initially frustrated because I tired so quickly. Once I slowed the pace, I could run further, longer and was much more satisfied.

KEY TO SUCCESS

Log your miles. Whether you use a pen and notebook or a GPS (eg, Garmin Forerunner 10, £89.99, wiggle.co.uk), you'll draw confidence from seeing the miles rack up.

Take your pulse. Measure your resting heart rate first thing in the morning; as you become fitter, you'll see this get lower. "This shows your body is responding to the training," says Susan Paul.

Practise patience. Many of the positive changes happening to your body won't yet be visible, but don't panic – this process takes time. The weight loss *will* come.

Plan	MON	TUE
Week 1	Walk 5 mins; run 3 mins/walk 2 mins for 20 mins; walk 5 mins	Walk 5 mins; run 3 mins/ walk 2 mins for 30 mins; walk 5 mins
Week 2	Walk 3 mins; run 3 mins/ walk 1 min for 20 mins; walk 2 mins	Walk 5 mins; run 3 mins/ walk 1 min for 28 mins; walk 5 mins
Week 3	Walk 5 mins; run 4 mins/ walk 1 min for 25 mins; walk 2 mins	Walk 5 mins; run 4 mins/ walk 1 min for 30 mins; walk 5 mins
Week 4	Walk 4 mins; run 6 mins/ walk 1 min for 28 mins; walk 3 mins	Walk 5 mins; run 6 mins/ walk 1 min for 35 mins; walk 5 mins
Week 5	Walk 3 mins; run 7 mins/ walk 1 min for 24 mins; walk 3 mins	Walk 5 mins, run 7 mins/ walk 1 min for 32 mins; walk 5 min
Week 6	Walk 5 mins; run 9 mins/ walk 1 min for 30 mins; walk 5 mins	Walk 5 mins; run 9 mins/ walk 1 min for 40 mins; walk 5 mins
Week 7	Walk 5 mins; run 15 mins/walk 1 min x 2; walk 3 mins	Walk 5 mins; run 12 mins/ walk 2 min x 3; walk 3 mins

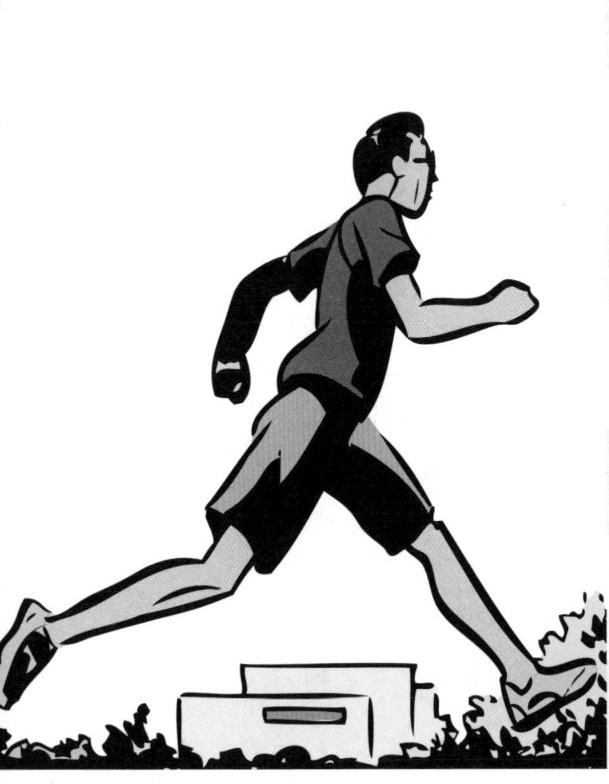

Stage 3

Run non-stop

Want to build your endurance and eliminate those walk breaks? This plan takes you from walking one minute for every two minutes of running, up to continuous running. Each run should be done at a conversational pace. If you're gasping, you're going too fast.

Length of plan Seven weeks
First workout 30 minutes; 20 minutes with a run/walk ratio of three minutes to two minutes.
Goal workout Run 3.1 miles (5K) continuously.
Are you ready? To begin this plan, you should have spent at least six weeks run/ walking for roughly 30 minutes, five days per week, running at least twice the amount of time you spend walking.
Room to manoeuvre There's flexibility: if it's too easy, skip ahead to the next week. If it's moving too fast, spend two weeks or more at each week, although ideally you'll complete the plan within 14 weeks.

WED	THU	FRI	SAT	SUN	Total
Rest or walk 20 mins	Walk 5 mins; run 3 mins/ walk 2 mins for 30 mins; walk 5 mins	20 mins cross-training	Walk 5 mins; run 3 mins/ walk 2 mins for 45 mins; walk 5 mins	Rest	160-180 mins
Rest or 20 mins cross-training	Walk 5 mins; run 3 mins/ walk 1 min for 28 mins; walk 5 mins	Rest	Walk 5 mins; run 3 mins/ walk 1 min for 40 mins; walk 5 mins	Rest	150-170 mins
Rest or 20-30 mins cross-training	Walk 5 mins; run 5 mins/ walk 1 min for 30 mins; walk 5 mins	Rest	Walk 5 mins; run 4 mins/ walk 1 min for 45 mins; walk 5 mins	Rest	165-195 mins
Rest or 20-30 mins cross-training	Walk 5 mins; run 6 mins/ walk 1 min for 35 mins; walk 5 mins	Rest	Walk 5 mins; run 5 mins/ walk 5 mins; run 10 mins; walk 5 mins/run 5 mins; walk 5 mins	Rest	165-195 mins
Rest or 30 mins cross-training	Walk 5 min; run 7 mins/ walk 1 min for 32 mins; walk 5 mins	Rest	Walk 5 mins; run 8 mins/ walk 2 mins; run 12 mins; walk 2 mins/run 8 mins; walk 5 mins	Rest	165-195 mins
Rest or 30 mins cross-training	Walk 5 mins; run 9 mins/ walk 1 min for 40 mins; walk 2 mins	Rest	Walk 5 mins; run 12 mins; walk 2 mins; run 12 mins; walk 2 mins; run 6 mins; walk 5 mins	Rest	175-195 mins
Rest	Walk 3 mins; run 12 mins/walk 2 mins x 3; walk 3 mins	Rest	Walk 5 mins; run 3.1 miles/5K continuously; walk 5 mins	Rest	175 mins

No more excuses!

THE EXCUSE It hurts!
BEAT IT Tuning out can help you, says US professor of kinesiology Christy Greenleaf: "Focus on something other than how your body feels." Try running with a friend or listening to music.

THE EXCUSE I'm just not a runner.
BEAT IT Runner-philosopher George Sheehan once said, "Everyone is an athlete. The only difference is some of us are in training." Focus on the fact that you're improving with *every* step.

KEY TO SUCCESS

Find your place. Map out a few safe, scenic, traffic-free routes you can cover in various weather conditions and times of day.

Find your pace. When you first start running, you want to be consistent enough to build strength and endurance, but slow enough to avoid injury. "A lot of runners try to run too fast; [otherwise] they feel like they're not a runner," warns coach Jeff Gaudette.

Stay flexible. It's OK to split workouts into two or three sessions at first. Three 10-minute sessions deliver the same health boost as a single 30-minute workout, says Blair.

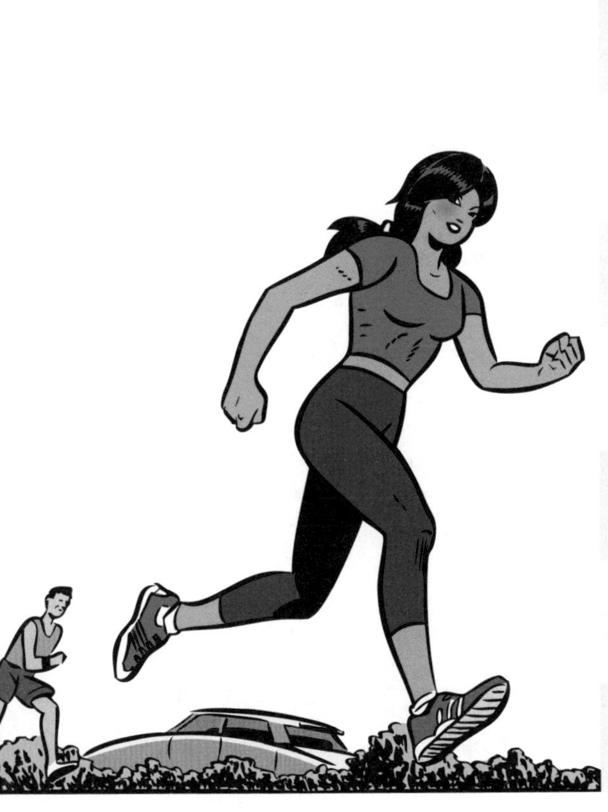

Plan	MON	TUE
Week 1	2 miles*	2 miles
Week 2	2 miles	2.5 miles, inc 8 x alternating 30 seconds of quicker pace with 90 seconds at usual pace
Week 3	2.5 miles	3 miles, inc 5 x 60 seconds of swifter pace alternating with 60 seconds at usual pace
Week 4	3 miles	2.5 miles, inc 8 x 30 seconds of quicker pace alternating with 90 seconds at usual pace
Week 5	3 miles	3 miles, inc 6 x 1 min at quicker pace alternating with 1 min at usual pace
Week 6	2.5 miles	3 miles, inc 4 x 2 mins at quicker pace alternating with 1 min at usual pace
Week 7	2.5 miles	3.5 miles, inc 10 x 30 seconds at quicker pace alternating with 60 seconds at usual pace

Stage 4

Run longer

You've done a nonstop 5K; now you want to run even further. This plan helps you develop the endurance to run a 10K, and build the strength to *race* a 5K. It includes some hills and loosely structured speedwork (fartleks) to build strength.

Length of plan Seven weeks
First workout Two-mile run
Goal workout Run six to seven miles continuously so you can either race a 5K or finish a 10K.
Are you ready? You should have been running for at least 30 minutes, five days a week for at least six weeks, and be able to run 5K without having to walk at all.
Room to manoeuvre If you're ready for a greater challenge, skip ahead a week. But don't rush things. It's better to build gradually so your body gets used to the extra load. If you feel the plan's moving too fast, you can repeat any week until you're ready to progress. Ideally, though, you'll complete this plan in 14 weeks.

WED	THU	FRI	SAT	SUN	Total
Rest or 20 mins cross-training	2 miles	Rest	3 miles	Rest	9 miles
Rest or 20 mins cross-training	2 miles	Rest	3.5 miles	Rest	10 miles
Rest or 30 mins cross-training	2 miles	Rest	4 miles (with 30-second breather at 2 miles if needed)	Rest	11.5 miles
Rest or 30 mins cross-training	2 miles, inc 4 x 30-45-second hill climbs with walk recoveries	Rest	5 miles (with 30-second breather at 3 miles if needed)	Rest	12.5 miles
Rest or 30 mins cross-training	2 miles, inc 4 x 30-45-second hill climbs with walk recoveries	Rest	5 miles	Rest	13 miles
Rest or 30 mins cross-training	2.5 miles, inc 5 x 30-60-second hill climbs with walk recoveries	Rest	6 miles	Rest	14 miles
Rest or 30 mins cross-training	2.5 miles, inc 5 x 30-60-second hill climbs with walk recoveries	Rest	6.5 miles	Rest	15 miles

*Warm up and cool down for 5 minutes before/after each session

'I went from smoking heavily to an ultramarathon'

Ken Thomas, 58

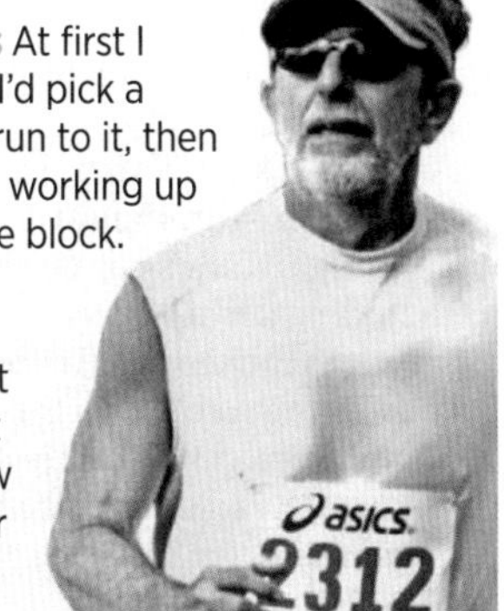

Secret of my success At first I nearly threw up, but I'd pick a lamppost and try to run to it, then walk to the next one, working up to running around the block.

I wish I'd known...
It's fun. It's not about speed; it's about just being out there. Slow as I go, I'm still faster than my sofa.

KEY TO SUCCESS

Think big. "At first, every run is going to be longer and faster, but at some point those wins get harder to come by," says Gaudette. Set long-term goals to give purpose to the short, easy runs.

Stick with the plan. At this stage, it takes discipline to hold back. "People get too excited and push it without thinking about accumulation of fatigue," says Gaudette.

Be alert. Watch for aches and pains that persist or worsen as you run or prompt you to change your gait.

Plan	MON	TUE
Week 1	2 miles	4 miles
Week 2	2 miles	4 miles, with hills
Week 3	3 miles	4 miles, with hills
Week 4	3 miles	4 miles, with hills
Week 5	3 miles	4 miles, with hills
Week 6	3 miles	4 miles, with hills
Week 7	3 miles	1 mile easy; 20 mins 'comfortably hard' with 3-min jog recoveries; 1 mile easy
Week 8	3 miles	1 mile easy; 20 mins 'comfortably hard' with 3-min jog recoveries; 1 mile easy

*After each repeat, jog for the same distance to recover. **About 8 out of 10 perceived effort

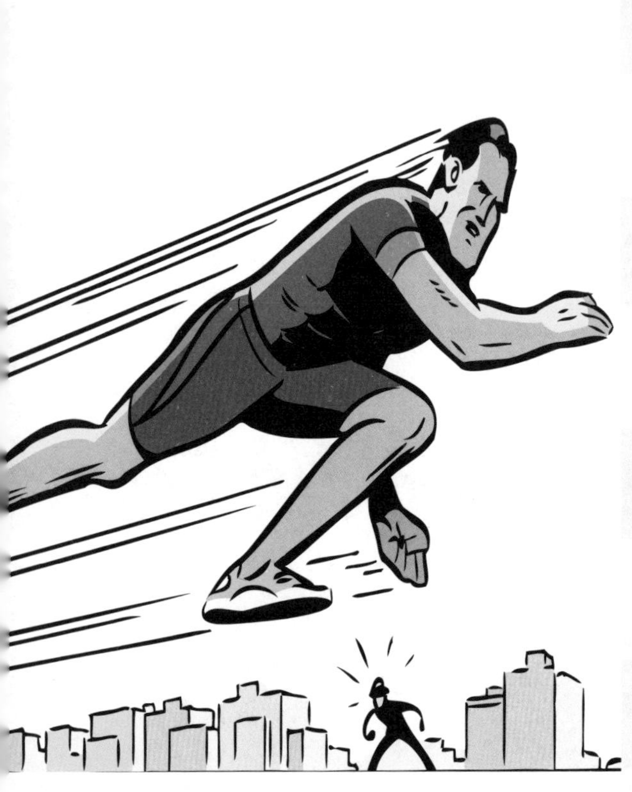

Stage 5
Get faster

This eight-week plan is for those who can already run five or six miles and want to boost their speed. It'll develop endurance, introduce you to speedwork to boost your leg and lung power, and develop 'pace awareness' to help you avoid going out too fast.

Length of plan Eight weeks
First workout Two-mile easy run
Goal workouts Eight-mile run; 4 x 800m at 5K pace.
Are you ready? This plan is for 'advanced beginners'. You should already be running 18 miles per week in total, including a five-miler.
Room to manoeuvre If you can only run four days a week, skip the shortest easy run of the week. Most people do long runs on the weekends, but you can shift days if it better suits your routine.

WED	THU	FRI	SAT	SUN	Total
2 miles	4 miles	Rest	6 miles	Rest	18 miles
2 miles	1-mile warm-up; 4 x 400m @ 10K goal pace;* 4 x 200m @ 10K pace; 2 x 100m @ 10K pace; 1-mile cool-down	Rest	6.5 miles	Rest	19 miles
2.5 miles	1 mile easy, then 2 x 1 mile at a 'comfortably hard' pace**, with 3 min jog between; 1 mile easy	Rest	7.5 miles	Rest	21 miles
2 miles	1-mile warm-up; 4 x 400m @ 5K pace; 4 x 200m @ 5K pace; 1-mile cool-down	Rest	5 miles	Rest	19 miles
2 miles	1 mile easy; 3 x 1 mile at a 'comfortably hard' pace, with 3-min jog recoveries; 1 mile easy	Rest	Walk 5 mins; run 8 mins/ walk 2 mins; run 12 mins; walk 2 mins/run 8 mins; walk 5 mins	Rest	22 miles
2.5 miles	1-mile warm-up; 2 x 800m @ 10K pace; 2 x 400m @ 5K pace; 2 x 200m @ 5K pace; 1-mile cool-down	Rest	8 miles	Rest	23 miles
2.5 miles	1-mile warm-up; 2 x 800m @ 5K pace; 4 x 400m @ 5K pace; 1-mile cool-down	Rest	5 miles (aim to be quicker than week 4)	Rest	21 miles
2.5 miles	1-mile warm up; 4 x 800m at 5K pace; 1-mile cool-down	Rest	8 miles	Rest	24 miles

'Running is thumbing my nose at my MS'

Jodi Edwards, 43

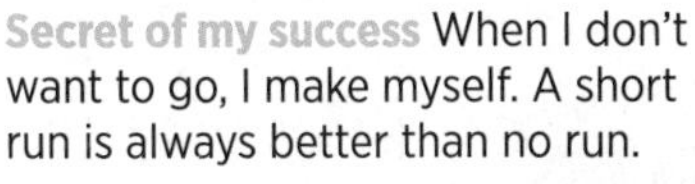

Secret of my success When I don't want to go, I make myself. A short run is always better than no run.

I wish I'd known... Don't compare yourself with others – just compete against yourself.

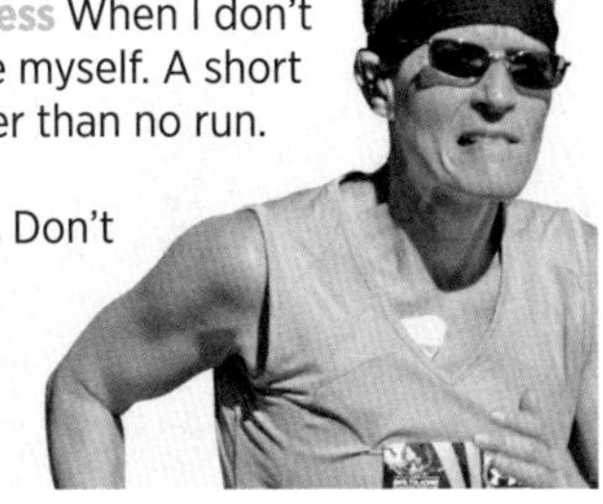

KEY TO SUCCESS

Get a baseline. Get your body fat measured so you track your progress, says coach Mindy Solkin. "Seeing tangible results really helps."

Don't cram. If you miss a day or two, don't risk injury by trying to cram in the extra miles.

Remember life stress. Exercise is a proven stress-reliever, but studies show that if you start your run frazzled (ill, sleep-deprived, anxious about work, etc) it *will* feel harder.

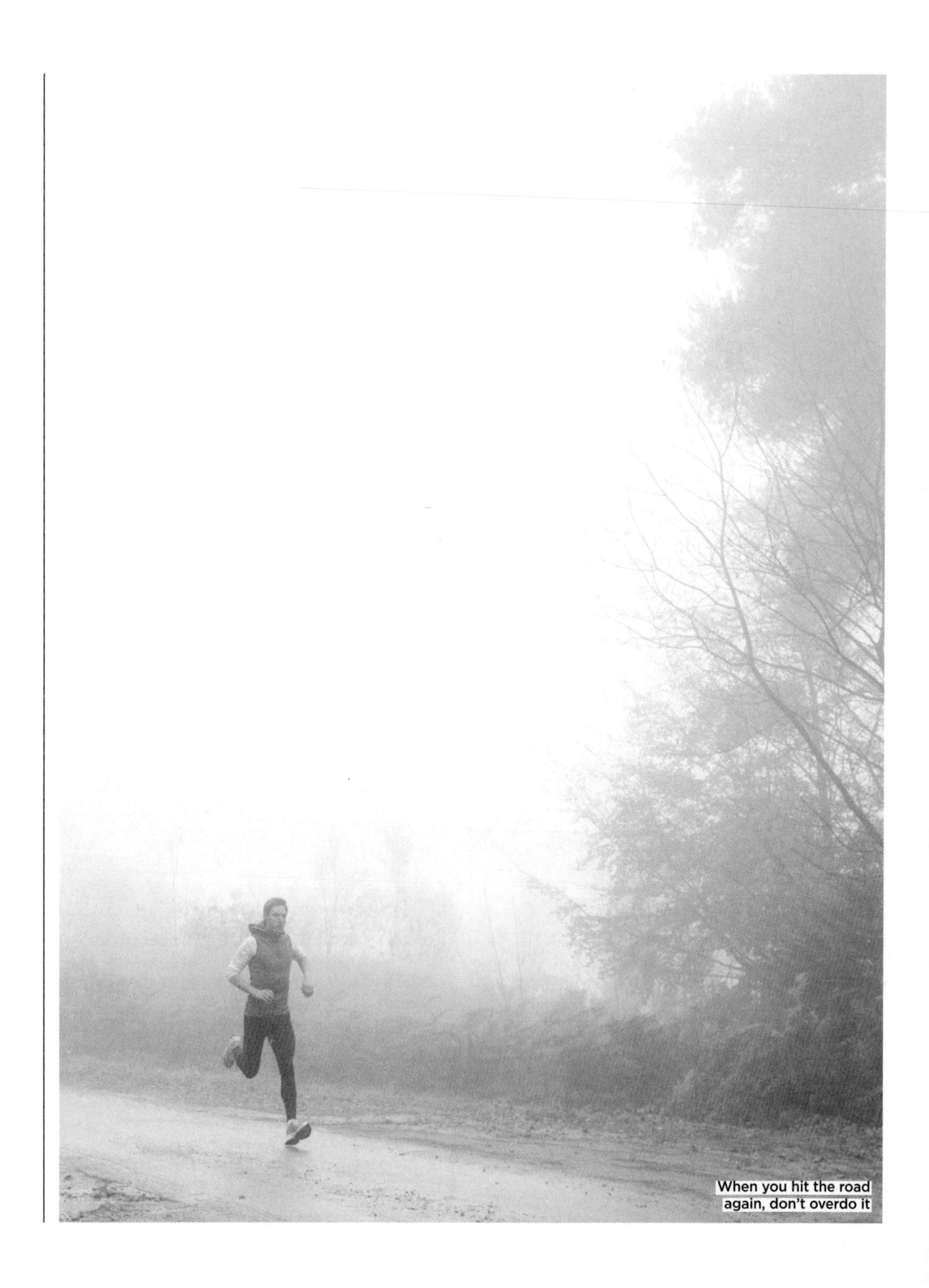

When you hit the road again, don't overdo it

23.

MAKING A COMEBACK

It happens to so many runners, and in all likelihood it's happened to you: you start running; you push your body faster, further and start to dream about PBs, six-pack abs and skinny jeans...

Then, WHAM! Something stops you right in your tracks. You get hurt. You get busy. You get burned out. And those gains in mileage, pace, fitness and confidence suddenly evaporate.

So how do you get moving again after being sidelined? The strategies below will help:

Get some perspective

What happens in your body when you stop running? There's a decrease in blood volume and mitochondria (the power plants in our cells), plus your lactate threshold falls, says coach and exercise physiologist Susan Paul. In general, the longer you've been training, the more quickly you'll be able to get back into it after a layoff, she says. So someone who's been running consistently for 15 years and then has a layoff of a year will have an easier time going back to it than someone who's been running a year and then is off for a year.

The longer you've been running, the bigger your foundation of aerobic strength, explains Paul. You'll have a much higher level of mitochondria to produce energy, more red blood cells to deliver oxygen to the running muscles and more metabolic enzymes. So while your fitness falls during a layoff, it won't drop as low as if you'd just begun running, since you're starting at a much higher fitness level. Also, you lose conditioning in your muscles, tendons, ligaments and connective tissues. It's difficult to assess how much conditioning you lose or how quickly you lose it, but it's the weakness in the musculoskeletal system that causes so many people to get injured when they return to running. This is why running more slowly, reducing mileage and allowing rest and recovery days are so important.

Walk before you run

Before returning to running, you should be able to walk for at least 45 minutes (without pain if returning from an injury), says Paul. Walking reconditions soft tissue (muscles, tendons, ligaments, fascia, connective tissue), preparing them for the more rigorous demands of running, she explains.

Start where you are

Don't just pick up where you left off; many runners try to do more than they should too soon after injury, and end up sidelined even longer. Even if you've been cycling, swimming or doing other cross-training to maintain your aerobic fitness, remember that, depending on the injury and the length of the lay-off, it can take weeks or even months for your body to get strong enough to handle running again.

Start with three or four short runs per week so you're running every other day. Try 5-10 minutes of running at a time, or alternate between running and walking, allowing your body to readapt to the stress of a workout. Use Susan Paul's guide (overleaf).

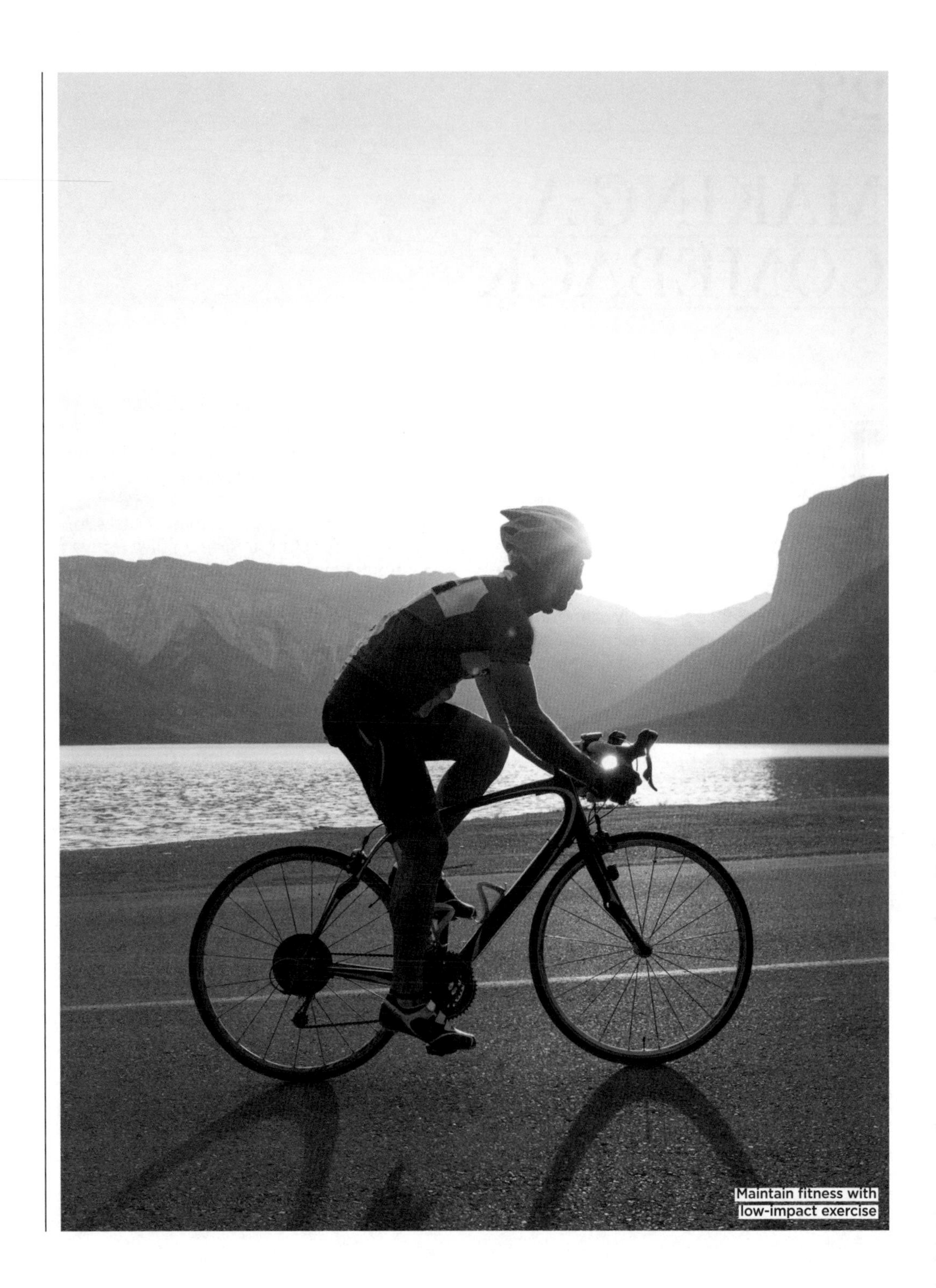

Maintain fitness with low-impact exercise

Comeback guide

IF YOU'RE OFF...	START RIGHT HERE
1 week or less	Pick up your plan where you left off
Up to 10 days	Start running 70% of previous mileage
15-30 days	Start running 60% of previous mileage
30 days to 3 months	Start running 50% of previous mileage
3 months+	Start from scratch

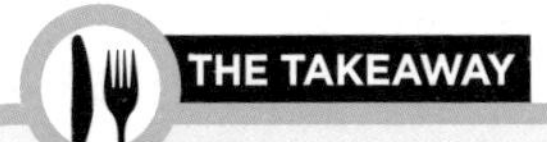

Practise patience.
Rushing back to the routine you maintained before your injury is a sure-fire way to reinjure yourself and even cause new injuries. Don't increase your mileage by more than 10% from week to week.

Mix it up.
Cross-train with exercises that work other parts of your body, don't aggravate your injury and give you a cardiovascular workout. Consult your doctor or a physiotherapist about which modes of exercise are safe and smart given your past injuries.

Be safe, not sorry.
As hard as it can be to rest when you'd rather run, remember that the cautious approach you take now will yield many happy, healthy miles later. If you restart your running and start to feel twinges of your old injury, it's best to take a rest day or do another activity.

Remember the 10% rule

If you've been off for three months or more, don't increase your weekly mileage or pace by more than 10% week over week. Increase it by even less if you need to.

Stay safe

You might consider avoiding the road, says Paul. Using an athletics track allows you to walk or run without being too far from your car in the event that you need to stop. It's a confined, flat, traffic-free area for a workout. Starting on a treadmill can be helpful too. The surface is forgiving, and you can control the pace and incline to suit your needs.

Cross-train

Working out every day will help speed up your cardiovascular fitness. But that doesn't mean you need to run. Add two or three days of cross-training to your routine, but check with your doctor to make sure the particular mode of working out – whether cycling, rowing on a machine, swimming or using an elliptical trainer – doesn't worsen any injury. Also, yoga, Pilates, weight training and core exercises can help you get stronger. That said, if you've done no exercise at all for three months, wait for two to three months before you cross-train; take rest days between your runs instead. That'll ensure that your aerobic system gets enough recovery between workouts.

Don't overmedicate

Over-the-counter painkillers might make you feel better in the short term, but they can mask pain that means you should stop. And for some, they can lead to gastric distress. If you can't run through pain, don't run. Walk or rest instead.

24.

BURN MORE CALORIES WHILE YOU WORK OUT

We runners tend to covet routine. When we start out, the regularity helps us exercise consistently so we can continue building our fitness and work toward our weight-loss goals.

But there's a fine line between a routine that grounds you and a rut that grinds you down. After you've been running for a while, it's easy to slog along at the same pace, at the same mileage, day after day. And while it may feel comfortable for a while, ultimately it can leave you sluggish, achy, bored and stuck on a weight-loss plateau. Even worse, you could start to gain weight instead of losing it.

High-intensity exercise burns calories *after* your workout

Why is that? Over time, your body adapts to any new stress you put on it. That's why running feels easier on your seventh day on the road than on your first day. It's why those five, 10 or even 26.2 miles that at first felt impossible to run, eventually become doable with training and experience. And it's why running at a speed that felt like torture at first eventually becomes your feel-great, I-could-run-all-day-at-this-pace.

"If all you do is run the same distance and terrain at the same effort day after day, you'll adapt to that," says exercise physiologist Janet Hamilton, founder of runningstrong.com.

The key to keep building your fitness – and losing weight – is to add intensity to your running routine. Research proves that when you ratchet up the intensity, you torch more calories on the road *and* after you've worked out. A study published in *Physiology Reports*[1] showed that runners who did high-speed interval work not only boosted their calorie burn during their runs but also upped their resting metabolic rate (the rate at which you burn calories while going about daily activities such as walking, working and cooking).

Further studies have shown that exercising for 45 minutes at vigorous intensity raises your calorie burn for 14 hours after you stop. And it's the 'vigorous intensity' that's the key to achieving this afterburn (known as EPOC: excess post-exercise oxygen consumption)[2]. What does that mean? Well, it's going to be different for everyone but, generally, equal to 70% of your VO_2 max – in other words a little faster than your everyday easy-run pace, so you're able to converse but only in short bursts, and are breaking a sweat.

And by dialling up the intensity, you're not only revving up your afterburn but you're also stimulating development of more fast-twitch muscle fibres – the same muscle fibres that tend to atrophy with age and a sedentary lifestyle, says Hamilton: "The more muscle fibres you have, the more calories you can burn, even when at rest."

And because it builds your fitness, over time you'll find that you get faster and are able to run stronger for longer. This will allow you to reach for more personal bests and burn more calories overall.

Getting fit without getting hurt

Upping the intensity of your workouts doesn't mean you should run as fast every single day. Your cardiovascular system adapts to new stresses much faster than your muscles, bones and joints do. It's important to take a very gradual approach when adding more intense workouts such as tempo runs and speed sessions. So buffer these tougher workouts with rest days and easy running so your body has a chance to adapt and get stronger.

It's also important to have a variety of more intense workouts to build full-body fitness. By mixing up the type of workouts you do – say, long runs one day, speedwork another day and tempo work another day – you're stimulating different parts of your physiology. And that's a mix recommended by many coaches; each one works the legs and lungs in a unique way. Tempo work promotes efficiency so you can push stronger for longer with less effort; a long run develops endurance, while speed sessions build aerobic power. Use the other days to recover with rest or low-impact cross-training (eg, cycling, yoga or strength training), and you'll build full-body fitness.

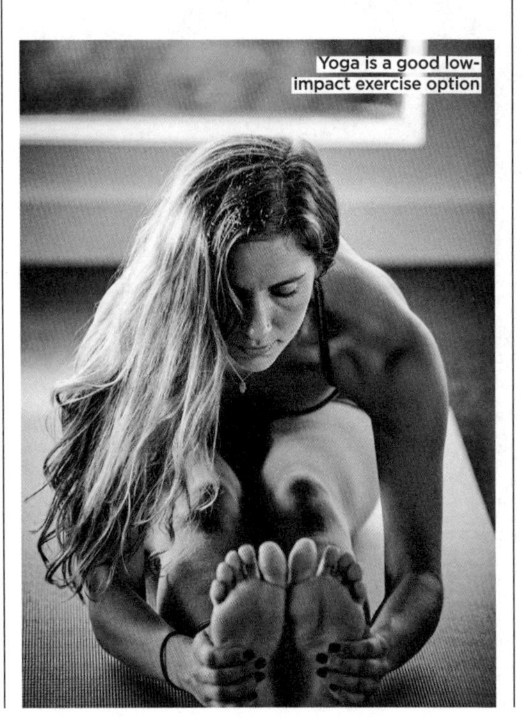
Yoga is a good low-impact exercise option

The good news? You won't have to find more time to work out. In fact, in many cases you'll get more results in less time. And if you equate running fast with pain, try not to worry. It's actually more fun: science has proved it. A study published in the *Journal of Sports Sciences* showed that runners enjoy higher-intensity intervals more than running continuously at a lower intensity.[3] That means you'll be more likely to stick to it.

If you replace three of your weekly easy runs with quality workouts, you can get fit fast without getting hurt. By including speed sessions, tempo runs and long runs, you can get maximum results with the time you have.

Four-day work week

Every week, do each of the following workouts, designed by Hamilton. On the other days, rest, cross-train or run easy. Don't do any of these workouts back to back; that could lead to injury.

TEMPO RUN

What it is Different coaches define a tempo run in different ways. Typically it means sustaining a faster-than-usual pace without breaking into an all-out sprint. This is roughly your 10K pace (to find yours, use the running calculator at runnersworld.co.uk/pacecalculator.)

Why it matters Tempo work improves efficiency so you can run faster for longer with less effort.

What to do Instead of running three to four miles at an easy pace, warm up with one mile of walking or easy running. Gradually speed up to your 10K pace and hold it for one mile. Then recover with three minutes' easy running. Repeat that cycle two more times, then cool down with 1 mile of easy running. If you're

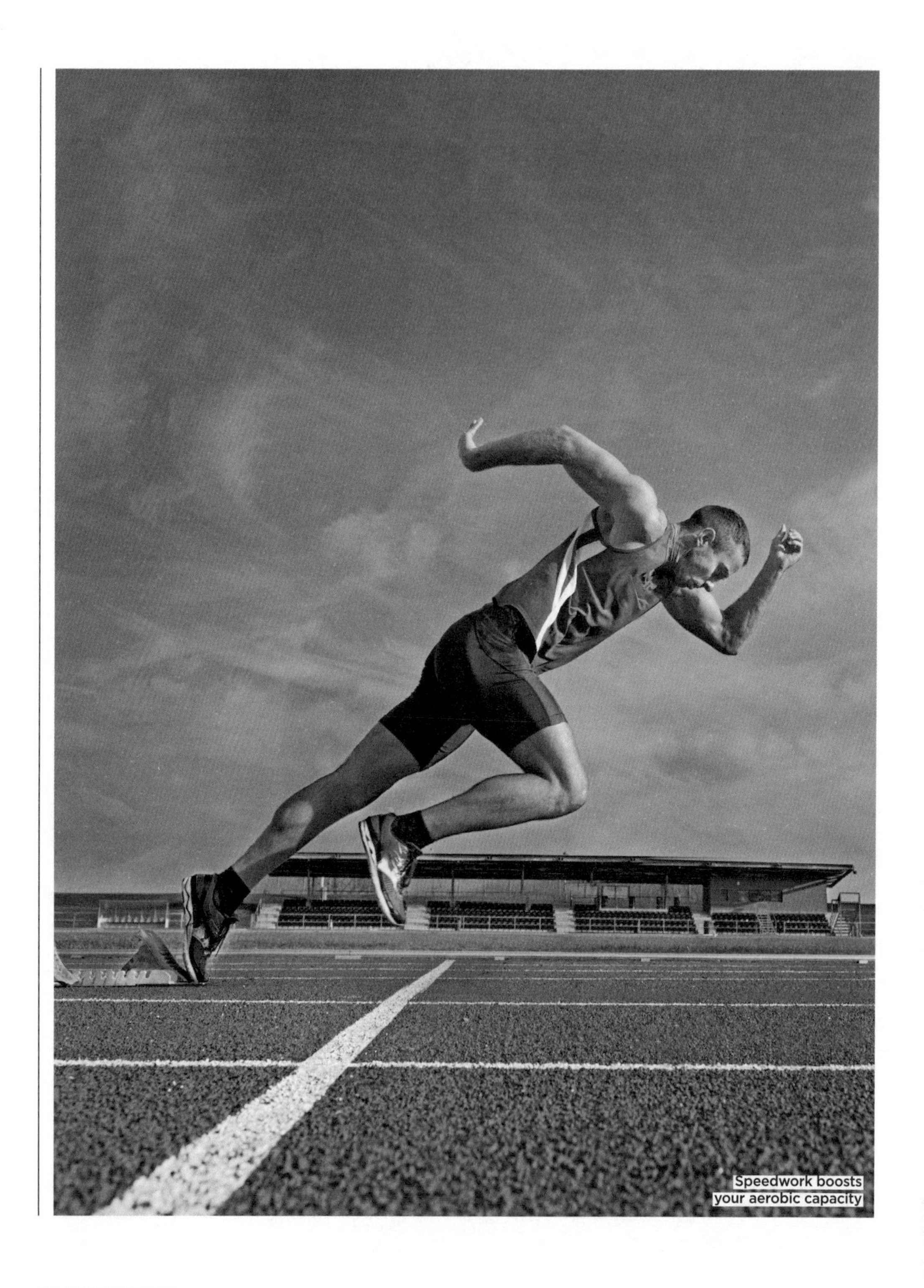

Speedwork boosts your aerobic capacity

more experienced, after a warm-up, start with 10-15 minutes at your 10K pace and build up to 20 minutes. Cool down.

How it feels While running at tempo, you should feel like you've stepped just outside your comfort zone – not actually huffing and puffing, but you should be able to feel the effort.

Keep it honest Every two to three weeks, lengthen the tempo segment of the run.

LONG RUN

What it is Any run longer than your usual ones.

Why it matters Long runs build your aerobic foundation, endurance and mental toughness. When you push your body further or longer than usual, you produce more mitochondria (the cells' powerhouses) and capillaries (which bring blood to the heart), and you train your heart to pump blood more efficiently.

What to do Start with a long run that's about one-third of your total weekly mileage. So if you typically run 15 miles a week, start with a five-mile run. If you're targeting a half marathon, you'll ultimately want to be able to tackle an 11-mile long run to comfortably complete the race. If you have a time goal for the race, your longest runs should be slightly further than the race distance – say, 15 miles for a half marathon or nine miles for a 10K. If you're training for a marathon and shooting for a time goal, you should have one or two 20- or 22-milers under your belt before race day.

How it feels Get into a comfortable, conversational pace you can sustain and finish feeling strong. You should be able to chat without getting out of breath. If you're able to belt out your favourite tune, step it up a bit.

Keep it honest Add one or two miles every three weeks. "It's helpful to hold your long run steady for a couple of weeks before you up it – you should feel like you've 'conquered' the distance before you progress," says Hamilton.

SPEEDWORK

What it is Sessions where you're alternating between bouts of very hard running (at 95% of your maximum effort) and recovery intervals. Typically these are done at your 5K pace.

Why it matters Improves aerobic capacity and helps you turn your legs over faster.

What to do Warm up with 10 minutes of walking and easy running. Then alternate between running at your 10K pace for 400m, then recovering with 400m of easy running.

How it feels During the bouts of hard work, you'll be running near your maximum effort. It should feel tough to say more than one or two words at a time. If you can ask the question 'Am I running fast enough?' without gasping for air, you're not. You should be able to say "this... (breath)... feels... (breath)... hard." The goal is to have enough recovery to be able to do the next speed interval. "Focus on matching your target pace, not beating it," says Hamilton.

Keep it honest Start with two 400m repeats, then move up to four to six 400m repeats, alternating that with 400m of easy running to recover. Once you're comfortable, start cutting the recovery intervals to 200m. If you want to switch things up, keep the recovery intervals at 400m but lengthen the bouts of hard work to 600-800m.

HILL WORK

Why it matters Hills build leg and lung strength, and give you the foundation of fitness you need to get faster.

What to do Once a week, incorporate into your run a variety of hills that take 30-60 seconds to climb. As you go uphill, try to stay relaxed. Keep your gaze straight ahead and your shoulders down, and envision your feet pushing up and and the road rising to meet you. On the way down, don't let your feet

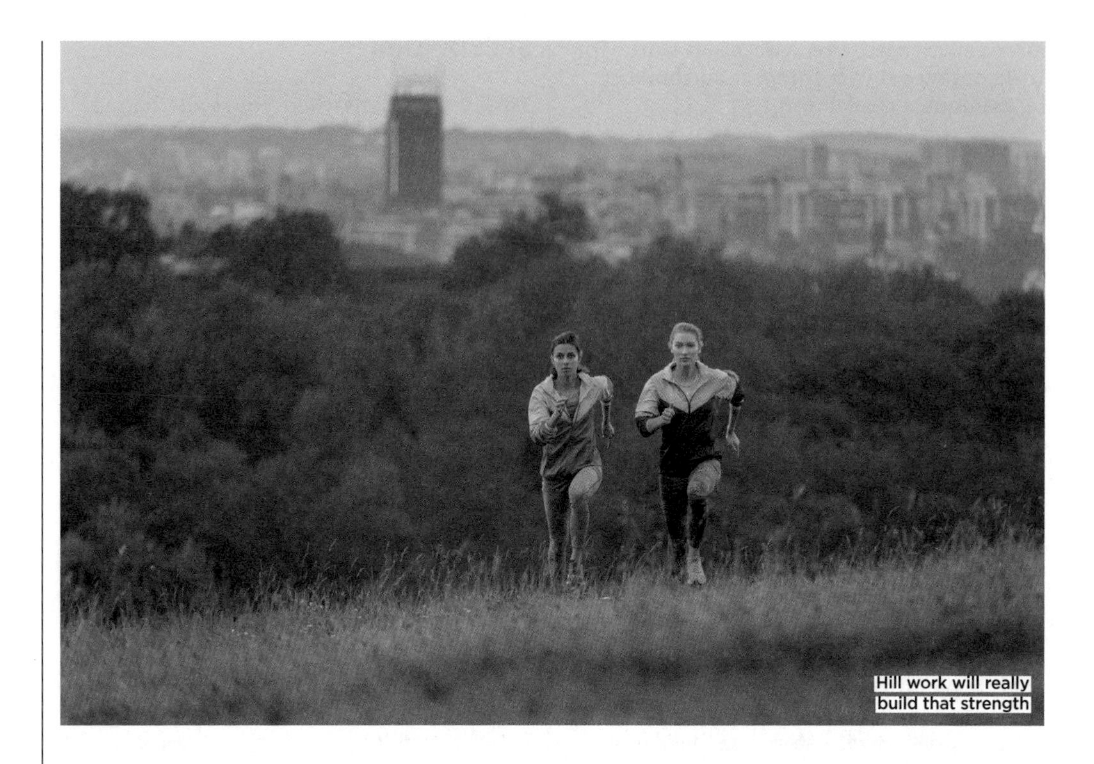

Hill work will really build that strength

slap the ground, and avoid leaning back and braking with the quads, as that will put you at risk of injury.

How it feels Try to maintain an even level of effort as you're ascending or descending. Avoid trying to charge the hill; you don't want to be spent by the time you get to the top.

Keep it honest As you get fitter, add tougher hills with a variety of gradients and lengths.

Keep it safe and effective

As you ratchet up the intensity, taking these steps will help you make the most of your time without getting injured.

Pick the right pace It's important to make sure you're doing your easy runs and your hard track workouts at a pace that's appropriate for your current level of fitness. To find your 5K or 10K pace, plug a recent race time into our training calculator at runnersworld.co.uk/pacecalculator. Don't have a recent race time? Run a 5K or do a time trial. Here's how: warm up with one mile of easy running. Then run four laps of a (400m) running track – or one mile on a flat stretch of road – and note your time. Run one mile to cool down. Plug the time of your fast mile into the training calculator to get the appropriate training paces.

Brush up on your track tactics Tracks are ideal for faster workouts; they're flat, usually traffic-free and the distance is measured. Haven't run on a track since you were at school? Don't be scared – here's what you need to know.

- Standard tracks are 400m long.
- 400m is about a quarter of a mile, so four laps around the track equals one mile.
- Many schools open their tracks to the public.

- No access to a track? You can do speedwork on a treadmill or any flat, traffic-free road.
- A 'repeat' refers to a bout of fast running. For example, in 4 x 100m at 10K pace, the 'repeat' is the 100m.

Don't cram Lots of people get hung up on running a certain number of miles per week and, if they miss a day or two, try to cram in extra miles. That's a recipe for injury. Stick to the plan as best you can, but when life gets in the way – or you feel fatigued or sore – it's OK to put the workout off until another day or skip it altogether. Remember: a single workout won't make or break your fitness; it's the accumulated impact of fitness you've built over the course of weeks or months that gets you in shape. But if you try to cram in miles in too short a period of time, you could get sidelined for weeks or months.

Stay well fuelled When you're running faster, and going longer, you must make sure you're well hydrated and fuelled before you go out. (See Chapter 17 on pre-run fuelling.) Running on empty doesn't aid weight loss; in fact, if you're energised, you'll be able to run faster (and burn more calories) and get fitter. To prevent GI distress, try to stay hydrated throughout the day. Each day, aim to drink half your body weight (in lbs) in fluid ounces. So if you weigh 200lbs (14st 4lbs), aim to consume 100 fl oz (2.8ltr) calorie-free fluids such as water; if you weigh 150lbs (10st 10lbs), aim for 75 fl oz (about 2.2ltr).

If you're going to be on the road for 75 minutes or longer, arm yourself with refuel carbs to keep you energised. A variety of energy gels and chews are available, or you can use sweets or real food. Aim for 30-60g carbs per hour while you're on the road. Even if you're not hungry or tired, to avoid hitting the wall, start fuelling 20-30 minutes into the run and refuel at regular intervals. Try different brands and flavours to find which foods give you a boost without leaving you with an upset stomach.

Don't discount your life stress While exercise is a proven stress reliever, if you start your workout frazzled or drained from your non-running life, the workout is going to feel harder. In fact, studies have shown that workouts feel tougher for people who are stressed than for those who aren't, even when they're working at the same level of effort.

Take good notes As you add speed to your routine, it's especially important that you keep a detailed training log, noting how far and fast you went, how you felt while you were out, the terrain, the route and what the weather conditions were. This will help you avoid injuries: if you see that your knee was achy a few days in a row, you'll know to take a break before it becomes a full-blown injury. It'll also help prevent burnout. Say you're starting to feel bored and less motivated to get on the road; you might see in your log that you've done that five-mile route for three months. You'll know it's time for a change. Also note when you buy your shoes: running shoes should be replaced every 300-500 miles: worn-out footwear is a common cause of injury.

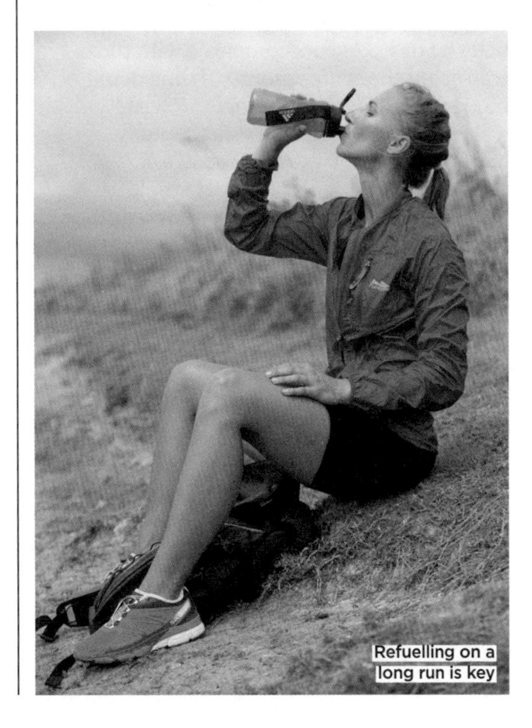
Refuelling on a long run is key

25.

STRENGTH TRAINING FOR WEIGHT LOSS

We runners tend to dread strength training and avoid it at any cost. After all, it's hard enough to find the time just to get the miles in. But research proves that weight training, when combined with running, can boost your calorie burn more than running alone.

In a 2014 study published in *Obesity*, researchers found that healthy men who did 20 minutes a day of weight training gained less belly fat over 12 years compared with those who spent the same amount of time doing moderate-to-vigorous aerobic activity.[1]

The 10-step workout in this chapter has been designed by *Runner's World* contributor and coach Jenny Hadfield, founder of jennyhadfield.com and co-author of *Marathoning for Mortals* and *Running for Mortals*.[2] These moves target strength, balance and mobility, so you can build more lean body mass, torch more calories and run faster.

"This total-body workout focuses on key exercises for a runner's needs, like glute and core strength, balance and stability," says Hadfield. "You don't have to train for an hour and a half at a gym with weights to develop balanced, lean muscle tissue. Like running, it's more about consistency, and this programme makes it too convenient not to do it anywhere."

And the best part? It can be done anytime, anywhere in less than 20 minutes. Add a warm-up and cool-down, and you can do it on days when you can't run. Use an interval timer (or a watch or phone with a suitable app) and set it up to repeat the interval at 75-second increments. Do the 10 strength moves back to back, performing each move for one minute. The goal is to keep your heart rate up by moving from one exercise to the next while fatiguing target muscle groups. (The 15 extra seconds allow for movement into the next exercise. If you find that you need less time, you can shorten the interval time.)

Repeat this sequence two or three times per week – after a run or as a standalone workout with an added warm-up and cool-down – for three to four weeks.

As you gain strength, you can easily tweak the sequence to ratchet up the intensity of the programme so you keep improving your fitness and strength. When you're ready, you can do the circuit in reverse. After three weeks, or whenever it feels suitable, change it up again, performing all the lower-body exercises consecutively, followed by the upper-body moves, then finishing up with the core work.

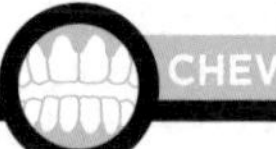

CHEW ON THIS

Because muscle weighs more than fat, when you start strength training you might find you're not losing weight as quickly as you'd hoped. But not only will you be getting more toned, your metabolic rate could increase by 15%, and for every extra lb of muscle you gain, your body will burn 50 more calories a week.

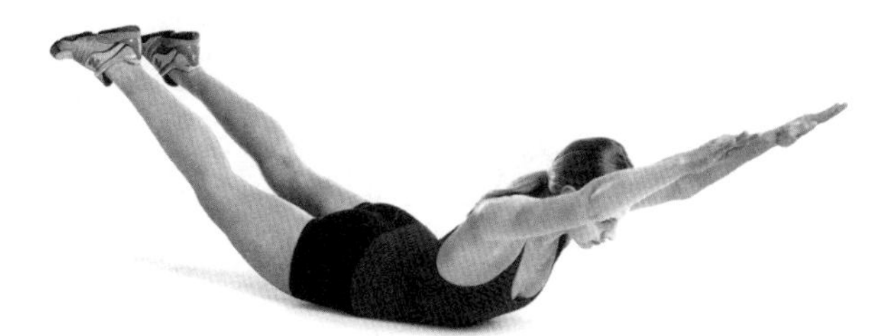

◂ Superman

Lie face down on the floor with your arms over your head and legs straight. Lift your arms and legs off the floor and hold for five seconds, then release. Repeat for one minute.

Press-up + plank hold ▸

Start in modified press-up position on your hands and knees (unless you perform press-ups regularly, on your toes). Press up and extend the arms straight, hold for five seconds with a neutral body alignment (plank), and lower slowly back down. Repeat for one minute.

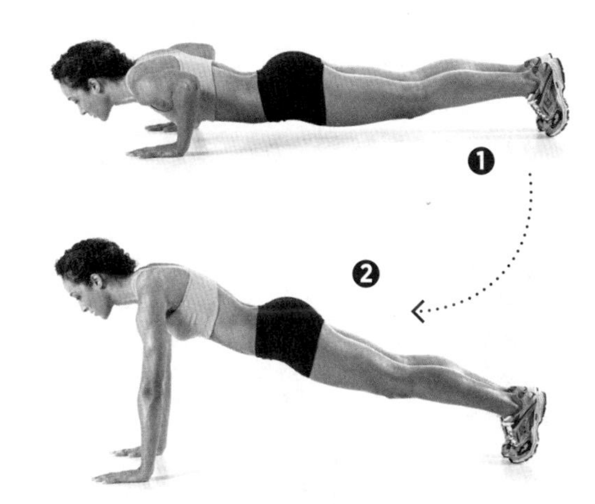

◂ Plank

Lie face down with your forearms on the floor. Push up so your elbows are under your shoulders and your arms are bent at 90 degrees. Hold your body in a straight line from your head to your feet for 30 seconds.

Side plank ▸

From plank position, shift to your side on your elbow and feet, and hold the side plank for 30 seconds. Repeat on the other side.

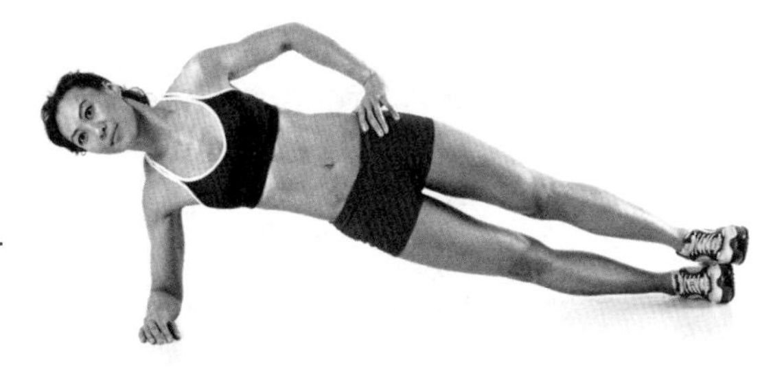

Photography: Beth Bischoff. **Sources:** 1. *Obesity*. 2. runnersworldonline.com.au/runners-strength-workout-can-done-anywhere/

Lunge ▸

Stand with your feet about hip-width apart. Take an exaggerated step forward. Keeping your core in good alignment, bend the front knee 90 degrees until your thigh is parallel with the floor. Make sure the knee is over the ankle and not beyond the toes. Pause and push through your front heel to return to the starting position and repeat for one minute. Do one minute on each leg.

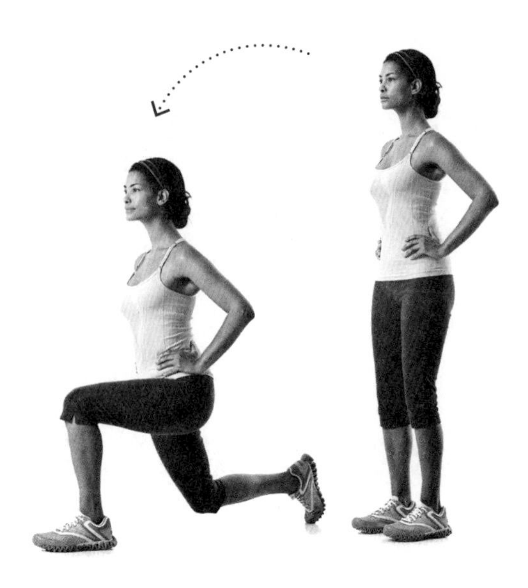

◂ Squat and calf raise

Standing with your feet hip-width apart, sit back and lower down into squat position, focusing on keeping your weight back over your heels. Press and extend your legs, then press up onto your toes for a calf raise. Lower and repeat slowly for one minute.

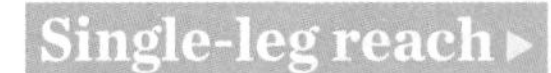

Single-leg reach ▸

Stand on your right leg and bend over, reaching your left hand towards your right toes. Stand up and bring your left knee high and right arm straight up. Repeat on both sides.

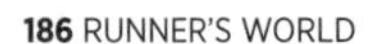

Bridge ▸

Lie on your back with your hands by your sides on the floor. Using your gluteal muscles, squeeze and lift your hips off the floor until you make a line from your knees to your hips and shoulders. Pause for a few seconds and then lower your hips back to the floor. Repeat for one minute.

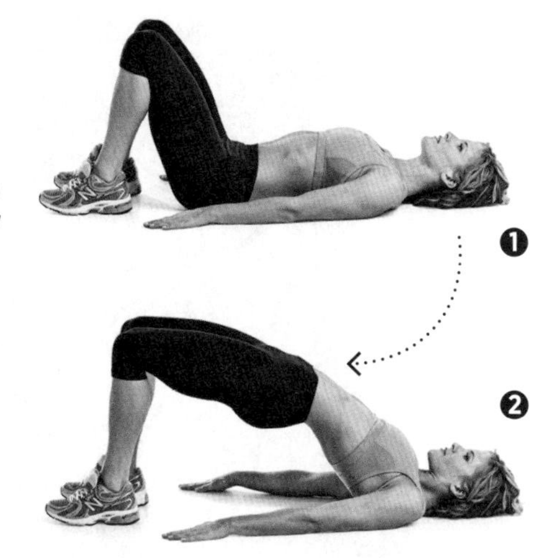

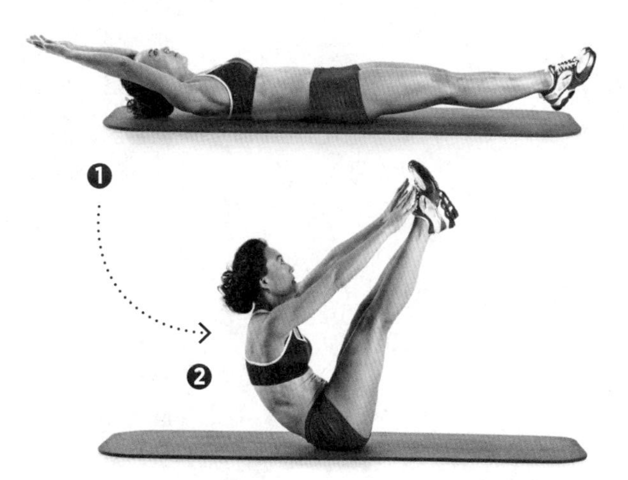

◂ Jackknife crunch

Lie on your back with your arms over your head and your legs bent, feet on the floor. Crunch and raise your legs slowly straight up towards the ceiling. Reach your hands towards your toes and slowly lower back down to starting position. Focus on keeping your core contracted and lower back on the floor. Repeat for one minute.

Fire hydrant ▸

On your hands and knees, slowly raise your right bent leg up to the side, pause, hold for two seconds, then slowly release down, for 30 seconds. Repeat on the left side.

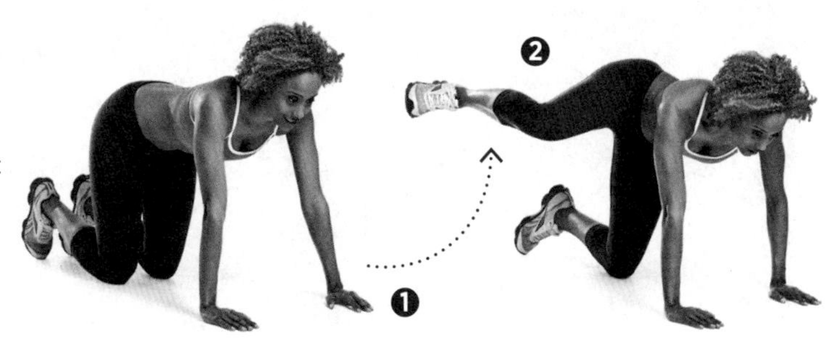

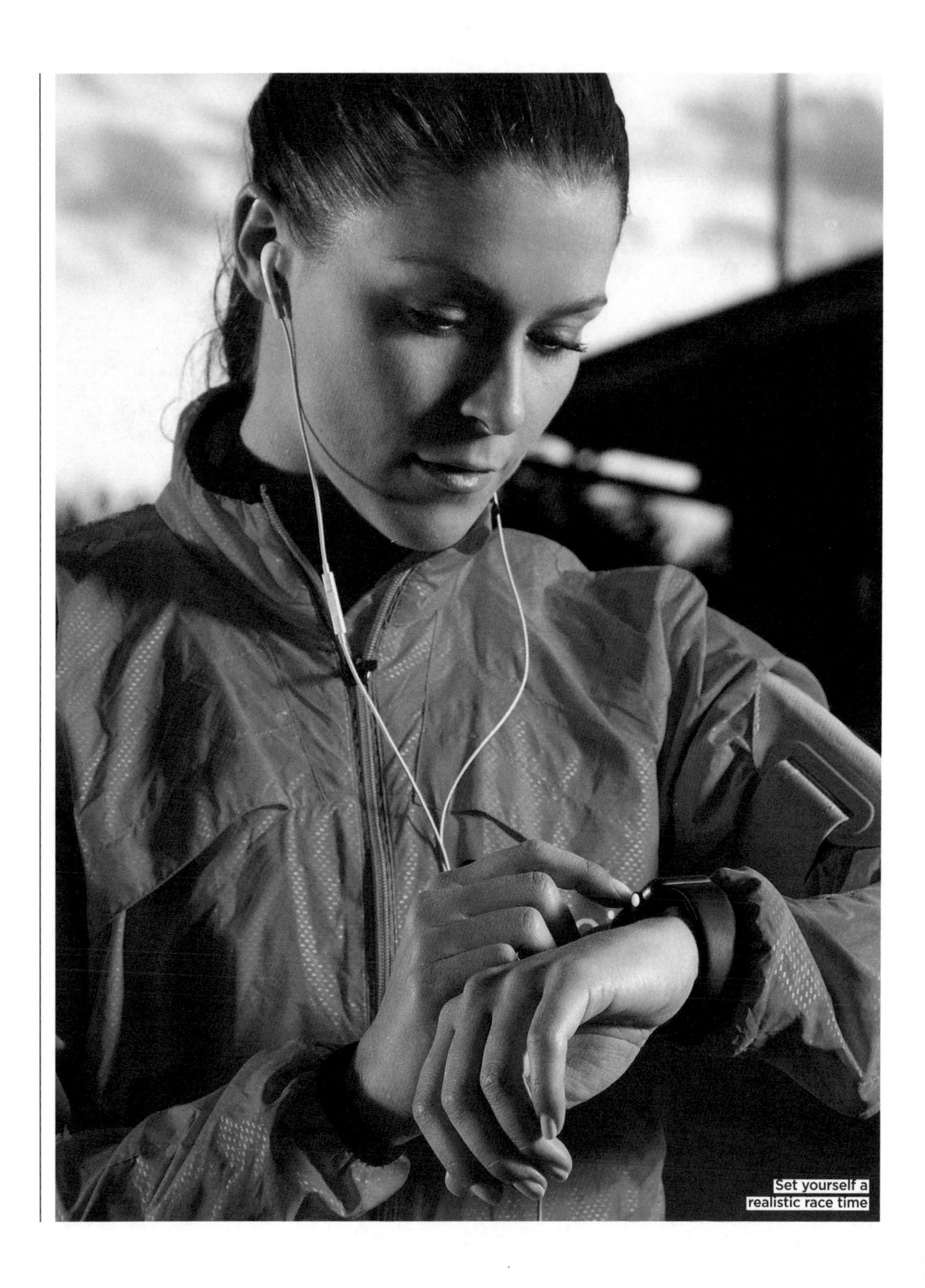

Set yourself a realistic race time

26.

SETTING SMART GOALS

Goals are critical. They drive us to be our best. They get us out of bed when we'd rather stay in; they help keep our fitness on track when it would be easy to make excuses and allow laziness into our routine.

But if your goals are going to help you unleash your potential, they've got to be the right fit for your lifestyle and temperament. If not, injury and disappointment are all but assured. Here's how to work out a goal that will set you up for success.

Make it personal

When it comes to choosing a goal, whether it's a certain distance, a finishing time, an ideal number on the scales or even what your abs should look like, make sure it's meaningful to *you*. Don't get swept up in what's trendy or what everybody else seems to be doing.

In our culture, many powerful influences try to tell us what our goals should be. Magazine covers and celebrities provide 'ideals' for what our bodies 'should' look like. We draw inspiration and motivation from the athletic accomplishments of our friends and family.

In recent years, half marathons and marathons have become wildly popular, and it's tempting to feel that if you run you have to go the distance. But these endurance events aren't for everyone. If it's not in sync with your fitness, experience or, most importantly, what you enjoy, you're setting yourself up for injury and burnout. Remember, a race takes just a day, but the training consumes months of your life and impinges on your work and family lives. If you're going to invest that kind of time and energy, make sure it's what you want.

How-to: Think about the kinds of distance and workout you enjoy most and pick a goal that will allow you to spend most of your time running that distance. If you want to target a half marathon, it's best to have at least six months' regular running experience before you start out; for a marathon, a year is preferable. And when it comes to picking a realistic finish time, you've got to start where you are. Do a 5K and plug your time into any of the many online fitness calculators.

Make sure the training fits your schedule

Whatever distance you intend to race, be sure you have the time to train for it. If you're training for a long distance, you'll need one to four hours at least once a week for an endurance-building long, slow distance run. And with most standard training plans, you'll need to run several days a week, plus make time for recovery, sleep and strength training.

If your schedule already feels jam-packed with work and family commitments, you might consider targeting a different goal. If the training begins to interfere too much with your lifestyle there's a good chance you'll burn out or give up before you reach the starting line.

How-to: Look at some standard training schedules for the distance you're considering. Map out how and when you'd do each workout

Don't train yourself to exhaustion

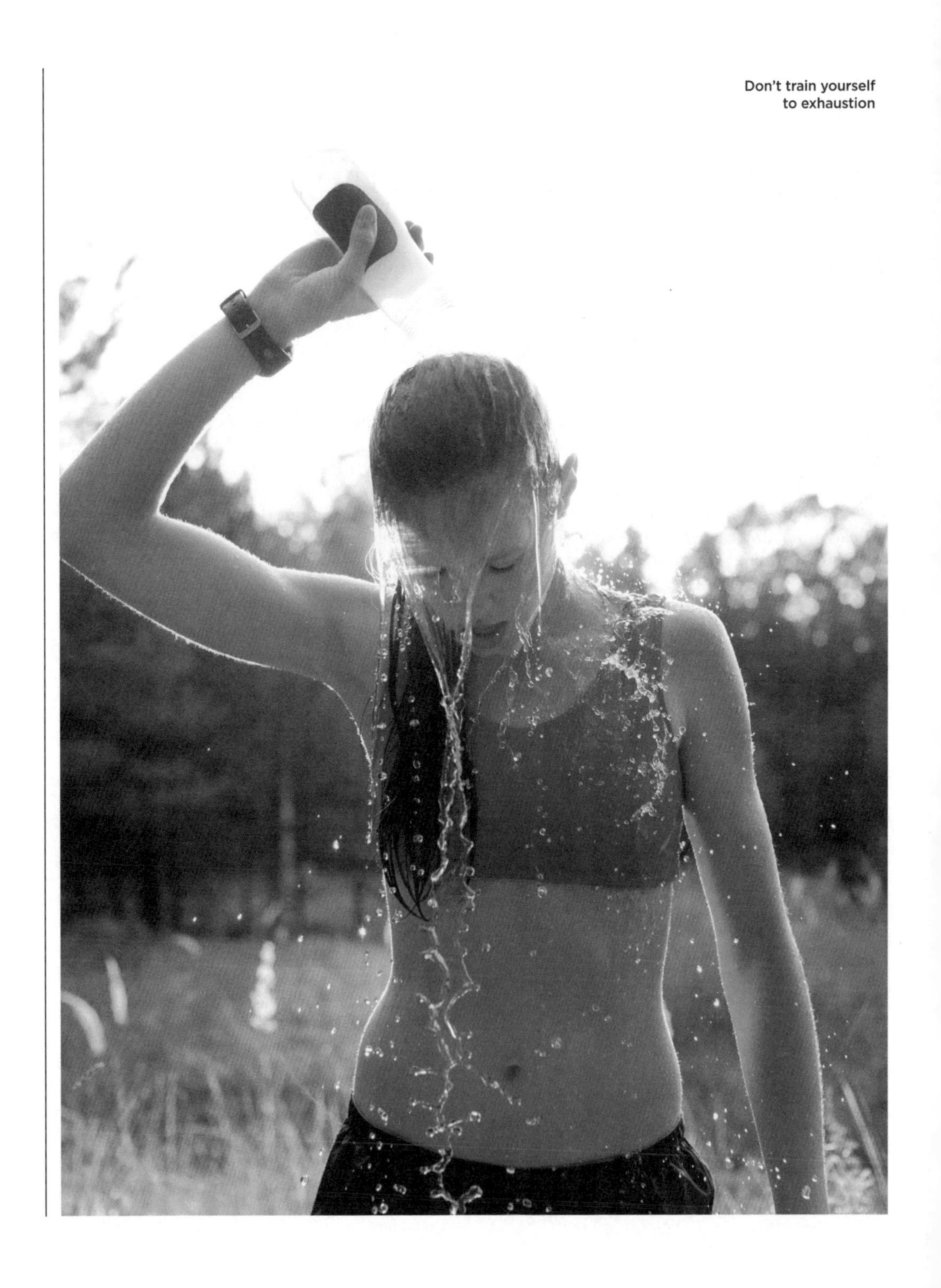

on each day of the week. Talk to your spouse, kids and boss to let them know you're considering training for an event and discuss how and when you'd fit the training in. If your first choice for a goal isn't going to work, target a different distance. You can build your fitness by racing at any distance: 5Ks will help you build speed so you can kick to the finish, while targeting 10Ks and half marathons will help you learn how to sustain a faster pace for a longer distance. All those skills will help you ultimately in longer-distance events.

Let the body be the boss

If you've made the mistake of overtraining, you know you can't just beat your body into submission. There's a huge difference between the general muscle soreness that goes along with pushing yourself further than you've gone before and the sharp, shooting, persistent pains that go along with injury. Each individual has their own unique orthopaedic threshold: ie, how many miles and how much intensity you can handle before your body breaks down. This is determined by age, genetics, gender, anatomy, biomechanics, history of injury, experience and a variety of other factors. Trying to train through pain will only turn short-term injuries into long-term problems that could haunt you for life.

How-to: Consider what types of workout and distance you can do without pain. Do cross-training and strength training help? Pick a distance and a goal that allow you to train within your pain-free sweet spot.

Get to the starting line with four goals

Even if your training goes perfectly, anything can happen on race day. If your satisfaction with your event is entirely contingent on reaching a single time goal, you're setting yourself up for upset. It's important to have four goals at the starting line: one for the ideal day; one you'd be happy with; one just to finish, and a process goal. A process goal has nothing to do with the outcome of the race; it's about what you do during the race to boost your chances of reaching your goal time. You might aim to execute your fuelling strategy perfectly, not walk up hills, or run a negative split (do the second half of the race faster than the first).

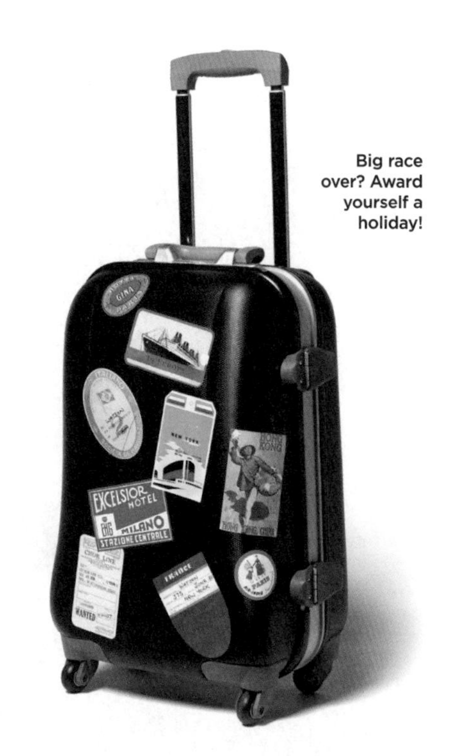

Big race over? Award yourself a holiday!

How-to: To set a realistic time target, schedule a tune-up race two to four weeks before your goal event to test your fitness. Put your finishing time into the *Runner's World* training calculator (runnersworld.co.uk/pacecalculator) to figure out a realistic goal for your big event. Aim for that time – not the one you targeted when you started training. Training requires months of preparation and anything can happen during that period – work, injuries and family commitments can all affect that original goal. You have to start each race where you are!

Think beyond the finish line

When training for an event, the preparation gets so intense and takes so long that it's easy to get consumed by the result, and to feel a little lost after it's all over. That's natural.

How-to: Schedule a race of a shorter distance, – or a holiday or a big event – in the weeks following your goal race. That way, no matter what the result, you'll have something to look forward to after you finish.

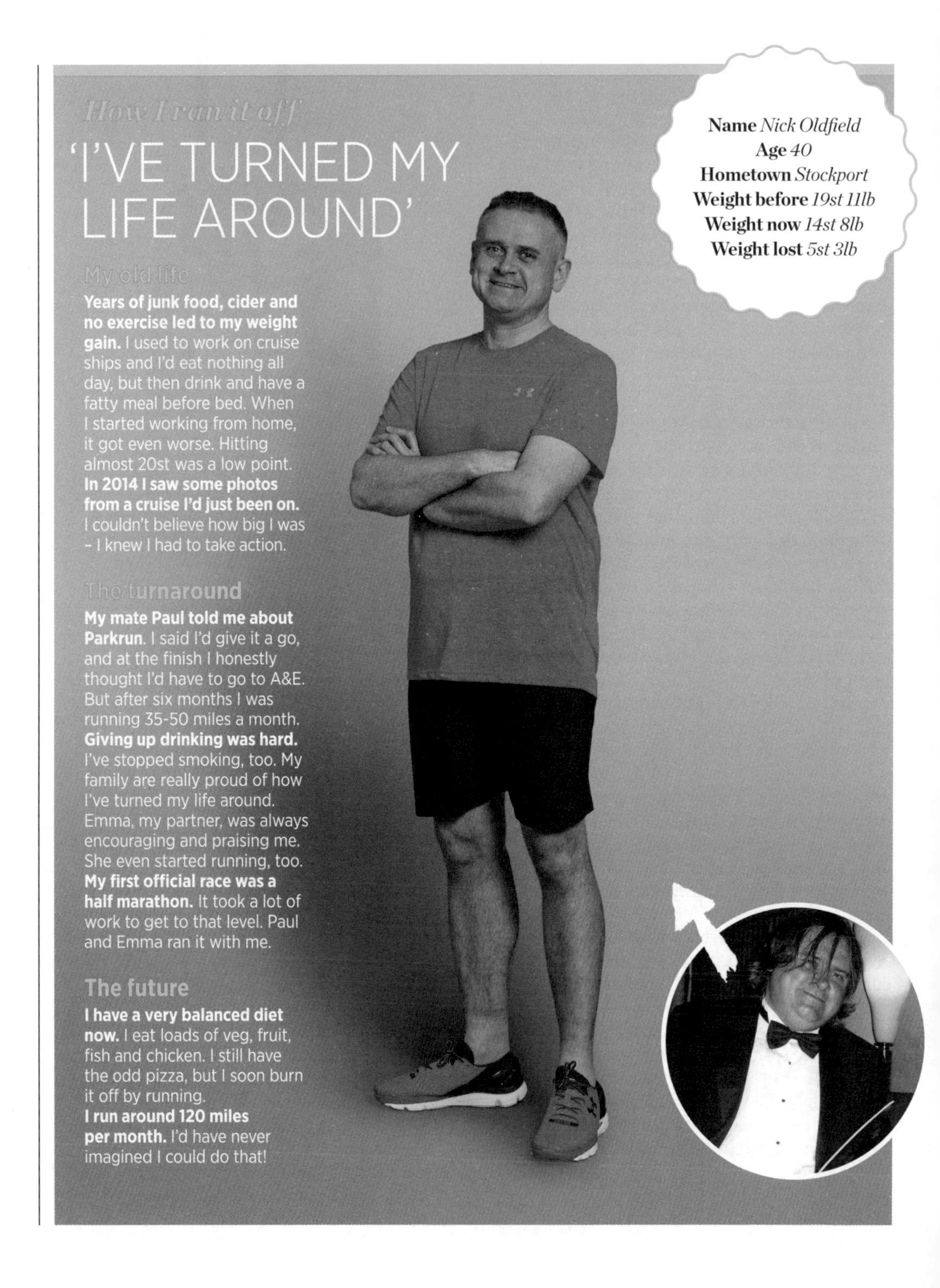

How I ran it off

'I'VE TURNED MY LIFE AROUND'

Name *Nick Oldfield*
Age *40*
Hometown *Stockport*
Weight before *19st 11lb*
Weight now *14st 8lb*
Weight lost *5st 3lb*

My old life

Years of junk food, cider and no exercise led to my weight gain. I used to work on cruise ships and I'd eat nothing all day, but then drink and have a fatty meal before bed. When I started working from home, it got even worse. Hitting almost 20st was a low point. **In 2014 I saw some photos from a cruise I'd just been on.** I couldn't believe how big I was – I knew I had to take action.

The turnaround

My mate Paul told me about Parkrun. I said I'd give it a go, and at the finish I honestly thought I'd have to go to A&E. But after six months I was running 35-50 miles a month. **Giving up drinking was hard.** I've stopped smoking, too. My family are really proud of how I've turned my life around. Emma, my partner, was always encouraging and praising me. She even started running, too. **My first official race was a half marathon.** It took a lot of work to get to that level. Paul and Emma ran it with me.

The future

I have a very balanced diet now. I eat loads of veg, fruit, fish and chicken. I still have the odd pizza, but I soon burn it off by running.
I run around 120 miles per month. I'd have never imagined I could do that!

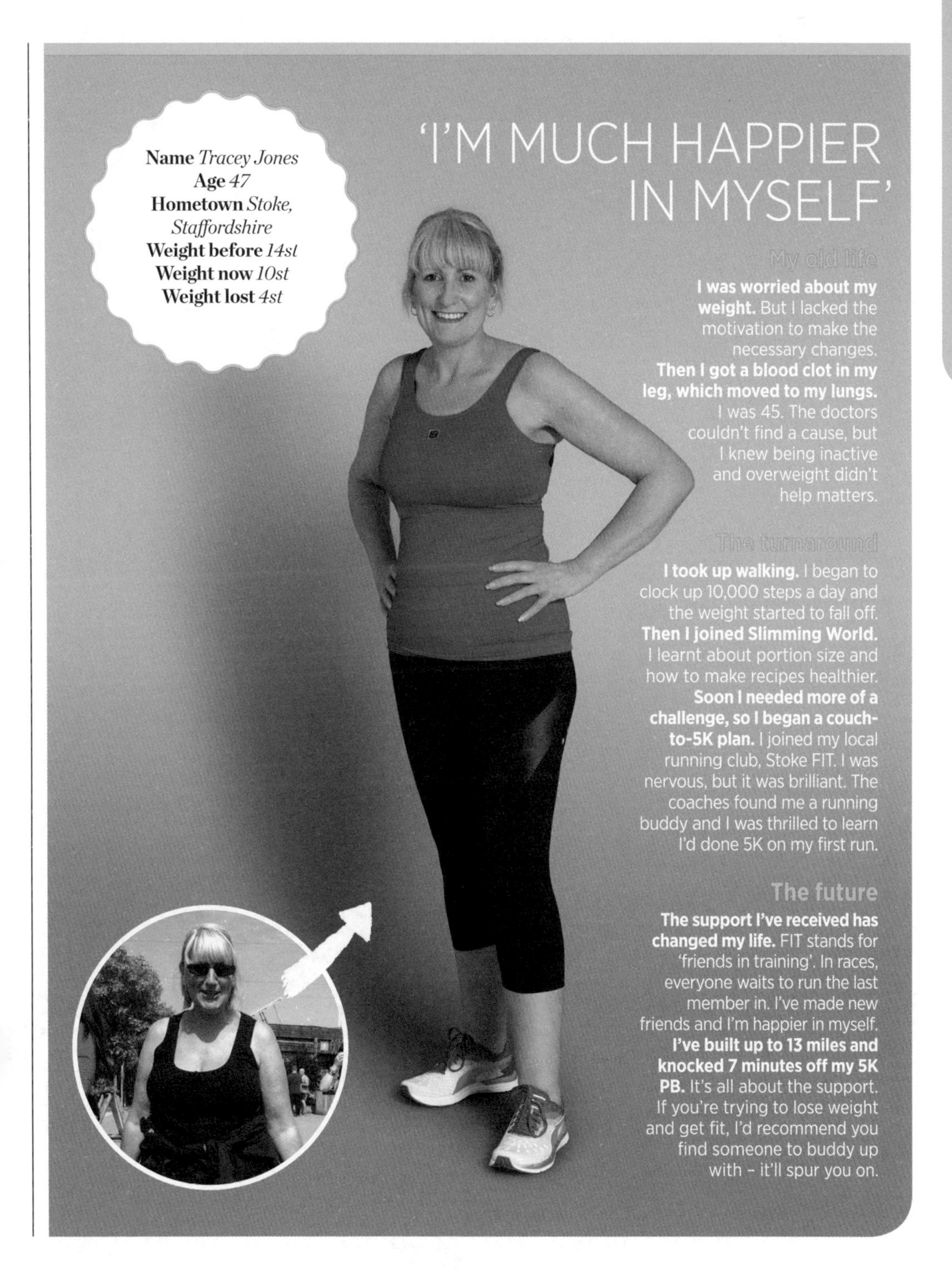

'I'M MUCH HAPPIER IN MYSELF'

Name *Tracey Jones*
Age *47*
Hometown *Stoke, Staffordshire*
Weight before *14st*
Weight now *10st*
Weight lost *4st*

My old life

I was worried about my weight. But I lacked the motivation to make the necessary changes. **Then I got a blood clot in my leg, which moved to my lungs.** I was 45. The doctors couldn't find a cause, but I knew being inactive and overweight didn't help matters.

The turnaround

I took up walking. I began to clock up 10,000 steps a day and the weight started to fall off. **Then I joined Slimming World.** I learnt about portion size and how to make recipes healthier. **Soon I needed more of a challenge, so I began a couch-to-5K plan.** I joined my local running club, Stoke FIT. I was nervous, but it was brilliant. The coaches found me a running buddy and I was thrilled to learn I'd done 5K on my first run.

The future

The support I've received has changed my life. FIT stands for 'friends in training'. In races, everyone waits to run the last member in. I've made new friends and I'm happier in myself. **I've built up to 13 miles and knocked 7 minutes off my 5K PB.** It's all about the support. If you're trying to lose weight and get fit, I'd recommend you find someone to buddy up with – it'll spur you on.

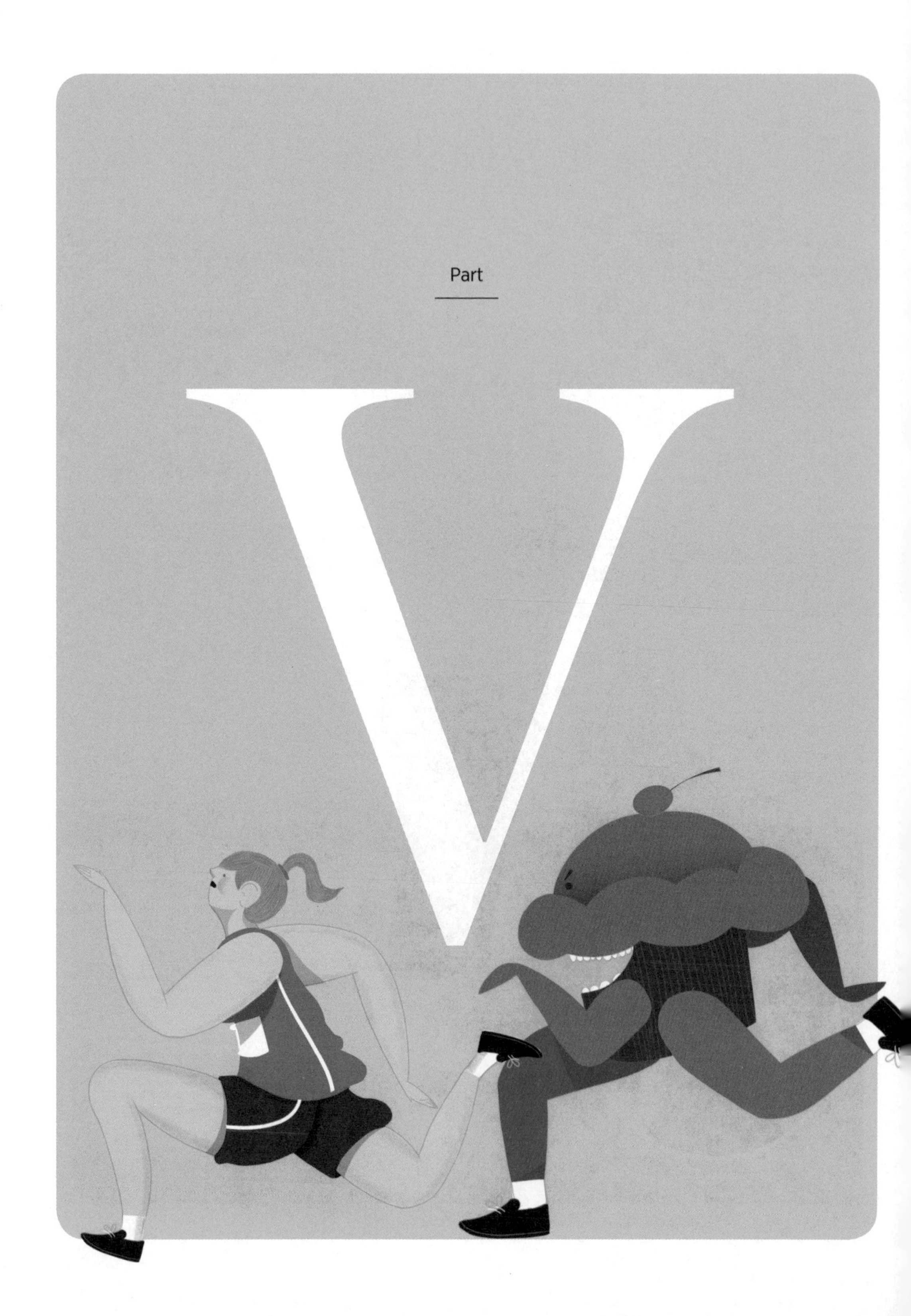
Part
V

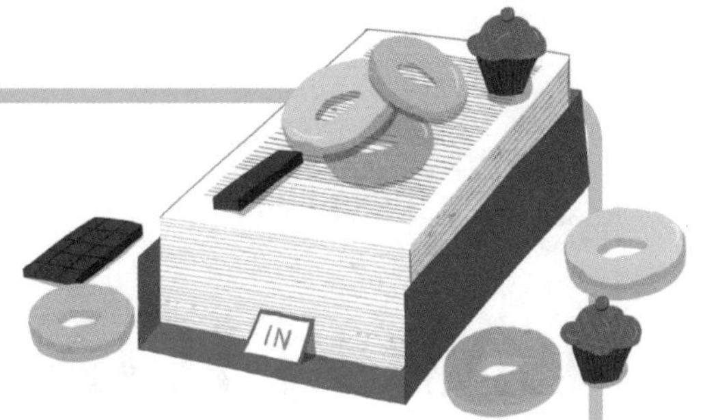

WHY WE EAT

Emotional and environmental triggers can drive much of our eating habits – from tucking into a tub of Ben & Jerry's because we're feeling a little down, to indulging in free cakes in the office, *because* they're free. But while these triggers can be beyond our control, the good news is that by learning how they shape your eating habits, you can design your personal *Run Your Belly Off* programme to make lasting changes and develop healthier habits that set you up for success. Read on to discover how to do just that.

27.

EMOTIONAL EATING

Often when we say, 'I'm hungry,' what we really mean is that we're longing for something else – relief from some other uncomfortable sensation, such as boredom, stress, loneliness, fear, anger, sadness, shock, depression, disappointment... or even a high-charged sense of elation.

In our culture, we're accustomed to getting instant gratification for our every desire and easy escapes from even the slightest tinge of emotional discomfort.

While legal substances such as alcohol and cigarettes, and illicit ones such as drugs, offer quick and easy ways to numb those discomforts, most people find such options not very compatible with their work or family lives – let alone a running regime. If you're meeting your mates for a 6am long run on Sunday, you can't risk a hangover by partying hard on Saturday night.

> 'It can be tricky to decide is it hunger or is it emotion?'

But given how cheap and available unhealthy foods are, and how heavily they're marketed (which we'll address in Chapter 30), it's no surprise that many of us – even weight-conscious runners – use food to anaesthetise ourselves from emotional discomfort.

Unhealthy snacks – from chocolate bars to cakes to fast food – are an easy, accessible, cheap, legal and socially acceptable form of self-medication. Compounding the problem: the sugar that many of these sweet treats contain is scientifically proven to be addictive. Studies have shown that sugar ignites cravings, tolerance and withdrawal just as drugs do. In *Current Opinion in Clinical Nutrition and Metabolic Care,*[1] researchers concluded that, 'Sugar and sweet reward can not only substitute to addictive drugs, such as cocaine, but can even be more rewarding and attractive.' (You can read more about sugar in Chapter 4.)

Given how addictive many sweet treats are, and how tightly food is yoked to comfort in our culture, it's often hard to distinguish between a growling stomach and an emotional hunger for something that can't be satisfied with food.

"It can be very confusing to sort out the signals and decide, is it hunger or is it emotion?" concedes Susan Albers, psychologist and author of seven books, including the *New York Times* bestselling *Eat Q: Unlock the Weight-Loss Power of Emotional Intelligence.*

The problem is, because sweet treats are not solutions or remedies for emotional problems (a chocolate chip cookie won't erase your stressors or your loneliness), no amount or type of food will ever offer a lasting sense of satisfaction. Once the momentary pleasure you get from that cookie fades, the stress and the loneliness are still there. And more often than not, the original problem is compounded by the guilt you have for indulging in a food that's off your diet.

Luckily, we're living in a time when researchers such as Albers have spent years studying the emotional drivers that shape

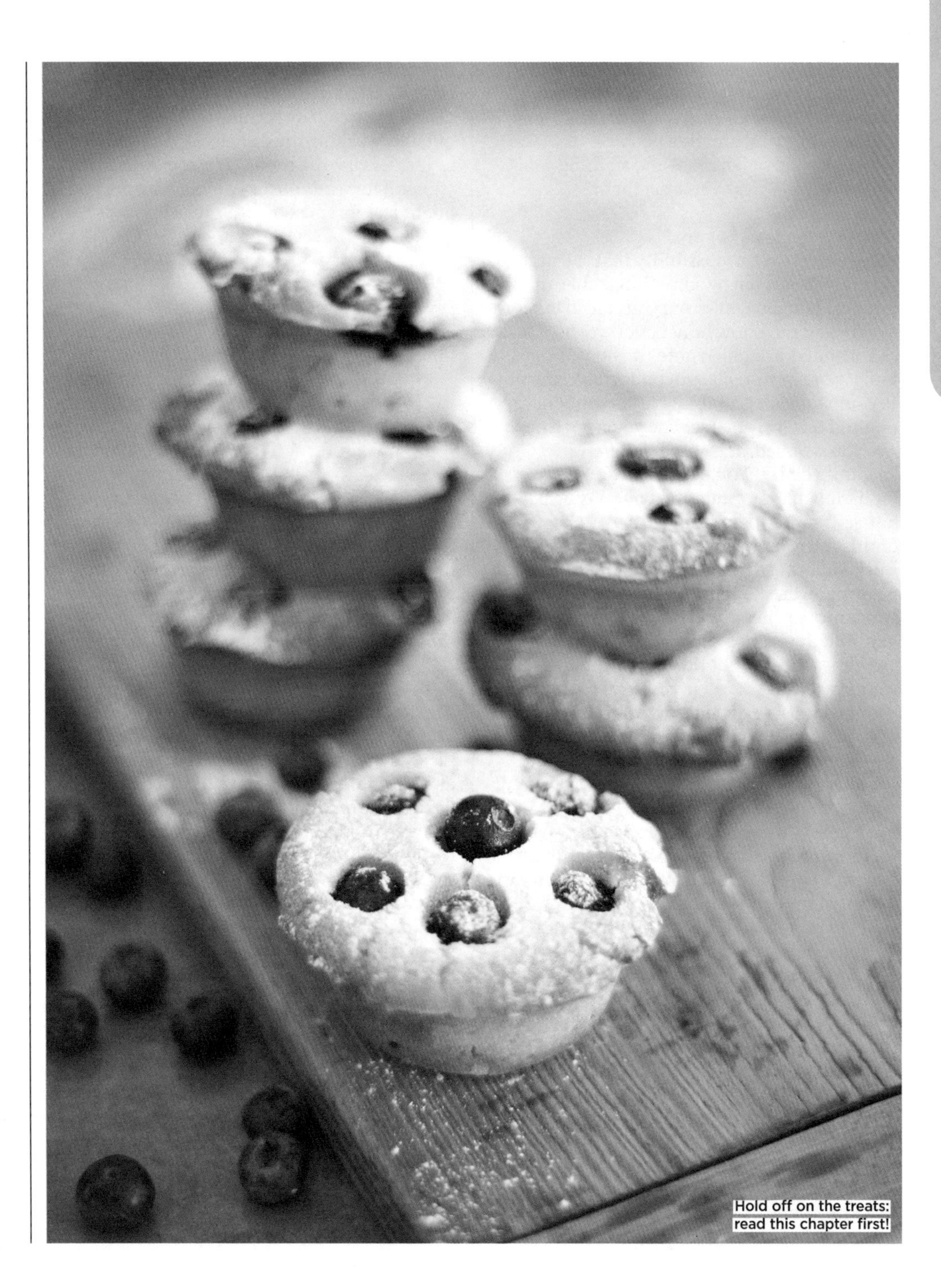

Hold off on the treats: read this chapter first!

what and how we eat. Albers suggests trying the following strategies: a) to identify the emotional drivers that are influencing your eating habits, and creating obstacles to reaching your weight-loss and training goals, and b) to find ways overcome them.

Question the urge to eat

First, entertain the possibility that the urge to eat could be driven by something other than physical hunger. One thing you can do is keep a diary and rank how hungry you are on a scale of 1-10, or take detailed notes on how physically hungry or emotionally uncomfortable you are. Is your stomach grumbling? Has your energy plummeted? Do you feel like you need a nap? Are you stressed, angry, sad or lonely? By keeping a diary, "You'll find there's a pattern both for your emotions and your physical hunger," says Albers. You may have a habit, for instance, of hitting the vending machine at work for a sweet treat after the daily 10am staff meeting, even though you ate breakfast just two hours earlier. If you keep a journal, you may find that your stomach isn't actually growling for food, but the meeting increases your stress level because you start to think about all the work you have to do; you feel the need to change your physical state so you can get temporarily distracted from that stress.

Wait two minutes

Next time you have the urge to eat, or you begin to reach into the food cupboard without even making a conscious decision to eat, don't try to stifle that urge then and there. Instead, give yourself permission to eat after two minutes have passed. By creating this gap between the urge and the deed, you're interrupting the momentum that leads so many of us to feel hijacked by our cravings. Suddenly we're on the couch, having emptied a family-size bag of crisps before we even know what hit us. That two-minute pause, says Albers, "allows you to explore what's happening." It gives you the chance to ask yourself if you are actually hungry. "The thought, 'I want to eat' and immediately answering that [by eating] is so reflexive," explains Albers. "Slowing that down does amazing things." The urge to eat can be powerful, and just two minutes can feel like an eternity to wait to satisfy it. You may need to distract yourself by turning on the TV, walking outside, washing the dishes, taking a shower or just leaving the room. "If you can distract yourself for a minute or two, chances are you might just forget about it," says Albers.

Understand the difference between hunger and a craving

If you're genuinely starving, you'll eat anything: celery, lettuce, lasagne... If you're longing for something to fulfil an emotional need – something crunchy, sweet, creamy or chocolatey – it's more than likely just a craving born out of habit or the association of that food with a feeling of comfort. "When you feel like you've got to have *barbecue* crisps – not just crisps," it's probably a craving, says Albers. "When you're really hungry, there are a lot of things that could fill that need."

'Let your mantra be "progress, not perfection"'

Be mindful of your body

Are you standing in front of the refrigerator in a daze? Scanning the cupboards restlessly? Picking food up and putting it in your mouth like a zombie? Zoning out? "If you're feeling a little bit numb, shift back into the moment and pay attention to what you're thinking and feeling," says Albers. "If you just can't get a sense of what it is that you want, often that's a clear sign of emotional eating."

Taking the following steps will help you pause, think about what you're eating and feel more satisfied from whatever you eat:

Sit down

Taking the time to find a place to sit down and eat will again help create a gap between the urge to eat and the act of consuming food, giving you time to consider what's driving that urge.

Slowly chew

When you slow down, you make the experience of eating – whether that be chocolate or an apple – last longer and feel more enjoyable. You also give your body a chance to register feelings of fullness. In addition, using your non-dominant hand can reduce how much you consume. It disrupts the automatic process of hand-to-mouth feeding that doesn't require thought.

Savour what you're eating

When you think about the smell, taste, texture and all the sensations that go along with whatever you're eating, you're more likely to enjoy it more and remember it later. You lower that feeling of deprivation that can ultimately lead to bingeing. A study in *Appetite* found that when people focused on the sensory qualities of their food, they ate less later.[2]

Be aware of entitlement eating

Runners often eat by way of reward for all the hard work they did on the road, and this is where they can easily go wrong: they overcompensate with calories post-workout. In a study published in the journal *Marketing Letters*,[3] Brian Wansink, director of Cornell University's food and brand lab, tested this dynamic. He had two groups of people take a 2km walk around a lake. One group was told the walk was exercise; for the other it was a 'scenic walk'. Those who 'exercised' ate 35% more chocolate pudding afterward than those who enjoyed a 'scenic walk'.

"Just be aware of the idea that there could be a sense of deserving [a treat]," says Albers. Yes, you need quality recovery food to bounce back for your next workout, but, she adds, "Take a good hard look at what you're saying to yourself." Plan ahead for what kinds of refuelling foods would be good, rather than just eating whatever you want. How to do it? Adjust your attitude to your workout – or even adjust your workout. If your run doesn't feel like torture, you're less likely to pamper yourself with calories afterwards. Download podcasts or movies as your 'reward'. Or make a date to work out with friends so it doubles as a social occasion. If you enjoyed your workout, you'll be much less likely to feel as if you 'need' a sweet treat to reward yourself for all the hard work you did. (See Chapter 20 to learn more about eating for recovery.)

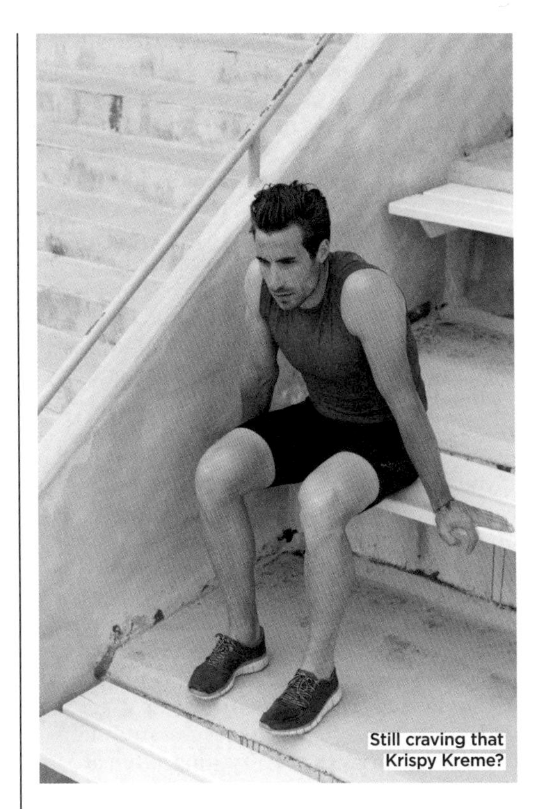
Still craving that Krispy Kreme?

Give yourself a break

"Let the mantra 'progress, not perfection' be your guide," says Albers. Focus on small victories, giving yourself credit instead of fixating on your failures. You know from running that the inner critic is a lot less motivating than a compassionate inner voice. Treat yourself just as you would a good friend who was struggling with unhealthy habits. Life is about making progress each day; it's not about being perfect all the time.

Get support

Reach out to a friend who shares or at least understands your struggle. Or connect with an online or on-the-ground group that can provide support, empathy and guidance.

Find healthy alternatives

Rather than trying to wrestle your willpower to the ground every time you have a craving, think about healthy alternative activities that will actually satisfy you when you have the urge to eat. When you're feeling sad or lonely, would it help to call or email a friend? If you tend to eat when you're in need of distraction or relief from boredom, keep plenty of magazines or books around the place. You might find relief from angry energy by playing a musical instrument. Rather than just trying to break bad habits, think about trying to develop new ones, Albers recommends. When you find a strategy for dealing with emotional discomfort that provides genuine relief, you'll be naturally inclined to stick with it.

Build an environment that supports your goals

If you've ever been on a diet or tried to stop eating a food you love – be it chocolate, crisps or sugar-laden cereal – you've probably noticed what scientists have now proved: when your diet feels like a daily struggle, it's not likely to last. Our modern world doesn't help matters. Food is everywhere. It seems you can't go to a cash register anywhere without being presented with sweets to grab and go. And many fast-food restaurants offer extra-large servings of everything, often at a discount, so you're encouraged to buy them. And those environmental triggers can be just as powerful as the emotional ones that are driving our eating decisions.

Over the past 25 years, researcher Brian Wansink has been probing the environmental cues that cause us to overeat the wrong things. He's found that even after people are made aware of cues that drive them to eat when they're not hungry, they still tend to fall back into bad habits. "Most people like to think they're too smart to get fooled," he says. "I guess we like to believe we're more in control of our lives than we are. And no one likes to be told they're wrong." In his book *Slim by Design: Mindless Eating Solutions for Everyday Life,* Wansink outlines easy steps anyone can take at home or work to eliminate or minimise those external cues to eat; to make living and office spaces more conducive to weight loss and active living. So to avoid mindless noshing, keep the food out of sight. Make it more convenient to grab and cook healthy foods, and avoid lounging around, watching TV, listening to music or working in the kitchen.

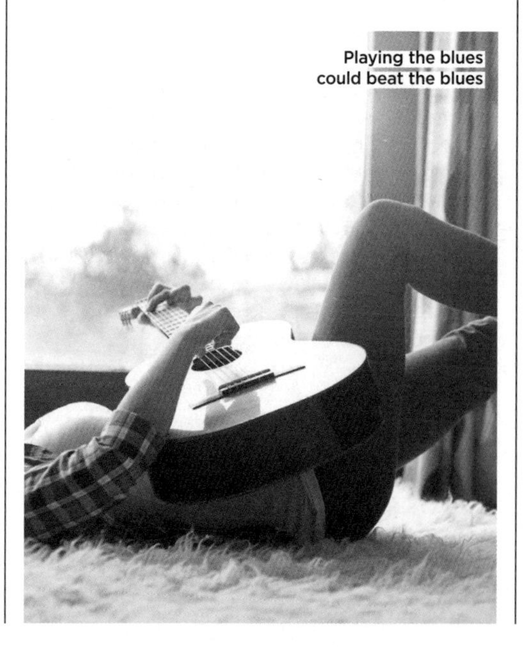

Playing the blues could beat the blues

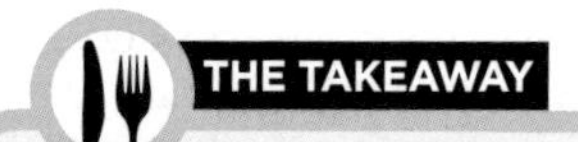

THE TAKEAWAY

Do a gut check.
The next time you reach for food, consider whether that urge is driven by a biological signal such as a rumbling empty stomach, or you're craving mental or emotional comfort.

Put on the brakes.
Slow down your eating so you can enjoy your food more, give your body a chance to register whether it's full and avoid consuming excessive calories. You could try the two-minute rule, sitting down before you eat or eating with your non-dominant hand.

List non-food forms of relief.
We all experience stress, mental anguish and emotional discomfort from time to time. Make a list of strategies that will genuinely provide relief from those states. List as many as possible so you have lots of options for a variety of different moods or circumstances.

28.

HOW STRESS AFFECTS YOUR WEIGHT AND RUNNING

Yes, it's stressful when you can't reach your feel-great weight or your finish-line goals. But there's pretty good evidence that chronic stress can also get in the way of your weight-loss goals.

Not only can it affect how many calories you consume, it can also hinder your ability to burn them. Stress can affect sleep, cause fatigue, compromise your form and endurance, and even put you at risk of injury. "All those things can have a profound effect on performance and injury risks," says Anthony Luke, a sports medicine doctor at the University of California, San Francisco (UCSF) Medical Center. "It's a pretty complex web."

Stress can dampen the immune system, too. In a study published in the journal *Neuroimmunomodulation*, the higher marathon trainees scored for factors such as anxiety and worry a month before their races, the worse off their immune systems were.[1]

Some of the impact of stress is driven by behaviour – for example, reaching for chocolate – and some of it boils down to biochemistry. Here's what you need to know about how your state of mind can affect your waistline and your race times.

Your body under stress

When we're stressed, our bodies perceive an imminent threat. In response, our glands release adrenaline and cortisol so we can fight or flee (hence the so-called fight-or-flight response). Cortisol tells the body to stockpile calories to contend with that threat and to store those calories where they're most likely to stick: deep within the belly.

That's why stress can rev up your appetite for sugary, fatty comfort foods – which deliver the biggest calorie punch per gram – and why those extra pounds are so problematic. Visceral belly fat, which is underneath the chest and abdominal walls, has been linked to a higher risk of diabetes and heart disease.

What's more, overexposure to cortisol can cause your muscles to break down at a faster rate than they do when you're not feeling stressed, according to Shawn Talbott, a nutritional biochemist who has completed more than 100 marathons and triathlons. When muscle breakdown is added to increased appetite and greater deposits of visceral belly fat, stress creates a 'triple

CHEW ON THIS

Being stressed may be worse for your race times – and your waistline – than any traditional overuse injury. In addition to derailing your sleep and sapping the energy you need to run, stress can drive you to eat – and may even amplify the ill effects of – sweet and salty foods.

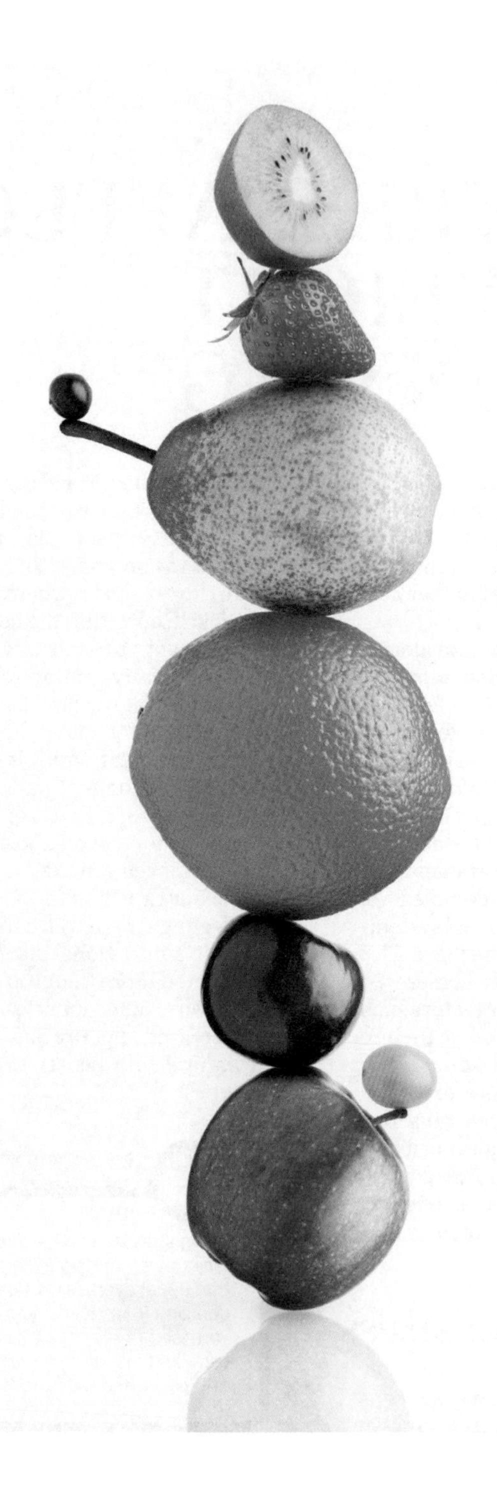

Make fruit part of your anti-stress armoury

whammy' for anyone looking to lose weight through running, Talbott says.

Recent research suggests that stress seems to worsen the effects of junk food. In a study published in 2014 in the journal *Psychoneuroendocrinology*,[2] researchers found that highly stressed people who eat a lot of fatty, sugary foods were more prone to health risks than unstressed people who ate the same food. Another study indicates – according to the lead author Kirstin Aschbacher from the department of psychiatry at UCSF – that when people are stressed, fat cells might grow faster in response to junk food than when they're not. However, so far this effect has only been shown in lab animals, not humans.[3]

Here are some proven strategies you can use to stress less and protect your body – and your waistline – from its most harmful effects.

Eat your fruit and vegetables

"The more stress you're under, the more varied your phytonutrient intake should be," says Talbott. Brightly coloured fruits and vegetables are known to have huge health benefits, but there's also emerging evidence that they can help shield your body from stress-related damage, he adds. "The more you get, the more you're going to protect yourself." Talbott is working on mapping out exactly how certain phytonutrients, such as green-tea extract, turmeric and resveratrol, can shield the body from the effects of cortisol and, he says, "how they can short-circuit that stress response at a cellular level".

Sleep

It's been proven to lower cortisol levels.[4] Lack of sleep is "probably one of the most underappreciated stress triggers out there", says Talbott. If you're working out hard, trying to lose weight and hitting a plateau, one of the problems may be that you're only getting six hours of sleep every night.

Be mindful

Research is now proving that mindfulness-based interventions for stress eating reduce both cortisol and visceral fat. A study published in 2011 in the *Journal of Obesity* found that increasing mindfulness and responsiveness to bodily sensations reduced anxiety, eating in response to external food cues and emotional eating. In the study, those who had the greatest reduction in stress lost the most fat.[5] One component of mindfulness training involves teaching people to become aware of the cues of hunger and satiety, rather than responding to automatic eating behaviours, says Frederick Hecht, a co-author of the study and a professor of medicine at UCSF. Another element is using mindfulness techniques to respond to stress and difficult emotions. "That may be easier to maintain than calorie counting for the rest of your life," he says. "I don't think it's going to be a magic bullet, but it is going to add to people's weight-loss strategies," says Hecht. (For more on mindful eating, see Chapter 27.)

> People who cut their stress levels the most lost more fat

THE TAKEAWAY

Stop the stress eating.
Even though sweet and salty foods beckon when you're feeling stressed, that's the time when junk food can wreak the most havoc on your waistline and your long-term health. Draw up a list of convenient and easy activities you can do when you're stressed to help you avoid junk food.

Get some sleep.
Aim for eight hours a night. Studies show that if you're chronically sleep deprived, you're going to be more prone to the damaging effects of stress.

Get quality meals and mileage.
The compounds in fruit and veg help reduce risk of chronic diseases that stress creates. When you're stressed, reach for a variety of fruits and vegetables to get the protective benefits their phytonutrients create.

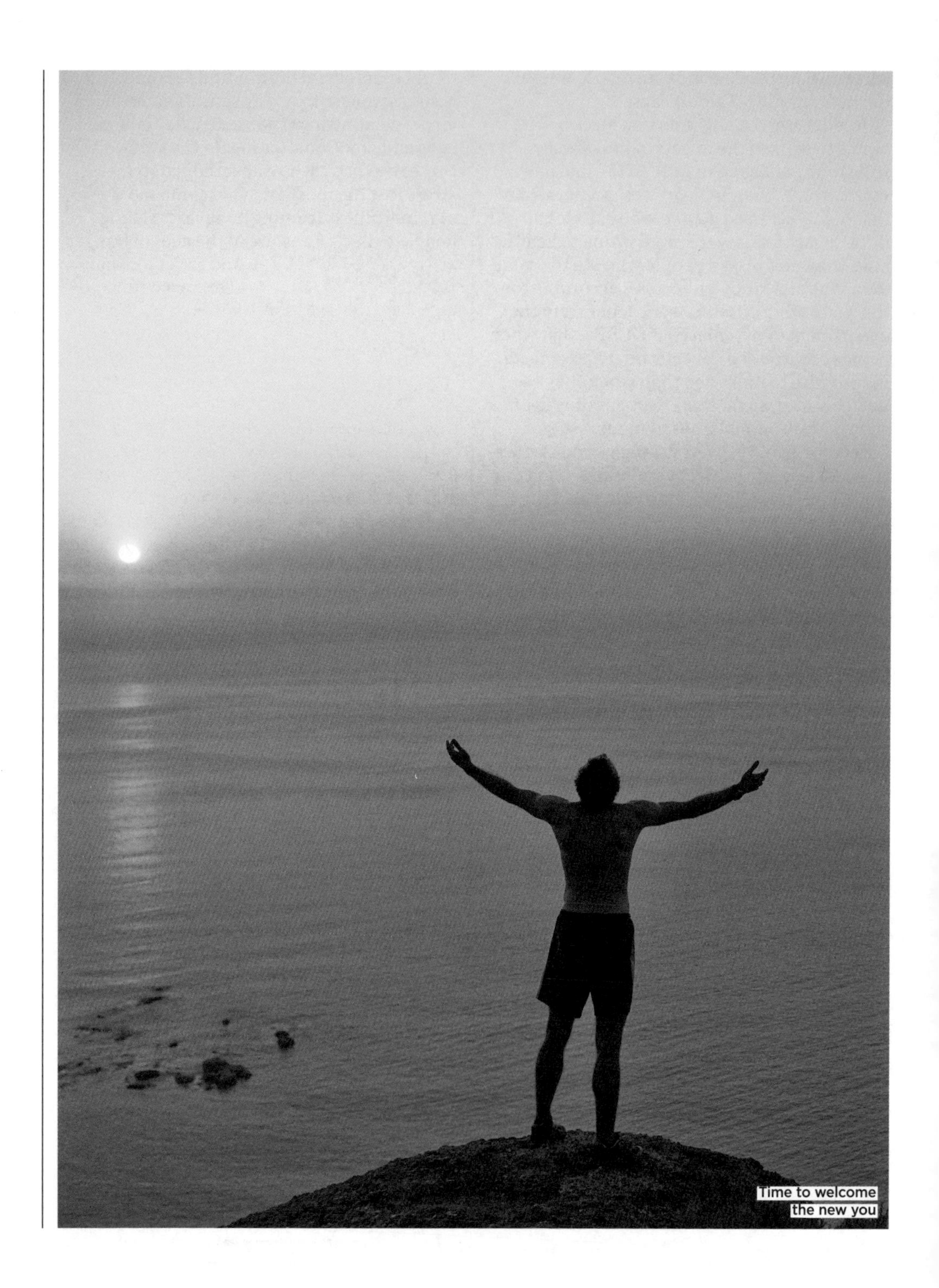

Time to welcome the new you

29.

HOW TO CREATE HEALTHY HABITS

Embarking on a new weight-loss plan is exciting, but the very idea can also be overwhelming. We know how much physical and emotional effort it requires to make lasting change. After all, most people assume that to achieve your feel-great weight, you'll have to exercise herculean feats of willpower and white-knuckle it through minefields that make healthy eating and exercise so very challenging.

Wouldn't it be great if we could just flip a switch in our brain that would force us to eat the healthiest foods in the right amounts and get the most effective workouts? That may be impossible, but forming good habits may be the next best thing.

Once you become aware of the emotional and environmental triggers coming between you and your goals and get some perspective on your own desires and temperament, you can use that information to create habits that set you up for success. By setting up a series of carefully crafted behaviours, you can put your healthiest eating and most effective training practices on autopilot.

Habit: a force of freedom

The word 'habit' has negative connotations; it implies servitude and obligation. It sounds downright unpleasant. But as Gretchen Rubin explains in her book *Better Than Before: Mastering the Habits of Our Everyday Lives*,[2] habits can actually liberate us from fretting about what to eat, when to exercise and how to reach and maintain our goal weight. "Habits are freeing and energising," she says. "They save us from the draining and difficult work of making decisions and exercising self-control."

Indeed, if you're constantly wondering, 'Should I eat that?' you're bound to exhaust your emotional energy, which is usually depleted when we need it most, she says. But each time you practise a healthy habit, it gets stronger and more automatic, so you don't have to muster up as much willpower to do it.

"Habits make it easier. Your behaviour goes on autopilot," explains Rubin. "The more you do it, the more you grease the wheels; you don't have to use up your decision-making. What's more, you'll have that precious resolve when you need it the most – to spend on the

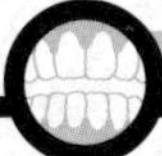

CHEW ON THIS

Investing the time to form healthy habits can pay off when you need it most. A study published in the *Journal of Personality and Social Psychology*[1] concluded that during times of high stress, when reserves of energy, willpower and self-control feel most depleted, you'll be likely to fall back on habits – whether they're good or bad.

2. *Better Than Before: Mastering the Habits of Our Everyday Lives*

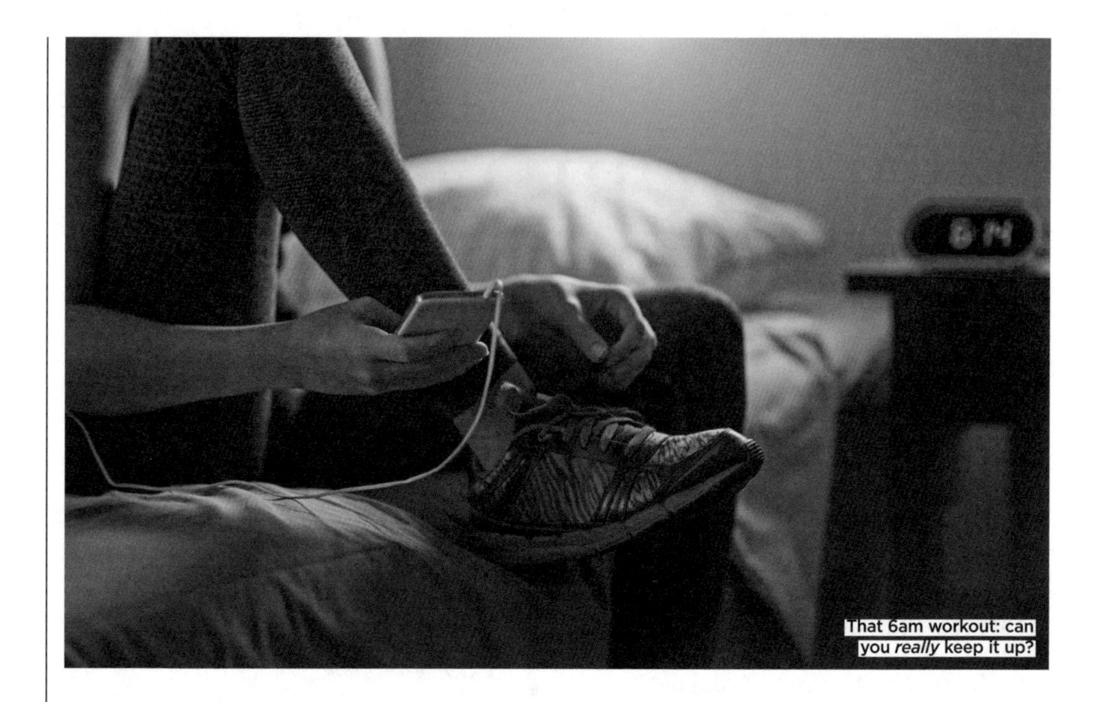
That 6am workout: can you *really* keep it up?

things you most care about. You haven't worn yourself down wondering, 'Should I go to the gym today?' You could spend the whole day fussing about it and never go."

The most effective habit-making habits

This isn't to suggest it's easy to adopt a whole new set of healthy habits – it's not. (There's a whole canon of self-help literature on the topic for a reason.) But here are some lessons about effective habit creation Rubin learnt that could help you reach your weight-loss and racing goals.

Respect yourself

This is probably the most important advice. "We can build our habits only on the foundation of our own nature," says Rubin. "You are who you are. You can be yourself." Change is definitely possible, but personality transplants are highly unlikely. So as you're setting up habits, do so with an honest understanding of your own nature. If you're a night owl, don't vow to start daily 5am workouts. If you have a rebellious nature, starting a diet that requires keeping a daily food diary isn't a good idea. Focus on changing the situation to suit *your* desires and inclinations: "That's much easier," notes Rubin.

Of course, it can take some time to figure out what those desires and inclinations are. An important part of this is understanding how you tend to respond to internal and external expectations, and into which of four categories that Rubin outlines you fall:

- Are you an upholder who responds readily to both external and internal expectations?
- Are you a questioner who challenges all expectations, unless you think they're justified?
- Are you an obliger who can easily meet someone else's expectations but not your own?
- Are you a rebel who resists all expectations, whether from yourself or other people?

Knowing and embracing your own nature will help you frame your habits in a way that is most helpful to you.

Show a little self-compassion

"A lot of people think that if they load themselves with guilt and shame, they'll energise themselves," says Rubin. "Research shows just the opposite." Usually people feel so bad about themselves that they turn to the very bad habits that got them into trouble. Treat yourself as you would a good friend, and you'll get the motivation to engage and try again. And don't try to pretend you're someone you're not, counsels Rubin.

Convenience matters

If you've ever attempted to drown your sorrows in a tub of ice cream, you know the danger of convenience: "Often with a bad habit, you're in the middle of it before you even notice it. We are extremely influenced by convenience and inconvenience," says Rubin. So if you don't want to indulge in cakes, don't buy them. Having to leave the house to get them will discourage you from doing so. And if you want to avoid eating a whole family-size bag of crisps, get single-serving bags. That way, if you want to eat more you'll have to think about opening a second pack, and that will interrupt the momentum of eating enough to make you stop in your tracks.

Treat yourself

Have a list of tasks that feel like treats for you, and make sure they don't have anything to do with eating, drinking or exercise. Treats are a critical part of life. "When we give ourselves a treat, we feel recharged and taken care of," says Rubin. "It's important give yourself a lot of healthy treats so that you don't feel deprived and depleted." The danger is, of course that the most popular forms of treats involve eating and drinking. When we're feeling low and in need of a lift, food is often our first thought. And it's no wonder: it's legal, and one of the cheapest and most convenient forms of aesthetic pleasure there is. In our culture, we're conditioned to think of certain foods as treats; in fact, many adults have few stress-relieving treats that *don't* involve food.

So make a list of fun things you can indulge in anytime you're feeling low and need a pick-me-up. Maybe it's a podcast, new music, a new book, a DVD, a manicure or an hour to wander through a camping store to ogle the gear. Rubin discovered that for a lot of people it's ironing. "Do whatever works for you," she says. "Just don't use food."

No one is an island

"We're enormously influenced by other people's habits," Rubin says. "If you want to adopt a particular behaviour, think carefully about what those around you are doing." If they're doing a good job, that's helpful. If they're not, or they're actively sabotaging your goals, plan how you'll contend with this. Be prepared for the 'frenemies' who tell you one muffin won't hurt that diet, or the food pushers at family meals who say you're obsessed because you're forgoing the pudding. Or what about the partner who gives you grief for getting up for that Saturday-morning run? You can have an iron will, but you can't be immune to other people around you.

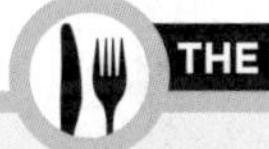

Know yourself.
As you make a list of healthy habits you'd like to adopt, think about your tendencies and desires and make sure they fit within that framework.

Make a list of non-food rewards.
Compile some pick-me-ups that don't involve eating, drinking or working out: walk the dog; call a friend; give yourself 30 minutes of Googling with abandon; play the piano; clean out a drawer; have a scented bath; revisit photos from a previous holiday... Do whatever gives you relief when you feel low. Write this list down and keep it in a place where you can easily access it.

Surround yourself with support.
Connect with others who are working on weight loss and exercise or struggling with the same obstacles. If it's tricky to meet them in person, connect online on a regular basis. That'll make you feel less self-conscious about your efforts and give you the support you need to stay on track.

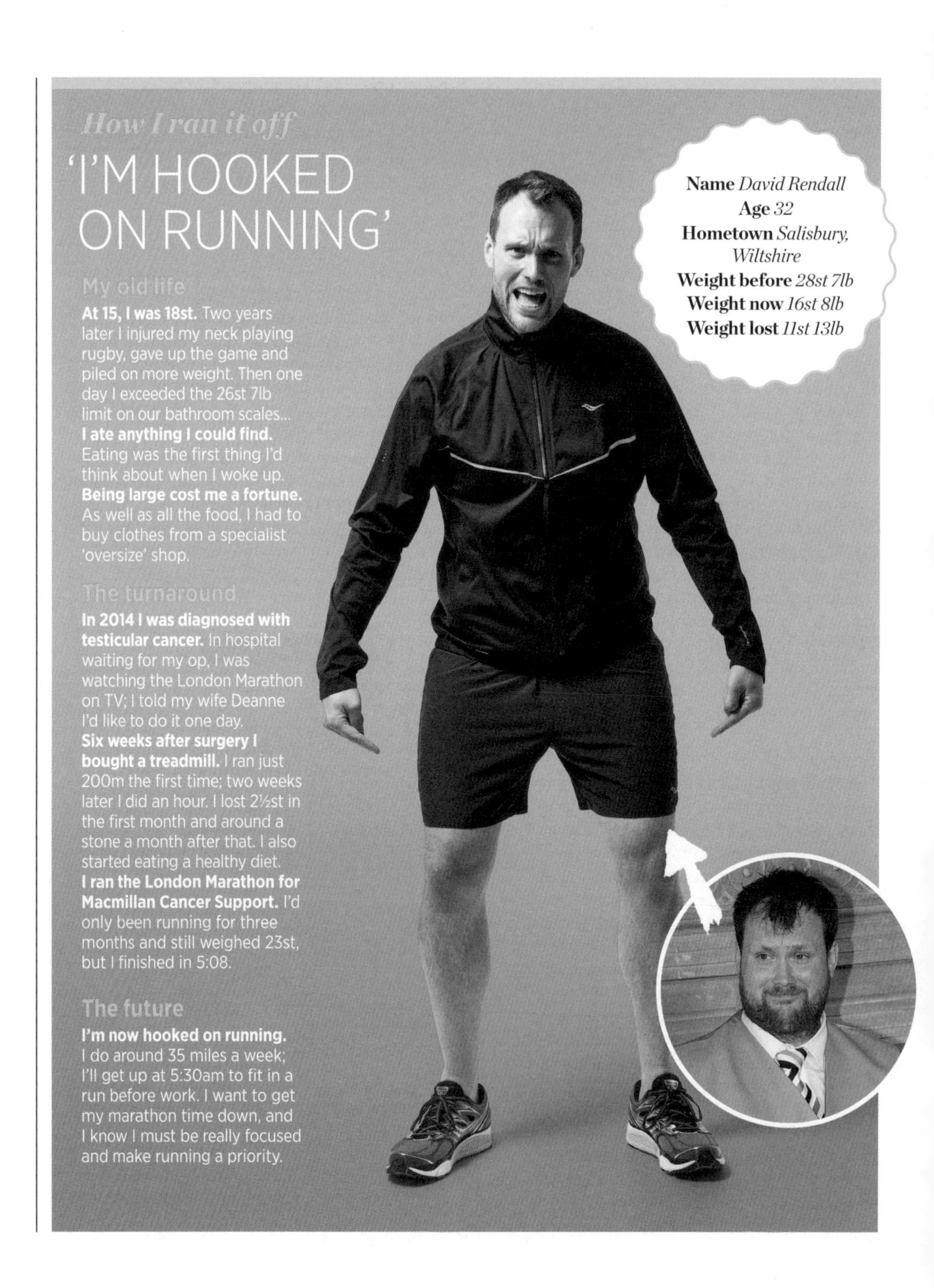

How I ran it off

'I'M HOOKED ON RUNNING'

Name *David Rendall*
Age *32*
Hometown *Salisbury, Wiltshire*
Weight before *28st 7lb*
Weight now *16st 8lb*
Weight lost *11st 13lb*

My old life

At 15, I was 18st. Two years later I injured my neck playing rugby, gave up the game and piled on more weight. Then one day I exceeded the 26st 7lb limit on our bathroom scales...
I ate anything I could find. Eating was the first thing I'd think about when I woke up.
Being large cost me a fortune. As well as all the food, I had to buy clothes from a specialist 'oversize' shop.

The turnaround

In 2014 I was diagnosed with testicular cancer. In hospital waiting for my op, I was watching the London Marathon on TV; I told my wife Deanne I'd like to do it one day.
Six weeks after surgery I bought a treadmill. I ran just 200m the first time; two weeks later I did an hour. I lost 2½st in the first month and around a stone a month after that. I also started eating a healthy diet.
I ran the London Marathon for Macmillan Cancer Support. I'd only been running for three months and still weighed 23st, but I finished in 5:08.

The future

I'm now hooked on running. I do around 35 miles a week; I'll get up at 5:30am to fit in a run before work. I want to get my marathon time down, and I know I must be really focused and make running a priority.

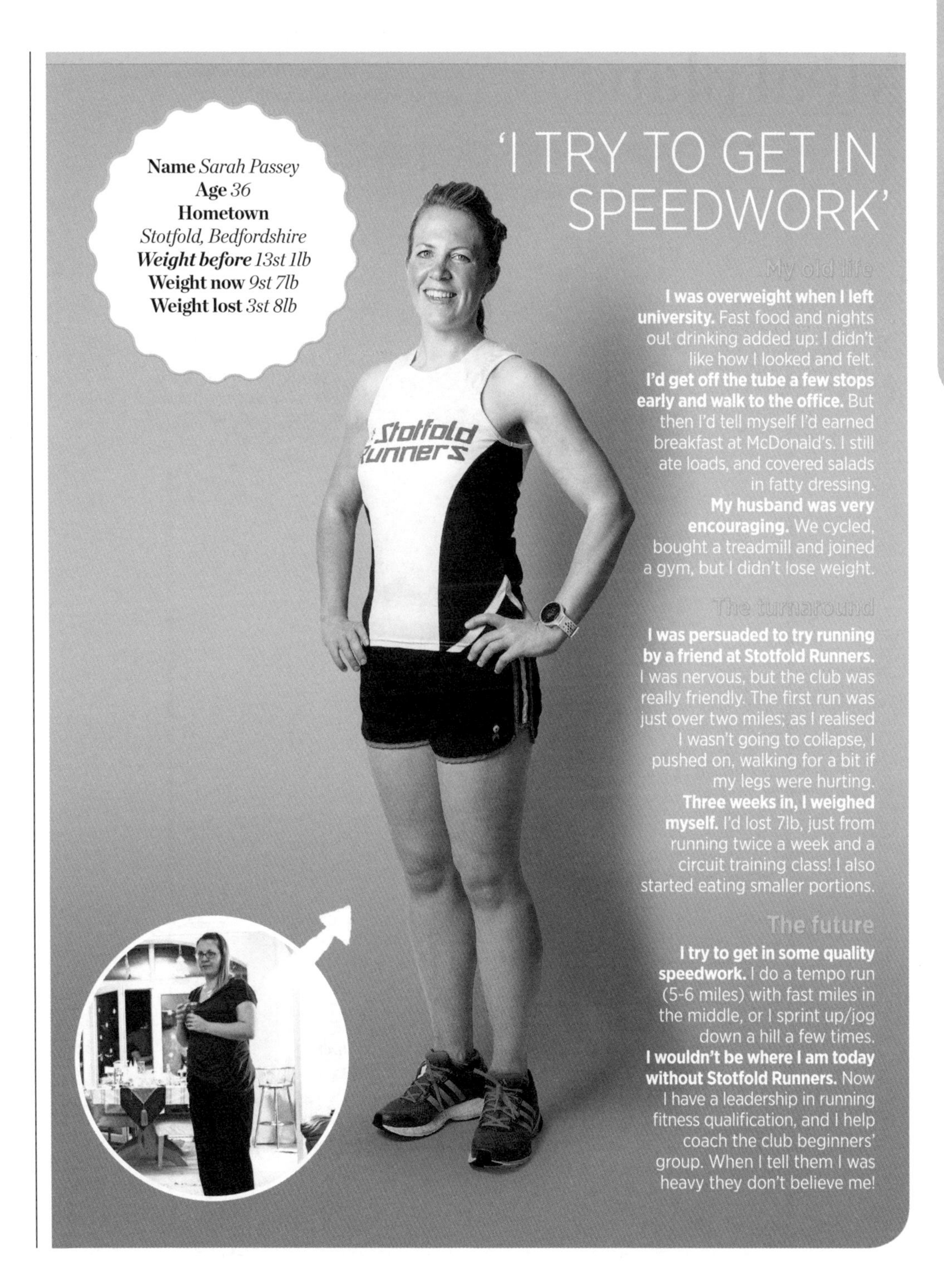

Name *Sarah Passey*
Age *36*
Hometown
Stotfold, Bedfordshire
Weight before *13st 1lb*
Weight now *9st 7lb*
Weight lost *3st 8lb*

'I TRY TO GET IN SPEEDWORK'

My old life

I was overweight when I left university. Fast food and nights out drinking added up: I didn't like how I looked and felt.

I'd get off the tube a few stops early and walk to the office. But then I'd tell myself I'd earned breakfast at McDonald's. I still ate loads, and covered salads in fatty dressing.

My husband was very encouraging. We cycled, bought a treadmill and joined a gym, but I didn't lose weight.

The turnaround

I was persuaded to try running by a friend at Stotfold Runners. I was nervous, but the club was really friendly. The first run was just over two miles; as I realised I wasn't going to collapse, I pushed on, walking for a bit if my legs were hurting.

Three weeks in, I weighed myself. I'd lost 7lb, just from running twice a week and a circuit training class! I also started eating smaller portions.

The future

I try to get in some quality speedwork. I do a tempo run (5-6 miles) with fast miles in the middle, or I sprint up/jog down a hill a few times.

I wouldn't be where I am today without Stotfold Runners. Now I have a leadership in running fitness qualification, and I help coach the club beginners' group. When I tell them I was heavy they don't believe me!

Meal plans

These sample recipe plans will help you achieve healthy, sustainable weight loss

1,600-calorie meal plan

Approximate daily intake Calories: 1,578; **total fat:** 45g; **saturated fat:** 9g; **trans fat:** 0g; **carbohydrate:** 194g; **protein:** 99g; **fibre:** 27g

Breakfast
- 30g bran flakes
- 180g light (reduced-calorie) low-fat yogurt
- 8 medium strawberries
- 250-500ml water

Morning snack
- 225g low-fat (1%) cottage cheese
- 1 medium apple,
- 250-500ml water

Lunch
Chopped chicken salad made from:
- 100g chopped grilled chicken
- 55g mixed salad leaves
- 35g each chopped green and red peppers
- 100g chopped tomatoes
- 50g goat's cheese
- 2 tbsp reduced-fat balsamic dressing
- 1 whole-grain bread roll
- 250-500ml water

Afternoon snack
- 1 digestive biscuit topped with 1 tbsp peanut butter
- 1 medium banana
- 250-500ml water

Dinner
- Pan-seared salmon with garlic and asparagus over rice:
  In a nonstick frying pan, heat 1 tbsp rapeseed oil. Once oil is hot, add 1 chopped clove garlic and 6 chopped asparagus spears and sauté for 1-2 minutes. Add 75g Atlantic salmon and cook until fish pulls apart easily with a fork. Serve on 200g cooked brown, long-grain rice.
- 250-500ml water

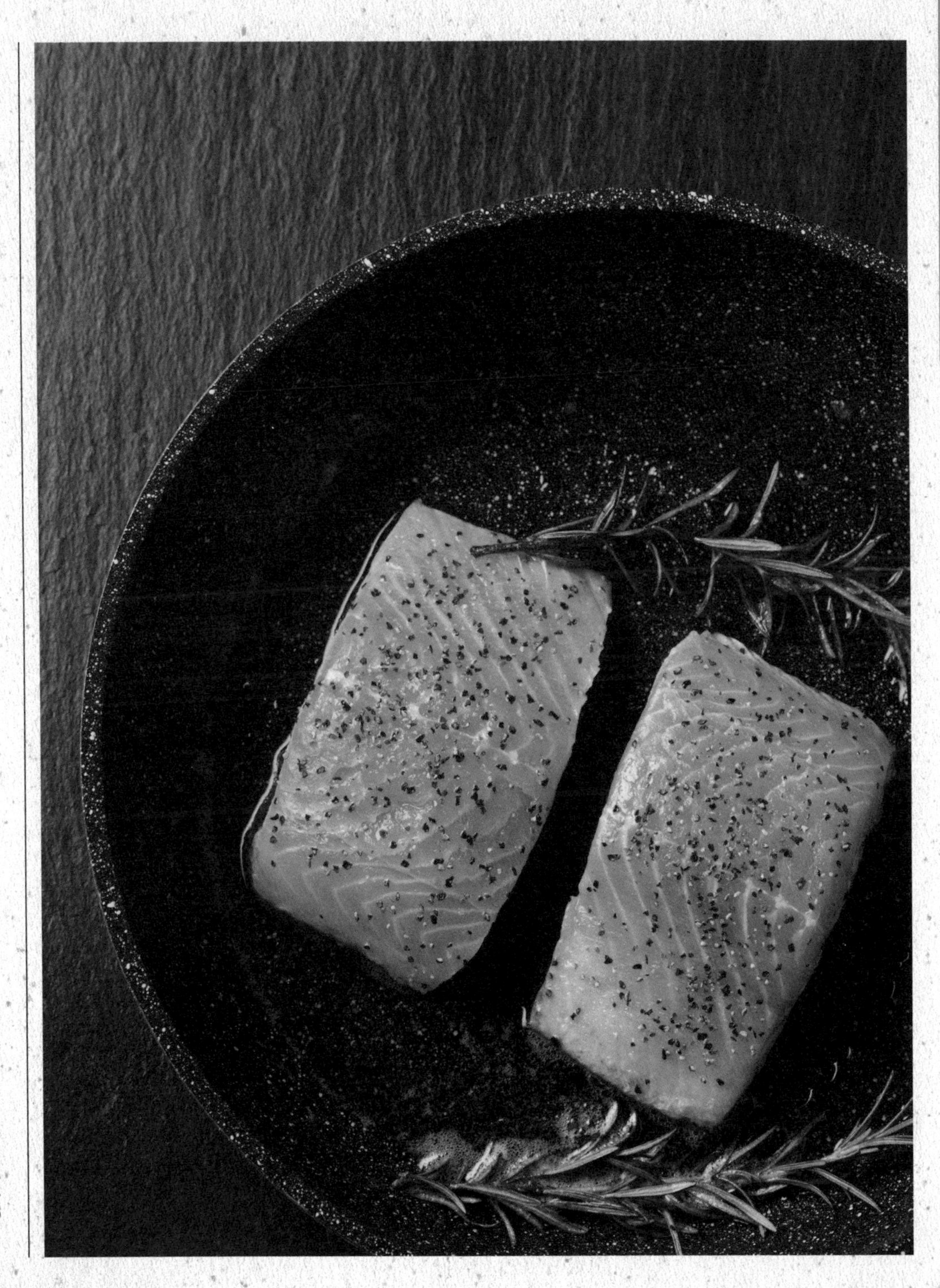

Photography: Getty

2,000-calorie meal plan

Breakfast
- 40g old-fashioned porridge made with 250ml skimmed milk
- 1 medium apple
- 250ml green tea with sliced lemon
- 250ml water

Morning snack
- 60g hummus
- ½ whole-grain pitta, toasted
- 125g baby carrots
- 250-500ml water

Lunch
- 1 turkey sandwich with 2 slices wholewheat bread and 50g low-sodium sliced turkey
- 50g chopped romaine lettuce topped with 2 tbsp low-fat vinaigrette
- 250g fat-free vanilla Greek yogurt
- 250-500ml water

Afternoon snack
- 15g high-fibre, high-protein cereal
- 1 medium banana
- 250ml skimmed milk
- 250ml green tea with sliced lemon

Dinner
- 75g baked salmon
- 200g (cooked weight) brown rice
- 150g steamed broccoli
- 250-500ml water

Evening snack
- 25g Cheddar cheese
- 6 wholewheat crackers
- 60g sliced cucumber

Approximate daily intake **Calories:** 1,990; **total fat:** 44g; **saturated fat:** 26g; **trans fat:** 0g; **carbohydrate:** 292g; **protein:** 108g; **fibre:** 46g

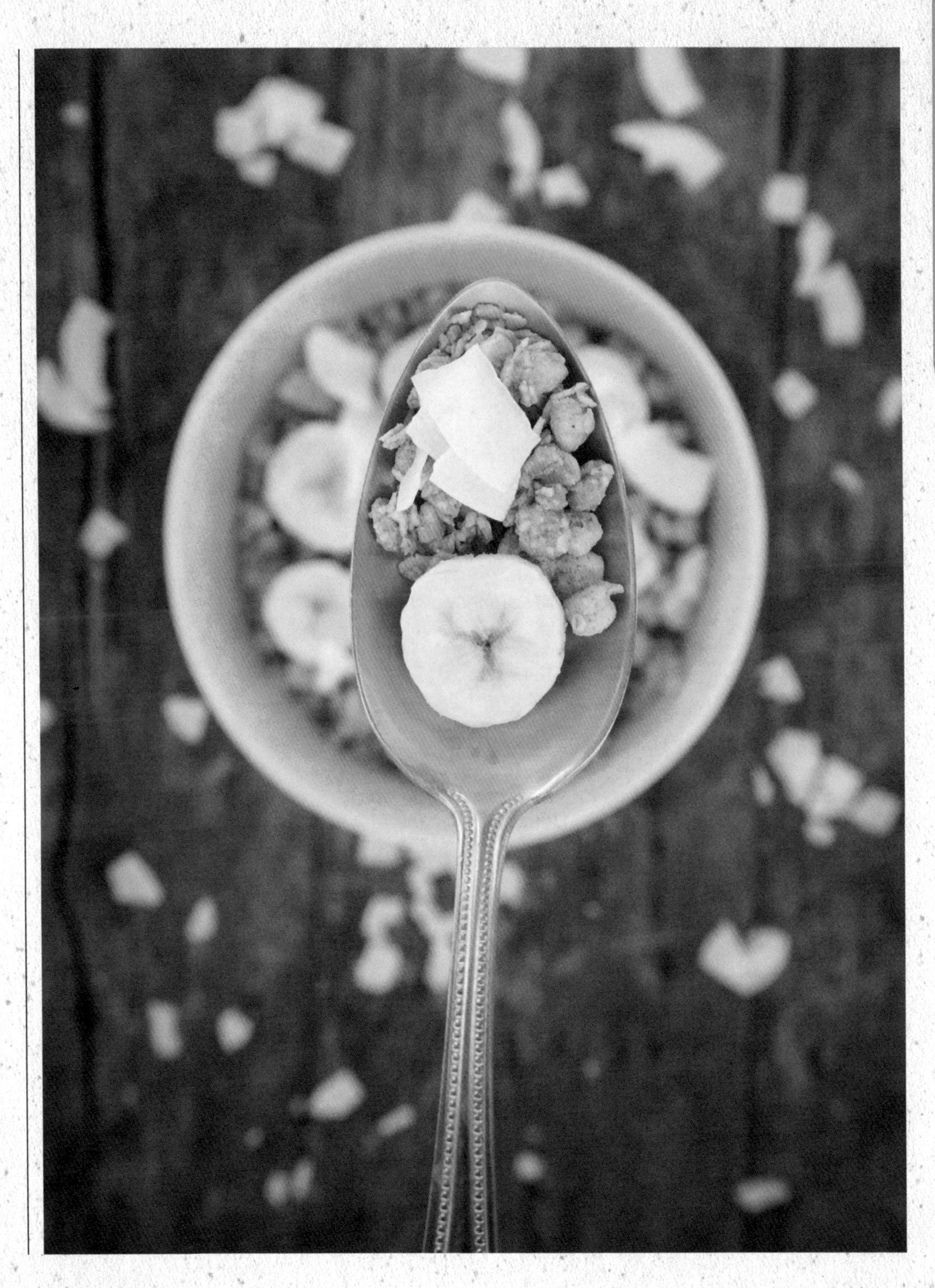

Photography: Getty

2,500-calorie meal plan

Breakfast

- 1 scrambled egg
- 180g cooked spinach
- 2 slices wholewheat bread
- 25g Cheddar cheese
- 250ml green tea,
- 250ml water with lemon

Morning snack

- 25g (49 kernels) dry-roasted pistachios
- 150g fresh mixed berries
- 250-500ml water

Lunch

- Salad with 100g shredded romaine lettuce, 2 tbsp low-fat vinaigrette, 75g canned chickpeas
- 150g couscous
- 1 wholewheat bread roll
- 75g grilled chicken breast
- 250-500ml water with lemon

Afternoon snack

- Smoothie made by blending 2 scoops 100% whey protein powder (chocolate), 1 medium banana, 250ml skimmed milk, and 150g ice

Dinner

- 75g roasted pork tenderloin
- 100g baked sweet potato
- 150g cooked broccoli
- 1 wholewheat bread roll
- 1 tbsp butter
- 250-500ml water

Evening snack

- 1 tbsp peanut butter
- 1 large apple
- 250-500ml water

Approximate daily intake **Calories:** 2,550; **total fat:** 84g; **saturated fat:** 20g; **trans fat:** 0g; **carbohydrate:** 288g; **protein:** 158g; **fibre:** 58g

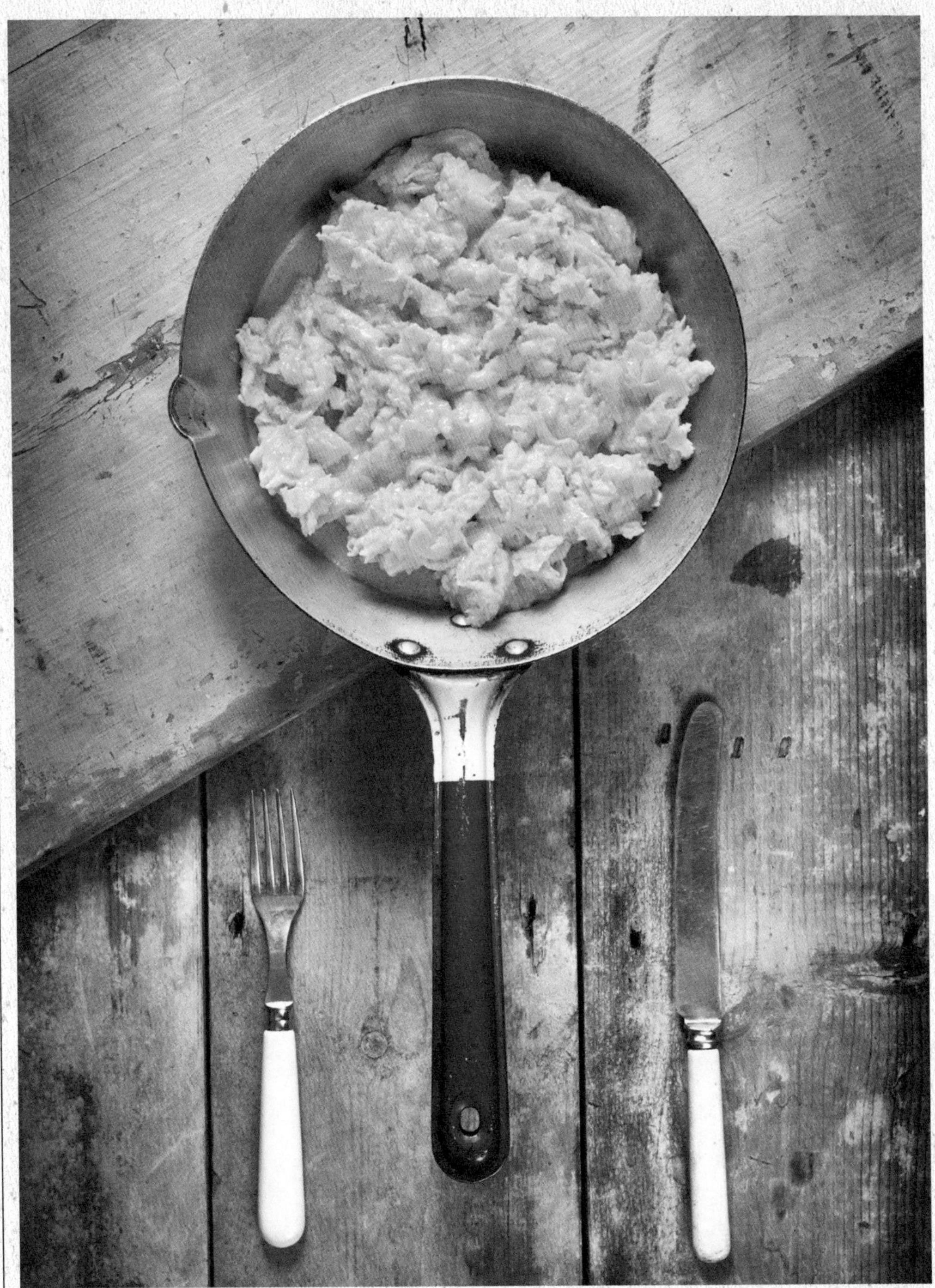

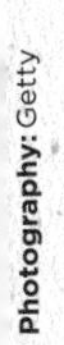
Photography: Getty

3,000-calorie meal plan

Breakfast

- 150g low-fat fruited Greek yogurt
- 150g fresh blueberries
- 60g granola
- coffee or tea, as desired

Morning snack

- 1 smoothie made with 2 scoops 100% whey protein powder, 150g baby spinach, 60g frozen blueberries, 250ml fat-free milk

Approximate daily intake **Calories:** 3,040; **total fat:** 80g; **saturated fat:** 21g; **trans fat:** 0g; **carbohydrate:** 400g; **protein:** 180g; **fibre:** 62g

Lunch

- Burrito bowl: 200g (cooked weight) brown rice, 120g low-salt black beans, 150g corn, 65g salsa, 175g grilled chicken
- 150g cooked broccoli
- 1 medium stone fruit (eg, apricot)
- 250-500ml water

Afternoon snack

- 1 rice cake topped with 1 tbsp almond butter
- 250-500ml water with lemon

Dinner

- Spaghetti and meatballs: 100g wholewheat pasta, 250g Italian-style tomato sauce, and 100g meatballs
- 125g green beans
- 25g Monterey Jack cheese
- 250-500ml water

Evening snack

- 25g roasted unsalted almonds
- 40g dried cranberries
- 250-500ml water

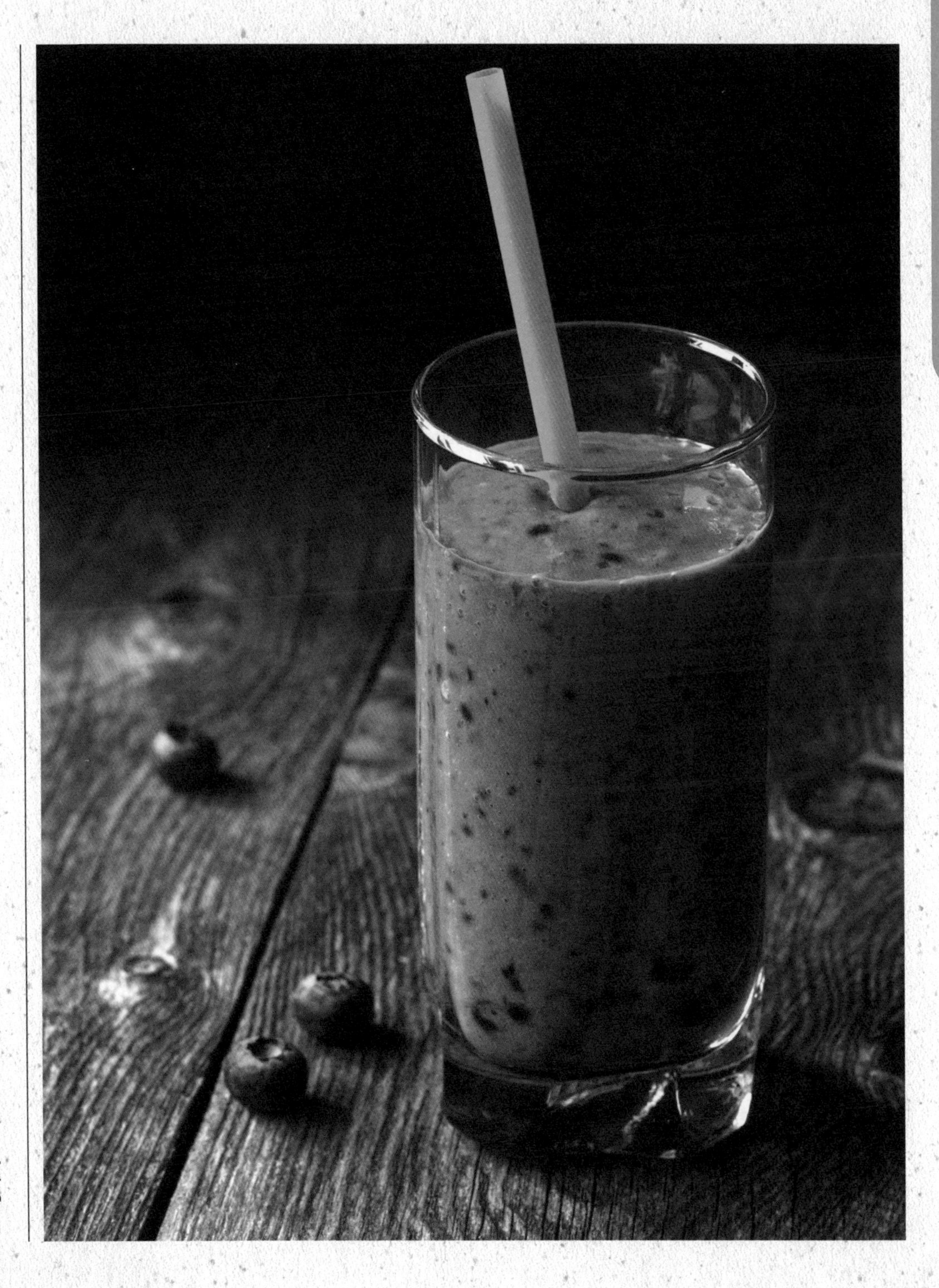

Photography: Getty

Rules of thumb

As you'll have realised by this point, *Run Your Belly Off* contains a huge amount of detailed information and advice designed to help you attain your running and weight-loss goals. Here we've distilled some of the key messages and lessons to take away with you, plus where you can go back and read about them in more detail.

Best balance of carbs, protein and fats

To fuel your running, at least 55% of your daily calories should come from wholesome carbohydrates (such as whole grains, fresh fruit and vegetables), and the balance should come from lean proteins and healthy fats. (See page 34 for more.)

Pack in the protein

Aim for 0.55-0.9g protein per lb of body weight per day to recover from workouts and continue to build strength and fitness. The more miles you're logging and the more strength training you're doing, the more protein you're likely to need. So if you weigh 9st 4lb, target 72-117g per day; a 14st runner will need to aim for 108-176g.

Stay hydrated every day

To avoid dehydration, which can drag down your running performance, fill up on calorie-free fluids until your urine is a light lemonade or straw colour. Many experts recommend you start with a goal of drinking about half your body weight (in lbs) in fl oz per day. (1 fl oz is about 30ml.) So if you weigh 200lb (14st 4lb), try to consume at least 100 fl oz (about 3ltr) calorie-free fluids each day. If you weigh 140lb (10st), aim for 70 fl oz (2ltr). Sip fluids throughout the day so you're not chugging huge amounts just before a run. (See page 76 for more.)

Get your fibre

To boost heart health and keep the GI tract running efficiently, have plenty of fibre. The Government recommends that adults consume 30g fibre per day. (See page 93 for more.)

Steer clear of sugar

To keep your sugar intake low, aim for less than 10g per serving in any food you eat. Look at the ingredients list: if sugar is among the first three, leave it alone. (See page 52 for more.)

Choose the right sports food at the right time

Whole foods are always the best choice. But when those are out of reach or your stomach won't tolerate them before a workout, a sports bar, shake or other engineered food can meet your needs. Whether you're choosing whole foods or sports foods, here's what to look for.

- Pre-run snack: for a run of 60 minutes or less at an easy effort, limit it to 200 calories or less, with less than 10g fat and 7g fibre.
- Mid-run refuelling: if you're going to be on a run for one to three hours at a time, you want to aim for a product that'll provide 30-60g carbs for every hour you're on the road.
- Post-run refuelling: after a speed session or a long run, have a protein shake,

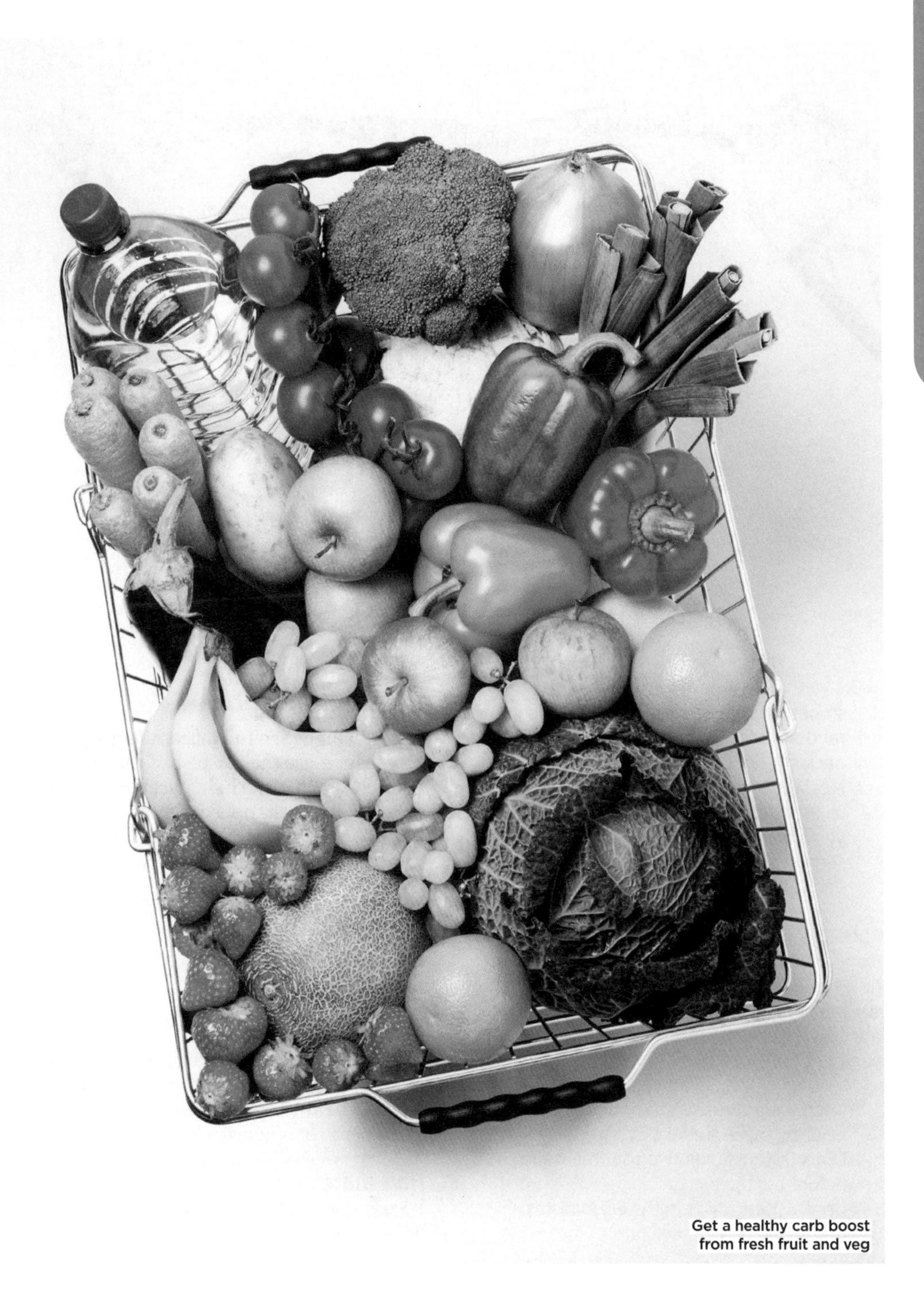

Photography: Getty

Get a healthy carb boost from fresh fruit and veg

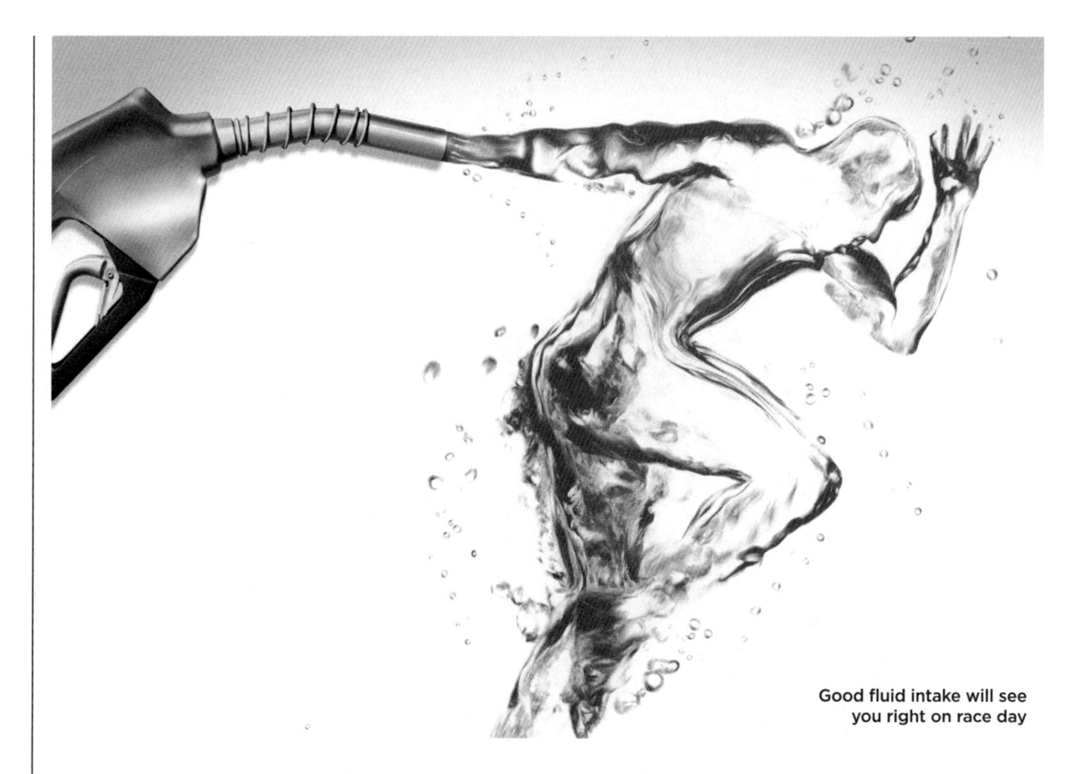

Good fluid intake will see you right on race day

smoothie, sports bar or snack with a 2:1 ratio of carbs to protein, to help you bounce back strong. For more, see Chapter 20.
- Meal replacement: make sure the bar or shake doesn't contain more calories than you'd have in a regular meal. Look at the serving size – some items have more than one serving per pack.

Race-day nutrition (for 5Ks and 10Ks)
Consume foods that are low in fat, fibre and protein. For each nutrient, aim for under 10g per serving unless you're sensitive to fibre; in that case, limit it to 7g or less. (See page 130 for more.)

- Keep your pre-race snack under 200 calories; make sure it's rich in carbs.
- Drink 600ml fluids two to three hours before the race.
- Drink 300ml fluids in the 20 minutes before the race.

When to carb-load
Carb-loading for a full marathon is the best way to increase the chances of running your best race. For a half marathon, it's only marginally necessary. For any race of less than 90 minutes, carb-loading is totally unnecessary and it may actually hurt your chances of running well on race day. (See page 131 for more.)

Calculated carb-load
See page 132 for more.

Marathons

7 days before the race Consume 2.3g carbs per lb of body weight each day.
1-3 days before the race Consume 3.6-5.5g carbs per lb of body weight each day.

Half marathons

1-3 days before the race Consume 2.5-4g carbs per lb of body weight each day.

Refuelling on the road

For a run of 75 minutes or more, refuel while on the go. Consume 30-60g carbs per hour, starting at the beginning of your run, before you risk becoming hungry or starved of energy. Then refuel at regular intervals throughout the run – say, every 15-30 minutes – to keep your energy levels stable. (See page 138 for more.)

Avoid unwanted pit stops on the run

To avoid GI distress, keep your pre-run meal or snack to these per-serving limits.

- Less than 7g fibre
- Less than 10g fat
- Less than 10g protein

The longer you go, the more you'll need to refuel

The longer the run, the more carbs you should consume per hour. If you're heading out for a 75-minute run, try 30g carbs per hour. If you're going to be running for 150 minutes, aim closer to 60g carbs per hour. For runs that last longer than three hours, aim for 90g carbs per hour. (See page 138 for more.)

Refuelling with sports drinks

If you're using sports drinks to refuel while you're on the road, stick with products that have less than 14-17g carbs per 250ml. However, runners with sensitive stomachs should aim for the lower end of this range or even less. For best tolerance, look for drinks with multiple sources of carbs – such as glucose, fructose, sucrose and maltodextrin – which your body will absorb better than a single source by itself. (See page 140 for more.)

Fuelling up with whole foods

When you're using whole foods to refuel on the road, go for products that are low in fat, fibre and protein – less than 3-5g of each per serving. Start there and see how you feel. Depending on how tough your gut is, you may be able to tolerate more. (See page 140 for more.)

Refuelling post-workout

Research has proved that carbs and protein are the most effective nutrients for helping the body recover after a workout. The carbs in your recovery meal restock your spent glycogen stores. Aim for approximately 0.5g carbohydrate per lb of body weight. So if you weigh 150lb (10st 10lb), have a recovery meal that packs 75g carbs. Adding a small amount of protein to a recovery meal will speed your muscle repair and recovery. Aim for at least 15-25g protein. (See page 145 for more.)

Rehydrating post-workout

How do you know if you're properly rehydrated after a tough workout? Do the sweat test. Weigh yourself naked before a run, then again afterwards, and determine how much fluid you lost through sweat. (Remember, 1lb equals approximately 450ml.) Then drink that same quantity of fluid (if you have another workout looming within 24 hours and need to rehydrate quickly, drink 700ml for each lb lost). If you don't have access to scales, you can simply drink until your thirst diminishes and your urine runs a light straw colour. (See page 145 for more.)

Returning to running after a layoff (See page 175 for more.)

IF YOU'RE OFF...	START RIGHT HERE
1 week or less	Pick up your plan where you left off
Up to 10 days	Start running 70% of previous mileage
15-30 days	Start running 60% of previous mileage
30 days-3 months	Start running 50% of previous mileage
3 months+	Start from scratch

Kitchen essentials

When you make your own meals, you'll be able to take the reins and more effectively achieve your weight-loss and racing goals. Yes, cooking at home is more time-consuming than microwaving a ready meal or picking up a sports-nutrition bar. But it doesn't have to consume your life. You probably already own basics (vegetable peeler, can opener, whisk, etc), but the following essentials can help you make healthy food fast.

Basic kitchen tools

TOOL	FUNCTION
Salad spinner	Centrifuge-type bowl that allows you to rinse, spin-dry and store your lettuce (or other salad ingredients). When you get home from the supermarket, wash, chop, and spin your salad ingredients. Store the leftovers in the spinner so you always have salad on hand.
Chopping board	Save your countertops by chopping and slicing food on chopping boards. Make sure you keep one exclusively for raw meat, poultry, fish and seafood, to avoid the risk of cross-contamination. Lightweight but sturdy boards are the best options. You might choose a plastic one that's dishwasher safe; if you'd prefer natural material, bamboo is a good choice.
Nonstick frying pan	While some home cooks shy away from Teflon coatings, when you're looking to cut calories and fat, a nonstick surface is your friend – in a frying pan it allows you to 'pan fry' your items with less oil or butter. If you're still worried about the health concerns around some nonstick coatings, go for a ceramic coating, as these are believed to be the safest option.
Kitchen knives	It's difficult to prepare any dish without a good set of knives. And while you might be hesitant to invest in a new set, if your knives are old and dull, as you put more effort into cutting, you risk cutting yourself. The most basic set should include chef's, paring, serrated and slicing knives.
Hand blender	Sometimes referred to as a stick or immersion blender, this is a handheld electric blender that purées food in the container in which it's being prepared (saving you the hassle of transferring your ingredients from bowl to blender/food processor and back again). It's especially useful for soups and smoothies.
Food scales, measuring jugs and spoons	Use these to accurately measure portions when cooking or baking (to make sure the recipe turns out as intended), to stick to the correct proportions of a diet or meal plan, or measure out a proper serving size (check a food's nutrition-information panel for the serving size in grams). It can be particularly useful to double-check portion sizes – when you first try a new food and then a few weeks later: you might notice that if you're estimating your portion sizes they can grow over time. These tools can help you remain honest and keep your waistline in check.

Recipe prep bowls/ ramekins	These small vessels are helpful when lining up ingredients prior to mixing. They can also be used for portion control of snacks and indulgent items. If using for portion control, check the serving size of the item and place only a single serving into the ramekin. Once it's empty, you've finished snacking.
Food storage containers	Choose ones that are dishwasher safe, durable, airtight and clear. It's a good idea to buy some masking tape so if you store leftover food in a container you can mark what it is and when it was made. Most leftovers should be consumed within a few days. If you date the item, there'll be no more debating how old it is.

Kitchen wish list: tools that are useful but not essential

TOOL	FUNCTION
Meat pounder	This is a handy item for tenderising and flattening meat (such as pork loin, chicken breast and low-fat beef, which can be tough). It also makes meat cook more quickly. And since you'll need to cut more pieces and take more bites, you'll be forced to eat a bit slower, too.
Mandoline/ julienne slicer	A mandoline is the perfect tool if you're looking to cut veg quickly and make them look attractive. Many have straight and wavy blades that can be set to different thicknesses to create cucumber slices, courgette matchsticks and more. Most also include a julienne blade that churns out carrot sticks. Look for one that has safety features such as a handle that keeps your hands out of the way of the blades, and blades that can be removed and easily washed.
Silicone brushes	These are handy for basting foods. Instead of drowning something in sauce or coating a pan with copious amounts of oil, use a silicone food brush (which is heat-resistant, durable and doesn't capture quite as much sauce as natural bristle brushes) to spread just enough oil and sauce on foods as you cook. You'll save on calories and ingredients.
Strainer/ colander	Ideal for washing fruit and veg, especially harder-to-clean items such as berries. This makes it easy to keep fresh food on hand for healthy snacking.
Fat separator	This device looks like a liquid measuring jug but has a spout at the bottom of the cup and a strainer at the top to catch solids. Since fat naturally rises to the top of items such as gravy, soup and broth when the liquid cools, you can pour out the liquid you want to keep, and leave the artery-clogging fat behind. Simply transfer the sauce or broth from the pot it's been cooking in and let it cool it in the fat separator. Once the fat rises to the top, pour off the liquid you want to keep, discarding the rest. To accelerate the process, put the sauce in the fridge, allow the fat to harden, then pour off (and keep) the lower-calorie sauce, broth or soup.
Meat thermometer	A meat thermometer lets you know whether meat or poultry has been cooked long enough that it's safe to eat, and it also helps you avoid overcooking it to the point where it's dry and tough.

Running essentials

When you're new to running, the array of high-tech kit available can be a little daunting. Rest assured though, while you can happily indulge a penchant for gadgetry and high-performance products as you progress, running remains a reassuringly simple and accessible sport. That said, there are some true essentials you must have in your kit bag as a new runner, and a few other items that could provide a lot of comfort and enjoyment for a relatively small investment. Use our guide to decide what to invest in now, and what to consider as you progress.

1 The *right* running shoes
Those Dunlop Greenflash lurking in the shed probably won't cut it. Get yourself fitted at a specialist running shop (eg, Sweatshop). Wearing the wrong shoes may contribute to injury, and will certainly lead to a less comfortable experience.

2 Specialist sweat-wicking running kit...
Cotton absorbs sweat, leaving clothing sopping and heavy. It's uncomfortable on the run and can irritate your skin. Kit that's made from moisture-wicking material transports sweat away from your skin, leaving you to run in comfort.

3 ... and socks
Splashing out on shoes and skimping on socks is a mistake. Basic cotton ones are far less comfortable and greatly increase your blister risk.

4 Running jacket
Sometimes our busy lifestyles and the British climate mean you'll find yourself running in less-than-glorious conditions. But if you have a good running jacket, cold and/or wet weather isn't a disaster, and you can still enjoy a comfortable run. Look for weatherproofing plus breathability, a slim ergonomic fit and stretch in the fabric so it moves well as you run.

5 GPS watch
Not essential when you start out, but definitely helpful as you progress, it uses satellites to record your distance and display lots of useful data, from simple pace at entry level, to cadence and ground contact time as you move up the price points. Smartphone apps such as Strava and RunKeeper also track distance and pace, but phones are heavier, and harder to look at on the run.

6 Water bottle/hydration pack
You won't need one on every run, but when you start covering longer distances, particularly in warm weather, it's important to stay hydrated. Find a bottle that's shaped to fit comfortably in your hand. Or if you'd rather go hands-free, try a running-specific hydration pack.

7 Compression tights/socks
Not necessary for beginners but when you progress to more intense sessions such as speedwork and tempo runs, these can help your muscles recover faster post-run. Graduated pressure enhances blood flow, bringing extra oxygen and speeding the process of removing post-exercise waste products.

8 Runner's lube
Apply it pre-run to chafing-prone spots, to prevent friction. And don't let the term 'lube' worry you: these sports-specific products won't lead to embarrassment on purchase. They often look like sticks of deodorant, and application is mess-free.

9 Foam roller
If you don't have a personal sports masseuse, a foam roller is one of the best DIY methods to stave off overuse injuries. They come with instructions, but be warned, they can be a bit painful.

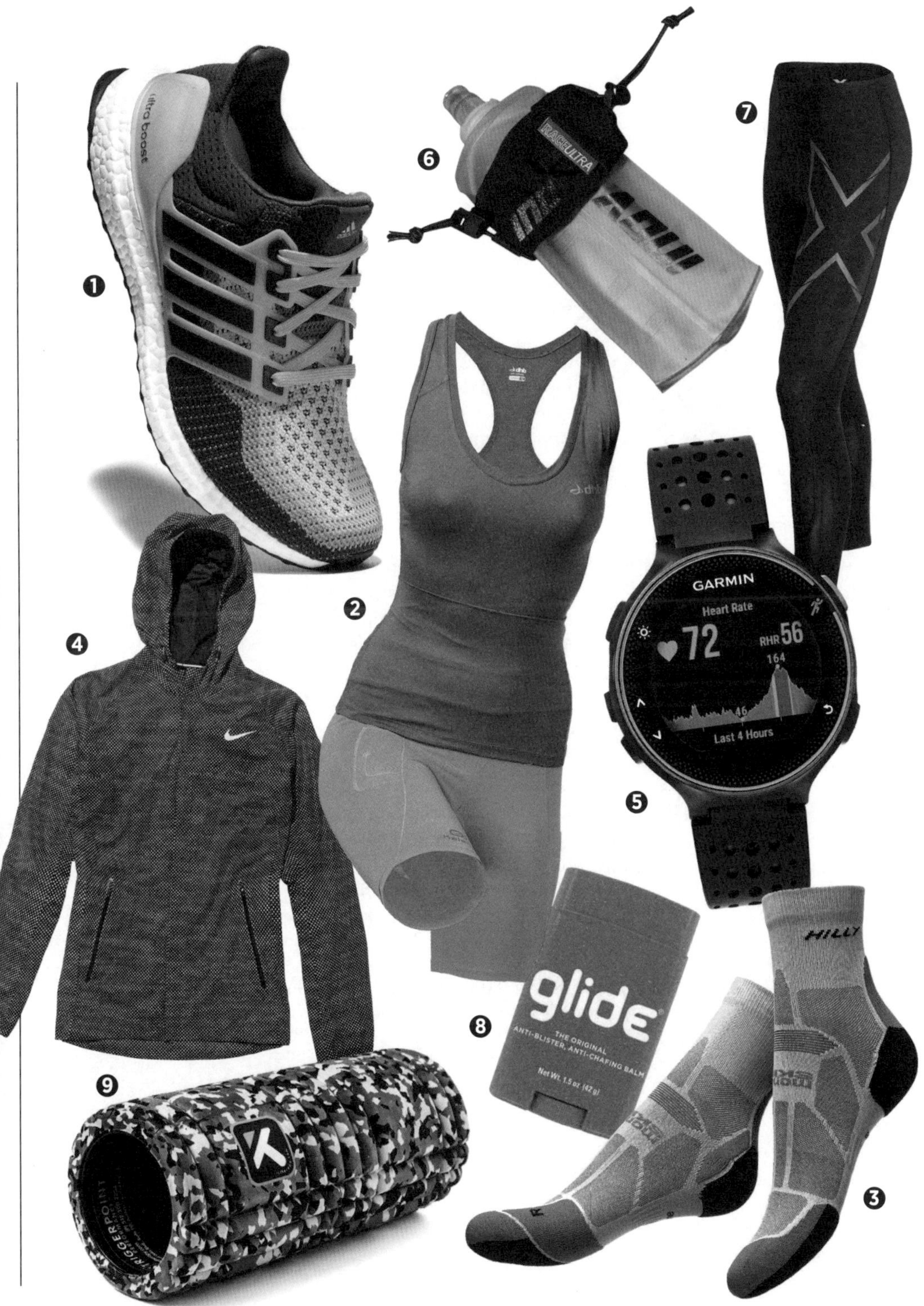
1
2
3
4
5
6
7
8
9
ultra boost
RACEULTRA
GARMIN
Heart Rate
72
RHR 56
164
46
Last 4 Hours
glide
THE ORIGINAL
ANTI-BLISTER, ANTI-CHAFING BALM
Net Wt. 1.5 oz (42 g)
HILLY
TRIGGERPOINT

About the authors

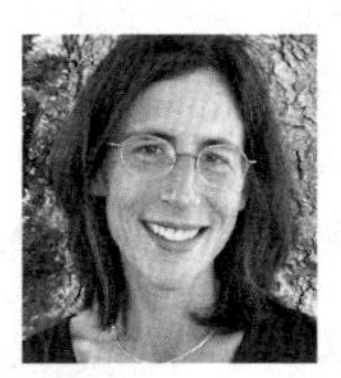

Jennifer Van Allen is a freelance writer and running coach certified by USATF and RRCA. A former special projects editor for *Runner's World* USA, Van Allen has finished 49 marathons and ultramarathons.

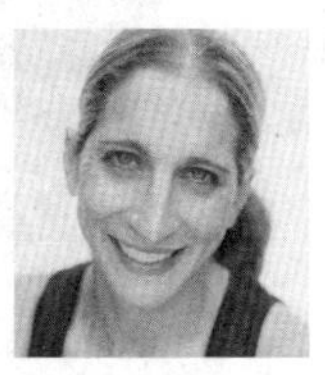

Pamela Nisevich Bede, RD, CSSD, is a sports nutrition expert and co-owner of Swim, Bike, Run, Eat!, LLC, a nutrition consulting firm.

Also by Jennifer Van Allen & Pamela Nisevich Bede:
The Runner's World Big Book of Marathon and Half-Marathon Training; The Runner's World Big Book of Running for Beginners

To Jason, Miller, Hunter, Noah, and Peter.
For all your love and support.